PROSTATE CANCER SCREENING

CURRENT CLINICAL UROLOGY

Eric A. Klein, SERIES EDITOR

Prostate Cancer Screening, edited by **Ian M. Thompson, Martin I. Resnick, and Eric A. Klein,** 2001

Bladder Cancer: Current Diagnosis and Treatment, edited by **Michael J. Droller,** 2001

Office Urology: The Clinician's Guide, edited by **Elroy D. Kursh and James C. Ulchaker,** 2001

Voiding Dysfunction: Diagnosis and Treatment, edited by **Rodney A. Appell,** 2000

Management of Prostate Cancer, edited by **Eric A. Klein,** 2000

PROSTATE CANCER SCREENING

Edited by

IAN M. THOMPSON, MD

*The University of Texas Health Science Center at San Antonio
San Antonio, TX*

MARTIN I. RESNICK, MD

*Case Western Reserve University
University Hospitals of Cleveland
Cleveland, OH*

ERIC A. KLEIN, MD

*Cleveland Clinic Foundation
Cleveland, OH*

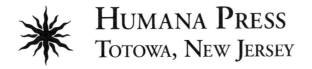

HUMANA PRESS
TOTOWA, NEW JERSEY

© 2001 Humana Press Inc.
999 Riverview Drive, Suite 208
Totowa, New Jersey 07512

For additional copies, pricing for bulk purchases, and/or information about other Humana titles, contact Humana at the above address or at any of the following numbers: Tel: 973-256-1699; Fax: 973-256-8341; E-mail: humana@humanapr.com or visit our Website at http://humanapress.com

All articles, comments, opinions, conclusions, or recommendations are those of the author(s), and do not necessarily reflect the views of the publisher.

Due diligence has been taken by the publishers, editors, and authors of this book to ensure the accuracy of the information published and to describe generally accepted practices. The contributors herein have carefully checked to ensure that the drug selections and dosages set forth in this text are accurate in accord with the standards accepted at the time of publication. Notwithstanding, as new research, changes in government regulations, and knowledge from clinical experience relating to drug therapy and drug reactions constantly occurs, the reader is advised to check the product information provided by the manufacturer of each drug for any change in dosages or for additional warnings and contraindications. This is of utmost importance when the recommended drug herein is a new or infrequently used drug. It is the responsibility of the health care provider to ascertain the Food and Drug Administration status of each drug or device used in their clinical practice. The publisher, editors, and authors are not responsible for errors or omissions or for any consequences from the application of the information presented in this book and make no warranty, express or implied, with respect to the contents in this publication.

This publication is printed on acid-free paper. ∞
ANSI Z39.48-1984 (American National Standards Institute)
Permanence of Paper for Printed Library Materials.

Cover Design: Patricia F. Cleary

Photocopy Authorization Policy:

Printed in the United States of America. 10 9 8 7 6 5 4 3 2 1

Library of Congress Cataloging-in-Publication Data

Prostate cancer screening / edited by Ian M. Thompson, Martin I. Resnick, Eric A. Klein.
        p.   ;cm.—(Current Clinical Urology)
    Includes bibliographical references and index.
    ISBN 0-89603-901-3 (alk. paper)
    1. Prostate–Cancer–Diagnosis. 2. Medical screening. I. Thompson, Ian M. (Ian Murchie), 1954–
II. Resnick, Martin I. III. Klein Eric A., 1955– IV. Series.
    [DNLM: 1. Prostatic Neoplasms–diagnosis. 2. Mass Screening. 3. Prostate-Specific Antigen. WJ
752 P96554 2000]
    RC280.P7 P75985 2000
    616.99'463075–dc21   00-044884

PREFACE

Perhaps no other subject in medicine has prompted such discussion, often with some animosity and certainly always with animation, as has the subject of screening for prostate cancer. Prior to the development of prostate specific antigen, screening was only a curiosity—an anecdote periodically due to the haphazard application of digital rectal examination. With PSA, however, screening was not only possible, but many men were found with the disease. The rate of increase in prostate cancer diagnoses in the late 1980s and early 1990s was unsurpassed by any other tumor in the history of modern public health statistics.

We may never know all the "right" answers regarding prostate cancer screening. We are currently awaiting the completion of very large clinical trials in Europe and the United States, designed to answer the question. However, for the man at risk for the disease and for his physician, be it urologist, internist, or family physician, the issue is: *What to do now?*

Prostate Cancer Screening is designed to help answer many of these questions. A balanced set of discussions is included that will provide an excellent, in-depth understanding for the physician and for the patient who strive to understand as much as possible about the disease and screening. This book is also designed for health care organizations that are struggling with the application of varying recommendations from medical specialty organizations.

There is no right answer, only choices. The premise of *Prostate Cancer Screening* is that, armed with information and augmented by personal priorities and expectations, both patients and physicians can make informed choices. If that is achieved, we have attained our goal.

Ian Thompson, MD
Martin I. Resnick, MD
Eric A. Klein, MD

CONTENTS

CONTRIBUTORS

ZINELABIDINE ABOUELFADEL, MD • *Division of Urology, University of Colorado Health Sciences Center, Denver, CO*

PETER C. ALBERTSEN, MD • *Division of Urology, University of Connecticut Health Center, Farmington, CT*

JOSEPH BASLER, PhD, MD • *Division of Urology, University of Texas Health Science Center, San Antonio, TX*

MICHAEL K. BRAWER, MD • *Northwest Prostate Institute, Seattle, WA*

OTIS W. BRAWLEY, MD • *Assistant Director, National Cancer Institute, National Institutes of Health, Bethesda, MD*

JOHN P. CAMPBELL, MS • *Systems Analyst, Litton/PRC, San Antonio, TX*

BERNARD CANDAS, PhD • *Prostate Cancer Clinical Research Unit, Department of Medicine ad Oncology and Molecular Endocrinology Research Center, Laval University Hospital (CHUL), Quebec, Canada*

EVELYN C. Y. CHAN, MD, MS • *Assistant Professor and Director, Clinical Bioethics, Division of General Internal Medicine, Department of Medicine, The University of Texas–Houston Health Science Center, Houston, TX*

E. DAVID CRAWFORD, MD • *Division of Urology, University of Colorado Health Sciences Center, Denver, CO*

LIONEL CUSAN, MD, PhD • *Prostate Cancer Clinical Research Unit, Department of Medicine ad Oncology and Molecular Endocrinology Research Center, Laval University Hospital (CHUL), Quebec, Canada*

RUTH ETZIONI • *Fred Hutchinson Cancer Research Center and University of Washington, Seattle, WA*

JOSÉ-LUIS GOMEZ, MD, PhD • *Prostate Cancer Clinical Research Unit, Department of Medicine ad Oncology and Molecular Endocrinology Research Center, Laval University Hospital (CHUL), Quebec, Canada*

ATANACIO C. GUILLEN, MS • *Systems Analyst, Litton/PRC, San Antonio, TX*

ISMAIL JATOI, MD, PhD, FACS • *Uniformed Services University of the Health Sciences, Bethesda, MD and Brooke Army Medical Center, Fort Sam Houston, TX*

FAIYAAZ M. JHAVERI, MD • *Northwest Prostate Institute, Seattle, WA*

ERIC A. KLEIN, MD • *Department of Urology, Cleveland Clinic Foundation, Cleveland, OH*

FERNAND LABRIE, MD, PhD • *Prostate Cancer Clinical Research Unit, Department of Medicine ad Oncology and Molecular Endocrinology Research Center, Laval University Hospital (CHUL), Quebec, Canada*

PAUL H. LANGE, MD • *Department of Urology, University of Washington School of Medicine, Seattle, WA*

MARK S. LITWIN, MD, MPH • *Departments of Urology and Health Services, University of California, Los Angeles, CA*

TILLMAN LOCH, MD, PhD • *Klinik und Poliklinik für Urologie und Kinderurologie der Universität des Saarlandes, Homburg, Germany*

CHRIS MAGEE, MD • *Division of Urology, the University of Texas Health Sciences Center at San Antonio, San Antonio, TX*

SCOTT A. OPTENBERG, PhD • *Professor, Department of Surgery, University of Texas Health Science Center at San Antonio, San Antonio, TX*

DAVID F. PENSON • *Fred Hutchinson Cancer Research Center and University of Washington, Seattle, WA*

KRISTEN A. REID, BA • *Departments of Urology and Health Services, University of California, Los Angeles, CA*

MARTIN I. RESNICK, MD • *Chairman, Department of Urology, School of Medicine, Case Western Reserve University, Cleveland, OH*

WAEL A. SAKR, MD • *Department of Pathology, Wayne State University, and the Karmanos Cancer Institute, Detroit, MI*

FRITZ H. SCHRÖDER, MD, PhD • *Professor and Chairman, Department of Urology, Erasmus University and Academic Hospital Rotterdam, The Netherlands*

DAVID L. SHEPHERD, MD • *Division of Urology, Department of Surgery, University of Texas Health Science Center at San Antonio, San Antonio, TX*

AARON SULMAN, MD • *Department of Urology, School of Medicine, Case Western Reserve University, Cleveland, OH*

GREGORY T. SWEAT, MD • *Senior Associate Consultant, Department of Family Medicine, Mayo Medical School, Mayo Clinic, Rochester, MN*

IAN M. THOMPSON, MD • *Professor and Chief, Division of Urology, The University of Texas Health Science Center at San Antonio, San Antonio, TX*

INGRID VAN DER CRUIJSEN-KOETER, MD • *Department of Urology, Academic Hospital and Erasmus University Rotterdam, The Netherlands*

CLARA WARD, MD • *Department of Pathology, Wayne State University, and the Karmanos Cancer Institute, Detroit, MI*

1   Epidemiology of Prostate Cancer

Wael A. Sakr, MD and Clara Ward, MA

CONTENTS

INTRODUCTION

The approach we followed to review the epidemiology of prostate cancer was to divide this chapter into three major sections. The first section provides a brief summary of the prevalence, incidence, and mortality data worldwide and in the United States. These data are compared for different geographic areas and among different ethnic groups, with an attempt to address how suspected risk factors for prostate cancer may relate to the observed global discrepancies with respect to incidence and mortality rates. The data provided in the first section pertain primarily, although not exclusively, to clinically evident prostate cancer. As it is becoming increasingly recognized that prostatic neoplasia covers a wide biological spectrum, the second section reviews available epidemiological data on the early "phases" of the diseases, specifically precursor lesions and preinvasive neoplasia, and the category of preclinical or the so-called "latent" prostate cancer. Finally, the third section highlights some of the changes in the clinicopathological profile of prostate cancer diagnosed in the prostate-specific antigen (PSA) era of the 1990s: During the last decade, the Western Hemisphere in particular has witnessed significant changes in the profile of both the patients diagnosed with prostate cancer and the characteristics of their tumors.

From: *Current Clinical Urology: Prostate Cancer Screening*
Edited by: I. M. Thompson, M. I. Resnick, and E. A. Klein
© Humana Press Inc., Totowa, NJ

1

These changes include the mode of diagnosis and the age by which the disease is detected, the downward stage migration, and, possibly, certain biological attributes that could affect the progression potential of a newly diagnosed prostate cancer.

Global Prevalence and Incidence and Mortality of Prostate Cancer

Worldwide, prostate cancer is the sixth most common cancer, with nearly 400,000 new tumors diagnosed each year; comprising 9.2% of all cancers in men, prostate cancer is the fourth most common male cancer *(1)*. These data vary markedly across the globe, however, prostate cancer is more than three times as prevalent in industrialized nations as compared to developing countries *(2)*. Several reasons could contribute to this disparity: the suspected and unknown risk factors are likely to vary by environment, geography, and ethnicity, the unavailability or lack of application of diagnostic techniques, and, possibly, the possibility of underreporting as a result of the lack of established tumor registries and documentation in some developing countries. Approximately 80% of prostate cancer cases are diagnosed in individuals 65 and older *(1)*, although the age distribution of the disease has been shifting toward younger men, at least in some countries, throughout the last decade *(3,4)*.

North America has the highest incidence of prostate cancer with 92.39/100,000 cases per year, nearly double the reported incidence in Australia and New Zealand, the second most afflicted region. Incidence rates for Europe range from 14.06/100,000 for Eastern Europe to 39.55/100,000 for Western Europe *(2)*. The Caribbean has the third highest incidence, with rates of 42.35/100,000 *(2)*. In Kingston, Jamaica, however, where the population is primarily of African-Caribbean descent, the prostate cancer incidence has been reported to be 304/100,000, the highest documented anywhere in the world *(5)*.

Prostate cancer incidence in men on the African continent has been historically reported to be low, especially when compared to African-Americans *(6)*. Recent reports indicate, however, that prostate cancer is the most common cancer in Nigeria (46.1% of all cancers diagnosed). Although the most recent estimate on the incidence of the disease in a country like Nigeria, (127/100,000) is considerably higher than previously reported figures, it continues to be significantly lower than the incidence in African-American men *(7)*. Prostate cancer represents the second most common malignancy in Uganda and a quarter of all cancer cases in Zambia *(8)*.

Central and South American nations occupy a moderate range of 22.86–28.05 per 100,000. The Middle East, the Far East, and Asia report exceptionally low rates: China has an incidence of 1.08/100,000 per year, and all other parts of Asia and the Middle East report incidence in the single digits. A higher incidence of 21.22/100,000 is reported in the Pacific Island regions of Micronesia and Polynesia *(2)*. While incidence rates for Asian countries may be significantly lower than those of the United States, these numbers are increasing rapidly and are expected to double by the year 2000 *(9)*.

Compared to overall cancer mortality, prostate cancer on a global scale is not as significant a cause of cancer mortality, with 3.2% of total cancer deaths and 5.6% of male cancer deaths resulting from it *(2)*.

Prostate Cancer Prevalence, Incidence and Mortality in the United States

With its diverse ethnic populations, the prevalence and incidence of prostate cancer in the United States largely reflects the global variations of the disease. In 1999 over 1.2 million new invasive cancer cases were expected in the United States, approximately half of which were diagnosed in males *(1)*. These figures represent a decline from those of 1993, the year that witnessed the highest recorded incidence (approximately 250,000). Prostate cancer comprises approximately 30% of all cancer cases diagnosed among Native Americans and Asian-Americans, 37% for Caucasian-Americans and Hispanic Americans, and half of all cancers in African-Americans *(1)*.

In the United States, an individual's overall chance of developing prostate cancer within their lifetime is 1 in 6. This prediction, however, is markedly influenced by age: males 39 yr old or younger have a less than a 1 in 10,000 chance, males 40–59 yr old have a 1 in 55 likelihood, and men 60–79 yr old, have a 1 in 7 chance of developing prostate cancer *(1)*. Although early neoplastic changes of the prostate begin at the microscopic level as early as the third decade of life *(10)*, the majority of clinically evident prostate cancer continues to be diagnosed in older men. African-American men have 60% higher incidence than Caucasian-Americans. The lowest rates are among Native American men, but all groups have lower rates than African-American men *(9A)*.

With respect to U.S. mortality, 37,000 of the 291,100 (12.7%) new cancer mortalities in 1999 will result from prostate cancer *(1)*. Accordingly, prostate cancer is a leading cause of cancer death, second only to lung cancer. Mortality rates in the United States vary in a fashion that parallels the incidence variability observed among different U.S. ethnic groups. Prostate cancer accounts for 10–15% of cancer mortality among Asian-Americans, Native-Americans, and Hispanic-Americans. The corresponding cancer mortality ratio attributed to prostate cancer in

Caucasian-Americans and African-Americans are 15% and 25%, respectively with African-Americans twice as likely to die of prostate cancer than Caucasian-Americans *(1,9A)*. Within the two latter race groups, some authors have demonstrated a "crossover" disease-specific mortality phenomenon: African-Americans 65 yr of age or younger suffer twofold to threefold higher prostate cancer mortality compared to Caucasian-American men *(11)*. In the older age group however, Caucasian-Americans appear to have a worse prognosis *(12,13)*.

The discrepancy in prostate cancer incidence and mortality between African Americans and Caucasian-Americans in the United States continues to be a major health concern. The reason(s) for this disparity is not clear. Prior to reviewing the "traditional" suspected risk factors for the disease, it may be appropriate to briefly summarize the controversial role of socioeconomic factors as a potential contributor to the racial difference in the United States. Several studies suggested that by adjusting for socioeconomic status as indicated by income and educational level racial differences in cancer development were eliminated with these adjustments, except for African-Americans *(11,14,15)*. Studies conducted in equal-access military facilities have also found that pathologic differences persist unabated in African-Americans, suggesting that unequal access to medical care is not the impetus behind the high incidence and mortality rates *(15,16)*. Other culturally specific issues for the African-American community have been identified as impediments to prostate cancer prevention and treatment: fear and mistrust of the medical system, limited access to facilities, inadequate/inaccurate health information *(17–20)*, differential recommendations on the part of the physicians for less of aggressive treatment *(21)*, and rural–urban disparities *(22)*. Studies assessing cultural and psychosocial factors affecting health-related decision making and behavior could shape possible education and awareness interventions in efforts to promote early detection *(19–23)*.

Finally, although the migration effect may not be classified as a social/socioeconomic factor, the accompanying cultural, environmental, and, possibly, later genetic changes in subsequent generations can contribute to changing risk for incidence and/or mortality. This is evident in the epidemiologic trends of prostate cancer in the United States, which parallel global tendencies, suggesting that intracultural genetic factors may be at work, contributing to the lower incidence in Asians and a virtual epidemic in African-Americans. However, because of the effects of migration on populations and their susceptibility to prostate cancer as they assimilate, the argument can be made for genetic arrangements that are conducive to the genesis of prostate cancer *(24)*, whereas environmental exert control over clinical expression.

Japanese in their native country have a very low incidence of prostate cancer, whereas rates for US-born Japanese and Japanese immigrants to the United States and South America are approximately four times the rate of indigenous Japanese *(26,27)*. The incidence of prostate cancer among US born and immigrant Hispanics to the Los Angeles area was 50% higher than in their homelands *(26)*. In another study, immigrants to the United States from China, Japan, and the Philippines had half the incidence of prostate cancer than their American-born counterparts *(27)*. The age of immigration and the length of stay in the new country appear to be directly related to incidence rates *(27)*. Residence in the United States of Chinese immigrants for more than 25 yr more than doubles their risk for prostate cancer *(28)*.

RISK FACTORS

Among the numerous genetic and environmental exposures as risk factors for prostate cancer, we selected a few that have been more frequently implicated and studied. More data continue to accumulate, however, on a variety of other factors, including smoking, the effect of vasectomy, sexual and physical activity, insulin, obesity, and benign prostatic hyperplasia, among others.

Diet and Other Consumptions

Nutrition is one of the more researched areas with respect to prostate cancer prevention and etiology, specifically the consumption of particular foods reported to contain preventative nutritional benefits or elements suspected to alter prostate cancer risk. Several studies have suggested that high intake of animal fats leads to increased production of testosterone, a promoter of cell division and protooncogene activator, deactivating tumor suppressor genes *(29–32)*. These associations appear to be more significant in individuals whose cancer was diagnosed prior to the seventh decade *(26)*. The age of exposure may be important, as one group found that consumption during adult years is more significant than adolescent exposure *(33)*. Some immigration studies also support the notion that environmental changes late in life have a greater effect on prostate cancer genesis *(27)*. The positive associations of prostate cancer with certain dietary elements are inconclusive according to other researchers *(34,35)*. Furthermore, many potential negative relationships with prostate cancer mortality have also inconclusively been identified in foods, including cereals, nuts, oilseeds, fish, vegetables, crudites, tea, and soy products *(29,30,32)*.

ANTIOXIDANTS, ALCOHOL

In recent years, a large number of compounds particularly in the categories of micronutrients and antioxidants have been claimed to have a chemoprotective role with respect to prostate cancer development and/or progression. The list is long and includes selenium, β-carotene and vitamin A derivatives, vitamins E, D, and C, isoflavins, and lycopenes, among others. *(29,36–38)*. Selenium and vitamin E specifically are of particular interest because when each was used in prospective trials for other malignancies, there was a significant reduction in prostate cancer development in participants on the treatment arm compared to controls. Although the latter finding was identified as a secondary end point in both trials, the data were encouraging and have justified the initiation of two national prospective trials in the United States *(37,38)*. In an indirect relationship to heavy alcohol consumption it has been suggested that alcohol metabolites can interfere with the absorption of certain micronutrients presenting an increased risk for prostate cancer *(32)*. Data on the role of alcohol consumption as a risk factor, however, are both sketchy and controversial *(32,35,39,40)*.

Occupation

Farmers and men residing in rural areas appear to be at a greater risk of prostate cancer *(41–45)*. It has been suggested that the number of years of farming is directly proportional to one's risk for prostate cancer, whereas others have found that the risk is higher for farmers who apply their own pesticides and the exposure to agrochemicals, lubricating oil and greases, petrochemicals, and biological dusts *(42–46)*.

Other occupational areas that have been investigated for disproportionate rates of cancer trends include pesticide, rubber, and metal manufacturers, jobs involving exposure to heavy metals and hydrocarbons, newspaper printing, construction and utilities workers, and firefighters *(46,47)*. In cancer-related deaths of firefighters, differential mortality patterns between races were observed. Nearly one-quarter of cancers in African-Americans were of the prostate, compared to only 10% in Caucasian-Americans *(47)*. Overexposure to heavy metals, such as cadmium, are thought to inhibit the ability of zinc to conduct its normal metabolic functions in the prostate. Workers in the cadmium industry have a higher prevalence of prostate cancer and clinically more aggressive tumors *(48)*.

Familial and Hereditary Prostate Cancer

Non-hereditary familial clustering is estimated to account for 15–20% of prostate cancer cases *(55)*. Family history is the one variable that has shown a consistent correlation with increased risk of prostate cancer for men with first degree relatives afflicted with the disease *(49–55)*. Familial prostate cancer can involve a multitude of factors interacting to create an increased risk, by virtue of common environmental exposures or genetic events. First-degree relatives of men with prostate cancer have a threefold increased chance of developing it by age 70 compared to the average individual *(49–52)*. In families with two men diagnosed with prostate cancer, there is a 25% chance for males in the family to develop the disease between the ages of 60 and 80, five times the rate in the general population. (After 80, the relative risk decreases to three times the rate in the general population.) If one of the relatives is diagnosed before the age of 70, the risk climbs to 43% *(50,52)*. These observations suggest that the effect of family history appears to be related to age; Bratt et al, among others, found that the risk for prostate cancer increased with the decreasing age of the diagnosed relative *(50,52,54)*.

Hereditary prostate cancer defined as a nuclear family with three diagnosed with the disease occurring through three generations, with two or more of these relatives diagnosed before the age of 55. The phenomenon has been attributed to a transmittance of a single gene within a family *(49)*. The gene thought to be responsible for this increased susceptibility has been termed HPC1 (hereditary prostate cancer 1 gene), located on chromosome 1. There are indications, however, that multiple chromosomal loci are likely involved, as well as the *BRCA1* and *BRCA2* genes. Linkage at the site appears to account for only 5–10% of prostate cancer cases, particularly in individuals with early onset and male-to-male disease transmission. The mean age of diagnosis for individuals with heredity prostate cancer is 65 yr, compared to 67 and 71 yr for familial and sporadic prostate cancer, respectively. No differences have been found in pre-operative PSA and methods of diagnosis between patients with hereditary, familial, and sporadic prostrate cancers, however studies debate whether genetic linkages perpetuate a more virulent neoplastic pathway in patients with hereditary distribution of prostate cancer *(56)*. Finally, the proportion of males with hereditary prostate cancer appears to be similar among African-Americans and Caucasian-Americans *(57)*, as well as Asian-Americans *(58)*. Of interest, among Asian-Americans, those reporting a relative with prostate cancer were more likely to have been born in North America.

Hormones

Androgens are essential for the development and progression of prostate cancer, emphasized by the fact that castrated men and individuals with congenital hormone abnormalities are rarely afflicted with it. Studies have also arisen postulating racial differences in androgen production and metabolism *(59,60)*. Poor diet, obesity, and related conditions create high levels of insulin, which then inhibits sex-hormone-binding globulin (SHBG). When insulin levels are low and the SHBG is high, it binds to the testosterone, preventing it from affecting the prostate. Prostate–testosterone interactions are correlated with tumor growth. Consequently, a diet high in fat raises the levels of insulin, prohibiting the binding of SHBG to testosterone *(61)*. One of the potential benefits of soy is the presence of isoflavonoids and lignans that also competitively bind to hormone receptor sites, preventing the interaction of androgens with the prostate *(29,61)*.

EPIDEMIOLOGY OF EARLY PROSTATIC NEOPLASIA

In this section, we review data on the prevalence of suspected premalignant lesions of the prostate and summarize the associations linking them to prostate cancer. Subsequently, a brief review of preclinical "latent" prostate cancer diagnosed in the postmortem setting is also provided. The objective is to supplement and contrast the prevalence and, particularly, the incidence figures of clinically manifest prostate cancer with the extremely high prevalence of these forms of early neoplastic transformation. A major question in the complex natural history of this disease concerns the relationship between these different phases of prostatic neoplasia and the efforts aiming at predicting the progression potential of early neoplastic lesions.

Precursor Lesions

There is a wide spectrum of atypical epithelial proliferative processes that occur in the prostate. The terminology applied to these processes have been inconsistent and often confusing. This resulted in a limited understanding for the true prevalence of prostatic precursors, their natural history and evolution, and the relationship to both preclinical or "latent" and to clinically evident prostate cancer. Two major categories of suspected precursors have emerged in recent years; the first, atypical adenomatous hyperplasia (AAH), defines a morphological entity in which the atypia is mainly architectural, with proliferation and crowding of small glands and acini that are most often located at the edges of a hyperplastic nodule in the transition zone of the prostate *(62)*.

The second category of atypical epithelial lesions is characterized primarily by the cytologic atypia of the lining epithelium of prostate ducts and acini and has been termed prostatic intraepithelial neoplasia (PIN) *(63)*. Furthermore, PIN has been separated into low- and high-grade categories *(64)*. The high-grade lesion (HGPIN) is characterized by severe cytologic atypia of prostate ducts epithelium with these neoplastic changes, however, being confined within the lining epithelium and the boundaries of the ducts, therefore, the term *intraepithelial.*

The literature investigating the associations between putative precursor lesions of the prostate and adenocarcinoma is heavily tilted in favor of HGPIN, with numerous epidemiologic, clinical, and molecular links between this lesion and prostate cancer *(65–67)*. Accordingly, we will limit the epidemiologic review of prostate precursors to HGPIN. Most importantly, the identification of isolated HGPIN on needle biopsies of the prostate indicates an approximate 4–50% risk of having a diagnosis of carcinoma on subsequent biopsy *(68,69)*. In this respect, HGPIN serves as a risk marker for the presence of carcinoma in addition to its role as putative precursor of prostate cancer. Depending on the type of prostate tissue sample evaluated, the cohort studied, and to an extent, the diagnostic criteria, reported figures for the prevalence of HGPIN tend to vary significantly. HGPIN is more likely to be identified in prostates harboring carcinoma compared to benign glands. McNeal and Bostwick reported in an autopsy series of 436 step-sectioned prostates, an 82% prevalence of HGPIN in glands containing adenocarcinoma compared to 43% of benign prostates *(70)*. In smaller series of 37 autopsies reported by Oyasu et al. HGPIN was present in 38% and 94% of benign and malignant glands, respectively *(71)*. Data from a large contemporary autopsy study conducted at Wayne State University in Detroit supplement these findings by documenting the microscopic findings of step sectioned totally embedded prostate glands procured from men 20 yr of age or older who died from trauma *(72)*. In a recent update on this study, Sakr et al. reported the findings of 652 consecutive prostate glands in which HGPIN was found in 25% of prostates not harboring carcinoma compared to 63% of men whose glands contained tumor. The lower figures found in our study are attributed to the younger age range of the individuals in our series. Furthermore, when the authors classified HGPIN into three categories depending on the extent of prostate gland involvement by the lesion, they found that most prostates with extensive HGPIN (76%) contained prostate cancer compared to 51% for glands with multifocal HGPIN (the intermediate category) and there was a 36% chance of harboring carcinoma in prostate with only focal HGPIN (the category with least glandular involvement by the lesion) *(73)*.

Equally important in the Wayne State University series were the data reported on the age and racial distribution of this precursor lesion. These authors have indicated that there may be potential differences in the prevalence and distribution of HGPIN in African-American and Caucasian-American men. The results of their microscopic evaluation of 525 step-sectioned prostate glands from 314 African-American and 211 Caucasian-American men indicated a higher prevalence of HGPIN in African-Americans across the wide age spectrum studied (20–80 yr). The lesion was identified in 7%, 26%, 46%, 72%, 75% and 91% of African-American men in their third, fourth, fifth, sixth, seventh, and eighth decades, respectively. Caucasian-American men tended to have lower prevalence with corresponding figures of 8%, 23%, 29%, 49%, 53%, and 67% respectively *(74)*. Moreover, they found a lesion of HGPIN to be more extensive at younger age in African-Americans. Their data indicate that 2%, 6%, 12%, and 28% of the men in their third, fourth, fifth, and sixth decade, respectively harbored extensive HGPIN in their gland. Extensive glandular involvement by HGPIN was less common in Caucasian-American men whose prevalence for the same age group was compared to 0%, 2%, 5%, and 12%. Similar findings to the data generated in the previous North American study were reported from Brazil by Billis et al., who found in an autopsy series of 180 African-Brazilian and white Brazilian men 40 yr of age or older that the prevalence of HGPIN was similar in the two races (84.4%). The study showed that the more extensive and diffuse HGPIN in African Brazilians tended to appear at a younger age compared to whites *(75)*. He suggested that this observation may help explain the higher prevalence of HGPIN in men from African descent compared to Caucasian Brazilians. Reports concerning the prevalence of HGPIN in prostate biopsies are variable. The frequency of identifying the lesion in biopsies without carcinoma have ranged between 4% and 16%, *(76,77)*, although most large biopsy series support a prevalence of about 5% *(78,79)*. HGPIN prevalence in transurethral resection specimens is also in the range of 2–4% *(80–81)*.

Preclinical "Latent" Prostate Cancer

In spite of the marked increase in the incidence of clinically diagnosed prostate cancer in recent years, the prevalence of the preclinical form of the disease discovered in prostates of autopsied men remains remarkably higher. The histologic changes that fulfill the criteria required to designate a prostate epithelial lesion as cancer are alarmingly prevalent. Historically, this "phase" of prostate cancer, often referred to as "latent" cancer, has been repeatedly documented to be present in approximately 30% of men more than 50 yr of age upon postmortem examination *(82–85)*. More recently, however, data from Sakr et al. have indicated that this histologically evident malignant transformation starts as early as the third decade of life and that 25–30% of men less than 50 yr of age harbor foci of prostate cancer in their glands *(10)*.

The high prevalence of preclinical cancer appears to be universal, with relatively mild geographic and ethnic variability. Although the prevalence is reported to be highest in the Western Hemisphere, autopsy data derived from different geographic regions indicate a limited twofold to threefold variation worldwide *(86)*. This is in contrast to the sharp discrepancies concerning incidence and mortality of the clinically manifest prostate cancer. In addition to the lower geographic variations, the Wayne State University autopsy data found that there were no significant differences in the frequency of latent prostate cancer between African Americans and Caucasian-American men in the wide age range this study evaluated *(10,74)*. Furthermore, these authors found no significant differences in the volume or histologic grades of the discovered tumors.

CHANGES IN PROSTATE CANCER EPIDEMIOLOGY DURING THE PSA ERA

The dramatic increase in the incidence of prostate cancer in the late 1980s and the first half of the 1990s could be directly attributed to the wide application of measuring PSA in the serum of men screened for or suspected to have prostate cancer *(86–90)*. PSA is produced by the epithelial component of the prostate gland and its value in the serum reflects the "volume" of the glandular epithelium. As men age, PSA values secreted by benign prostatic epithelial cells increase minimally, doubling over a period longer than the average lifetime *(91)*. When prostate cancer develops and starts to grow, PSA values increase slowly initially and then exponentially, paralleling the pattern of uncontrolled cellular "epithelial" proliferation characteristic of neoplastic growth.

The steadily increasing proportion of prostate cancer cases triggered by an abnormal PSA has been accompanied by significant changes in the "traditional" profile of these cancers. These changes include aspects of incidence, mode of diagnosis, age and other demographics of men in whom new cancers are discovered, and, finally, the stage and possibly the pathobiological characteristics of cancers diagnosed via PSA testing.

With a highly prevalent disease such as prostate cancer, one of the expected functions of PSA as a screening test would be to initially create an increase in incidence as a large number of previously undetected cases are revealed *(92,93)*. Once a substantial proportion of the population is screened, the incidence rates will begin to decrease, plateauing at the actual incidence rate of the disease *(92)*. Because the screening test would be detecting cancers earlier, it is logical to expect the newly diagnosed patients to be younger and for their cancers to be less advanced *(94)*. Some details supporting these trends are provided in the following subsections.

Changes in Incidence Rates

Prostate cancer incidence in the United States has been increasing slowly since 1973; the sharp surge experienced in the early nineties, however, parallels the wide utilization of PSA testing. Subsequently, the incidence rates have been steadily declining, approaching levels seen in the pre-PSA era *(95)*.

From 1973 to 1991, the incidence of prostate cancer nearly tripled, from 64 to 178/100,000, with nearly half of this increase occurring after 1986 *(86)*. The Surveillance, Epidemiology and End Results (SEER) database began recording PSA screening in 1988 *(86)*. To account for the increasing incidence prior to 1988, it is important to consider the increase in utilizing the transrectal ultrasound technique to guide the obtaining of the needle biopsy specimens. These have increased eightfold between 1986 and 1988 *(86)*.

Between 1986 and 1992 for CH and 1993 for AAH, incidence rates increased by 108% and 102%, respectively. This increase was evident in all age groups, localized and regional stages, and primarily moderately differentiated tumors. Distant stage cancers declined by 56% between 1985 and 1995 *(9A)*.

The years 1990 and 1991 boast the largest annual increases in incidence, of 17% and 24%, respectively *(86)*. During this period, all stages of disease increased exponentially, with the exception of advanced cancer. Between 1988 and 1991, the number of men 65 and older undergoing PSA screening increased 12-fold, from 1430 to 18,000/100,000 *(86)*.

In a multiethnic study of PSA utilization in New Mexico, Gilliland et al. *(97)* found that after the adoption of PSA testing, incidence rates increased by 77%, 50%, and 27% for Caucasian-Americans, Hispanic-Americans, and Native Americans, respectively.

It is widely believed that the increase in incidence is the result of utilizing a more effective detection test, namely, PSA, and the true prevalence of prostate cancer has not changed. This diagnostic modality has led to the discovery of many cancers that would have remained undetected prior to the PSA era *(98)*.

Changes in the Mode of Diagnosis

In addition to PSA testing leading to the marked increase in prostate cancer incidence, this modality has changed the traditional "mode" of detecting the disease. Increasingly higher proportions of patients have been diagnosed with prostate cancer following an "abnormal" laboratory blood test, namely, PSA, as opposed to identifying a nodule or "palpable" disease via digital rectal exam (DRE) *(99)*. Furthermore, numerous studies have recently been published assessing the sensitivity and specificity of PSA, DRE, and the combination of information obtained by each in diagnosing prostate cancer *(100–102)*.

Other authors have found that DRE used in combination with PSA found 45–75% more cancers than DRE alone *(101–105)*. PSA alone detected 82% of the total tumors in the comparative study, whereas DRE alone detected 55% *(101)*. However, when the two methods were used in tandem, there was an 81% increase in the number of tumors detected over DRE alone *(101)*. Transrectal ultrasonography (TRUS) failed to detect 39% of the cancers in this study *(101)*.

Changing Trends Within Different Populations in the United States

The utilization of prostate cancer diagnostic procedures have not been uniform across the country or within different racial/ethnic groups. Whereas the benefits of PSA screening often in combination with DRE have been proposed to be more pronounced in African-American men than their Caucasian-American counterparts *(106,107)*, TRUS and PSA testing are reportedly performed on Caucasian-Americans consistently more often than on African-Americans *(94)*.

Prior to 1987, TRUS was performed four times as often on Caucasian-Americans. By 1991, the rate of PSA or TRUS was 35% higher for Caucasian-Americans compared to African-Americans, and the number of Caucasian-Americans screened in 1994 jumped 40-fold since 1988 *(99)*. In a study of screening knowledge, beliefs, and behaviors of African-Americans and Caucasian-Americans, Demark-Wahnefried et al. *(108)* reported that only 28% of African-American men reported physicians ever having discussed screening options with them and that they were less likely to have a regular doctor or have had a previous screening (either DRE or PSA) compared to Caucasian-Americans *(108)*. The gap between the two groups, however, is beginning to close, as the screening programs for African-Americans increase *(86)*. In another study comparing Caucasian-Americans, Hispanic-Americans, and Native Americans, 93% of men over 70 yr of age regardless of race, underwent DRE *(97)*. Despite the disparities in diagnostic technique utilization, the incidence rates have increased similarly for both African-Americans and Caucasian-Americans over this time period (76% and 84% ,respectively) *(86,109)*.

Changes of Age at Diagnosis

Prior to the PSA era, the mean age for prostate cancer diagnosis for Caucasian-Americans was 72 and 70 for African-Americans. In recent years, however, there is evidence of an "age shift," with more men presenting with prostate cancer at a younger age. The mean age for African-American men presenting with prostate cancer is 67 yr. A similar decline is evident for Caucasian-Americans in whom the mean age at presentation dropped to 69 yr *(4)*.

Changes in the Pathological Parameters

TUMOR STAGE

Compared to prostate cancer diagnosed prior to the PSA era, tumors detected by abnormal PSA are more likely to present at a younger age and be in an earlier clinical and pathological stage *(10,101,110–112)*. Indeed, a new stage category signifying prostate cancers diagnosed based on PSA abnormality in the absence of a palpable lesion by rectal exam had to be introduced. These nonpalpable cancers (stage T1C) increased in proportion by over seven-fold between 1988 and 1996, from 10% to 73% of all cancers detected *(101)*. Although stage T1C tumors translate to a wide spectrum of pathologic stages, in general, these tumors compare favorably to even the low-stage palpable cancers such as clinical stage T2 cancers. T1C tumors are more likely than clinical stage 2 cancers to be diploid, organ confined, and have a Gleason score less than or equal to 7. These factors translate to a better prognosis for prostate cancer patients diagnosed via abnormal PSA and no palpable lesion *(92,113–115)*. Stage distribution is similar across ethnic groups, however, distant stage disease is disproportionately represented among Native Americans and men of Filipino and Hawaiian descent. Grade is similarly distributed, with Filipino men having slightly poorer differentiated tumors *(9A)*. A corollary study of tumor ploidy in radical prostatectomy at the Mayo Clinic revealed that parallel to the increase in the proportion of nonpalpable tumors, nondiploid cancers fell from 38.3% in 1987 to 24.6% in 1995 *(116)*.

It is important to emphasize that the vast majority of nonpalpable tumors detected by PSA continue to be considered clinically significant cancers *(101,117–119)*. The risk of diagnosing clinically insignificant tumors has been estimated to range from 3.8% to 16% *(102,120)*.

The likely explanation is PSA, although more sensitive than DRE as a diagnostic method is unlikely to detect tumors small enough to be considered insignificant, as these lesions will not secrete enough PSA to raise levels to suspicious limits *(101)*.

Smith and Catalona found that nearly 40% of the tumors in their serial PSA-based screening protocol were nonpalpable. When PSA and DRE were combined, there was a 34% increase in organ-confined tumors detected over using PSA alone, and a 78% increase over using DRE alone *(101)*. The rate of organ-confined disease in unscreened men is only 30% compared to 70–85% in men screened by DRE and PSA *(101)*. Compared to DRE, PSA detected approximately 50% more organ-confined tumors *(101)*. Ninety-seven percent of the study cohort had stage T1 and T2 clinically localized tumors *(102)*. There are limited indications to suggest that screening for prostate cancer may have resulted in changes in tumor grade, although some studies have suggested that more patients are presenting with Gleason scores of 7 or greater, with carcinomas occurring in small foci of higher-grade cancer *(102,122–124)*. Additional pathologic characteristics of prostate cancer has also been gradually changing. In a recent report from Wayne State University, tumors in radical prostatectomy specimens have become smaller but more multicentric with more extensive high-grade PIN *(10)*. PSA levels at the time of diagnosis have also dropped considerably. In a Mayo Clinic study, the number of patients with levels over 20 ng/mL was reduced to only 9%, compared to 24% 8 yr earlier *(116)*.

A 25% decline in prostate cancer mortality in the United States occurred between 1988 and 1995, approx. 7 yr after its use as a screening tool became widespread, following the sharp climb in incidence *(125)*. Canadian data also indicate that prostate cancer mortality increased steadily prior to the adoption of PSA as a screening test in 1989, and then fell between 1991 and 1997 by 23% *(98,125)*. This trend was observed in all age groups, but most notably in men younger than 75.

An example of the changing features of prostate cancer in the 1990s is the recent report from the Wayne State University radical prostatectomy database. In a study summarizing the findings of 450 patients treated by this modality between 1991 and 1999 (the authors included the first 50,000 patients of every year), they found that the proportion of men 55 years or younger undergoing surgery increased from 7% in 1991 to 19% in 1995 and to 34% in 1999. For the same time interval, the percentage of patients who had abnormal finding on DRE decreased from 100% to 69% to 41% respectively and the mean preoperative PSA dropped from 23.9 to 9.5 to 8.2 ng/mL *(126)*. The same study shows that the proportion of organ-confined cancer increased from 38% to 49% to 62% of this patient population, and the mean tumor volume in the resected prostate gland decreased from a mean of 8.2 to 5.6 to 2.4 cc for the same time interval.

In summary, the most significant change associated with widespread PSA testing appears to be the significant increase in the proportion of organ-confined cancers, and the 50% drop in metastasis. Organ-confined tumors are expected to continue increasing, as advanced stage tumors are detected and removed *(107)*.

Although there are some preliminary indications that this effect may have a favorable impact on prostate cancer mortality, some authors believe that more time and additional large prospective studies are needed to reach this conclusion.

REFERENCES

1. Landis SH, Murray T, Bolden S, Wingo PA. (1999) Cancer statistics. *CA Cancer J Clin* 8–31.
2. Parkin DM, Pisani P, Ferlay J. (1998) Global cancer statistics. *CA Cancer J Clin* 33–64.
3. Farkas A, Schneider D, Perrotti M, Cummings KB, Ward WS. National trends in the epidemiology of prostate cancer, 1973 to 1994: evidence for the effectiveness of prostate-specific antigen screening. *Urology* 52:444–448.
4. Amling CL, Blute ML, Lerner SE, Bergstralh EJ, Bostwick DG, Zincke H. (1998) Influence of prostate-specific antigen testing on the spectrum of patients with prostate cancer undergoing radical prostatectomy at a large referral practice. *Mayo Clin Proc* 73:401–406.
5. Glover FE Jr., Coffey DS, Douglas LL, Cadogan M, Russell H, Tulloch T, et al. (1998) The epidemiology of prostate cancer in Jamaica. *J Urology* 159:1984–1987.
6. Jackson MA, Ahluwalia BS, Ghestimat MY. (1977) Characterization of prostatic carcinoma amongst blacks: a continuation report. *Cancer Treat Rep* 61:167–172.
7. Osegbe DN. (1997) Prostate cancer in Nigerians: facts and nonfacts. *J Urology* 157:1340–1343.
8. Kehinde EO. (1995) The geography of prostate cancer and its treatment in Africa. *Cancer Surv* 23:281–286.
9. Egawa S, Matsumoto K, Suyama K, Iwamura, M, Kuwao S, Baba S. (1999) Observations of prostatic specific antigen doubling time in Japanese patients with nonmetastatic prostate carcinoma. *Cancer* 86:463–469.
9A. Stanford JL, Stephenson RA, Coyle LM, et al. (1999) Prostate Cancer Trends 1973–1995, SEER Program, National Cancer Institute. NIH Pub. No. 99-4543. Bethesda, MD.
10. Sakr WA, Haas GP, Cassin BF, Pontes JE, and Crissman JD. (1993) The frequency of carcinoma and intraepithelial neoplasia of the prostate in young male patients. *J Urol* 150:379–385.
11. Powell IJ, Schwartz K, Hussain M. (1995) Removal of the financial barrier to health care: does it impact on prostate cancer at presentation and survival? A comparative study between black and white men in a Veterans Affairs system. *Urology*, 46:825–830.

12. Pienta KJ, Kau TY, Demers R, Montie JE, Hoff M, Severson, RK. (1995) Effect of age and race on the survival of men with prostate cancer in the metropolitan Detroit tricounty area, 1973-1987. *Urology*, 45:93–102.
13. Anon. (1999) Medical Memo: Race and prostate cancer, *Harvard Men's Health Watch*, 3:1.
14. Polednak AP. (1990) Cancer mortality in a higher-income black population in New York State: comparison with rates in the United States as a whole. *Cancer*, 66:1654–1660.
15. Robbins AS, Whittemore AS, Van Den Eeden SK. (1998) Race, prostate cancer survival, and membership in a large health maintenance organization. *JNCI*, 90:986–990.
16. Brawn PN, Johnson EH, Kuhl DL, Riggs MW, Speights VO, Johnson CF III, et al. (1993) Stage at presentation and survival of white and black patients with prostate carcinoma. *Cancer*, 71:2569–2573.
17. Stone BA. (1998) Prostate cancer early detection in african-american men: a priority for the 21st century. *JNMA*, 90:S724–S727.
18. Anscher MS. (1999) Prostate cancer in african-american men. *NCMJ*, 60:10–12.
19. Myers RE, Chodak GW, Wolf TA, Burgh DY, McGrory DT, Marcus SM, et al. (1999) Adherence by African American men to prostate cancer education and early detection. *Cancer*, 86:88–104.
20. Price JH, Colvin TL, Smith D. (1993) Prostate cancer: perceptions of african-american males. *JNMA*, 85:941–947.
21. Schapira MM, McAuliffe TL, Nattinger, AB. (1995) Treatment of localized prostate cancer in african-american compared with caucasian men: less use of aggressive therapy for comparable disease. *Med Care* 33:1079–1088.
22. Liff JM, Chow W, Greenberg RS. (1991) Rural-urban differences in stage at diagnosis: possible relationship to cancer screening. *Cancer*, 67:1454–1459.
23. Powell IJ, Gelfand DE, Parzuchowski J, Heilbrun L, and Franklin A. (1995) A successful recruitment process of African American men for early detection of prostate cancer. *Cancer* [suppl], 75:1880–1884.
24. Shiraishi T, Muneyuki T, Fukutome K, Ito H, Kotake T, Watanbe M, et al. (1998) Mutations of *ras* genes are relatively frequent in Japanese prostate cancers: pointing to genetic differences between populations. *Anticancer Research*, 18:2789–2792.
25. Tsugane S, Gotlieb SLD, Laurenti R, de Souza JMP, and Watanabe S. (1990) Cancer mortality among Japanese residents of the city of Sao Paulo, Brazil. *Int J Cancer*, 45:436–439.
26. Cook LS, Goldoft M, Schwartz, SM, and Weiss NS. (1999) Incidence of adeno-carcinoma of the prostate in Asian immigrants to the United States and their descendants. *J Urology*, 161:152–155.
27. Shimizu H, Ross RK, Bernstein L, Yatani R, Henderson, BE, Mack TM. (1991) Cancers of the prostate and breast among Japanese and white immigrants in Los Angeles County. *Br J Cancer*, 63:963–966.
28. Whittemore AS, Kolonel LN, Wu AH, et al. (1995) Prostate cancer in relation to diet, physical activity, and body size in blacks, whites, and Asians in the United States and Canada. *JNCI*, 87:652–661.
29. Herbert JR, Hurley TG, Olendzki BC, Teas J, Ma Y, Hampl, JS. (1998) Nutrition and socioeconomic factors in relation to prostate cancer mortality: a cross-national study. *JNCI* 90:1637–1647.

30. Sung JFC, Lin RS, Pu Y, Chen Y, Chang HC, Lai M. (1999) Risk factors for prostate carcinoma in Taiwan: a case-control study in a Chinese population. *Cancer* 86:484–491.
31. Le Marchand L, Kolonel LN, Wilkens LR, Myers BC, Hirohata T. (1994) Animal fat consumption and prostate cancer: a prospective study in Hawaii. *Epidemiology*, 5:276–282.
32. Jain MG, Hislop GT, How, GR, Burch JD, Ghadirian P. (1998) Alcohol and other beverage use and prostate cancer risk among Canadian men. *Int. J. Cancer*, 78:707–711.
33. Slattery ML, Schumacher MC, West DW, Robison LM, and French TK. (1990) Food-consumption trends between adolescent and adult years and subsequent risk of prostate cancer. *Am J Clin Nutr* 52:752–757.
34. Schuurman AG, van den Brandt PA, Dorant E, Goldbohm RA. (1999) Animal products, calcium, and protein and prostate cancer risk in the Netherlands cohort study. *Brit J Cancer* 80:1107–1113.
35. Groenberg H, Damber L, Damber J. (1996) Total food consumption and body mass index in relation to prostate cancer risk: a case-control study in Sweden with prospectively collected exposure data. *J Urol* 155:969–974.
36. Eichholzer M, Staehelin HB, Lueden E, Bernasconi F. (1999) Smoking, plasma vitamins C, E, retinol, and carotene, and fatal prostate cancer: seventeen-year follow-up of the prospective Basel study. *The Prostate* 38:189–198.
37. Clark LC, Dalkin B, Krongrad A, et al. (1998) Decreased incidence of prostate cancer with selenium supplementation: results of a double-blind cancer prevention trial. *Br J Urol*, 81:730–734.
38. Hartman TJ, Albanes D, Pietinen P, et al. (1998) The association between baseline vitamin E, selenium, and prostate cancer in the alpha-tocopherol, beta-carotene cancer prevention study. *Cancer Epidemiol Biomarkers Prev*, 7:335–340.
39. Hayes RB, Brown LM, Schoenberg JB, Greenberg RS, Silverman DT, Scwartz AG, et al. (1996) Alcohol use and prostate cancer risk in US blacks and whites. *Am J Epid*, 143:692–697.
40. Lumey LH, Pittman B, Wynder EL. (1998) Alcohol use and prostate cancer in US whites: no association in a confirmatory study. *Prostate*, 36:250–255.
41. Parker AS, Cerhan JR, Putnam SD, Cantor KP, Lynch CF (1999) A cohort study of farming and risk of prostate cancer in Iowa. *Epidomology*, 10:452–455.
42. Van der Gulden JWJ, Kolk JJ, Verbeek ALM. (1992) Prostate cancer and work environment. *J Occup Med*, 34:402–409.
43. Acquavella JF. (1999) Farming and prostate cancer. *Epidomology*, 10:349–351.
44. Fincham SM, Hanson J, and Berkel J. (1992) Patterns and risks of cancer in farmers in Alberta. *Cancer*, 69:1276–1285.
45. Morrison H, Savitz D, Semenciw R, Hulka B, Mao Y, Morison D, et al. (1993) Farming and prostate cancer mortality. *Am J Epid* 137:270–280.
46. Aeronson KJ, Siemiatycki J, Dewar R, Gerin M. (1996) Occupational risk factors for prostate cancer: results from a case-control study in Montreal, Quebec, Canada. *Am J Epid* 143:363–373.
47. Ma F, Lee DJ, Fleming LE, Dosemeci M (1998) Race-specific cancer mortality in US firefighters: 1984–1993. *J Occup Environ Med* 40:1134–1138.
48. Elghany NA, Schumacher MC, Slattery ML, et al. (1990) Occupation, cadmium exposure, and prostate cancer. *Epidemiology*, 1:107–115.
49. Carter BS, Bova GS, Beaty TH, Steinberg GD, Childs B, Issacs WB, et al. (1993) Hereditary prostate cancer: epidemiologic and clinical features. *J Urol* 150:797–802.

50. Bratt O, Kristoffersson U, Lundgren R, Olsson H. (1999) Familial and hereditary prostate cancer in southern Sweden: A population-based case-control study. *Eur. J. Cancer* 35:272–277.
51. Spitz MR, Currier RD, Fueger JJ, Babaian RJ, Newell GR. (1991) Familial patterns of prostate cancer: A case control analysis *J Urol* 146;1305–1307.
52. Groenberg H, Wiklund F, Damber J. (1999) Age specific risks of familial prostate carcinoma: A basis for screening recommendations in high risk populations. *Cancer* 86:477–483.
53. Ghadirian P, Howe GR, Hislop TG, Maisonneuve P. (1997) Family history of prostate cancer: A multi-center case-control study in Canada. *Int. J. Cancer* 70:679–681.
54. Lesko SM, Rosenberg L, Shapiro S. (1996) Family history and prostate cancer risk. *Am J Epid* 144:1041–1047.
55. Valeri A, Azzouzi R, Drelon E, et al. (2000) Early-onset hereditary prostate cancer is not associated with specific clinical and biological features. *Prostate* 45:66–71.
56. Groenberg H, Isaacs SD, Smith JR, Carpten JD, Bova GS, Freije D. (1997) Characteristics of prostate cancer in families potentially linked to the hereditary prostate cancer 1 (HPC1) Locus. *JAMA* 278:1251–1255.
57. Hayes RB, Liff JM, Pottern LM, Greenberg RS, Schoenberg JB, Schwartz AG. (1995) Prostate cancer in U.S. blacks and whites with a history of cancer. *Int J Cancer* 60:361–364.
58. Whittemore AS, Wu AH, Kolonel LN, John EM, Gallagher RP, Howe GR. (1995) Family history and prostate cancer risk in black, white, and asian men in the United States and Canada. *Am J Epid* 141:732–740.
59. Ross RK, Bernstein L, Loro RA, Shimiz H, Stancyzk FZ, Pike MC, et al. (1992) 5-alpha-reductase activity and risk of prostate cancer among Japanese and US white and black males. *Lancet* 339:887–889.
60. Santner SJ, Albertson B, Zhang GY, Zhang GH, Santulli M, Wang C, et al. (1998) Comparative rates of androgen production and metabolism in caucasian and Chinese subjects. *J Clin Endocrin Metabol* 83:2104–2109.
61. Tymchuk CN, Tessler SB, Aronson WJ, Barnard RJ (1998) Effects of diet and exercise on insulin, sex hormone-binding globulin, and prostate-specific antigen. *Nutrition and Cancer* 31:127–131.
62. Grignon DJ, Sakr WA. (1996) Atypical adenomatous hyperplasia of the prostate, A critical review. *Eur Urol* 30:206–211.
63. Bostwick DG, Brawer MK. (1987) Prostatic intra-epithelial neoplasia and early invasion in prostate cancer. *Cancer* 59:788–794.
64. Drago JR, Mostofi FK, Lee F. (1992) Introductory remarks and workshop summary. *Urology*, 39:suppl:2–8.
65. Montironi R, Pomante R, Diamanti L, Hamilton PW, Thompson D, Bartels PH. (1996) Evaluation of prostatic intraepithelial neoplasia after treatment with a 5-alpha-reductase inhibitor (finasteride). A methodologic approach. *Anal Quant Cytol Histol* 18:461–470.
66. Drachenberg CB, Ioffe OB, Papadimitriou JC. (1997) Progressive increase of apoptosis in prostatic intraepithelial neoplasia and carcinoma: comparison between in situ end-labeling of fragmented DNA and detection by routine hematoxylin-eosin staining. *Arch Pathol Lab Med* 121:54–58.
67. Sakr WA, Macoska JA, Benson P, Grignon DJ, Wolman SR, Pontes JE, et al. (1994) Allelic loss in locally metastatic, multisampled prostate cancer. *Cancer Res* 54:3273–3277.

68. Langer JE, Rovner ES, Coleman BG, et al. (1996) Strategy for repeat biopsy of patients with prostatic intraepithelial neoplasia detected by prostate needle biopsy. *J Urol* 155:228–231.
69. Fleshner NE, O'Sullivan M, Fair WR. (1997) Prevalence and predictors of a positive repeat transrectal ultrasound guided needle biopsy of the prostate. *J Urol* 158:505–508.
70. McNeal JE, Bostwick, DG (1986) Intraductal dysplasia: a premalignant lesion of the prostate. *Hum Pathol* 17:64–71.
71. Oyasu R, Bahnson RR, Nowels K, Garnett JE. (1986) Cytological atypia in the prostate gland, frequency, distribution and possible relevance to carcinoma. *J Urol* 135:959–962.
72. Sakr WA, Grignon DJ, Crissman JD, Heilbrun LK, Cassin BK, Pontes JE, et al. (1994) High grade prostatic intraepithelial neoplasia (HGPIN) and prostatic adenocarcinoma between the ages of 20-69: an autopsy study of 249 cases. *In Vivo* 8:439–443.
73. Sakr WA. (1999) Prostatic intraepithelial neoplasia: A marker for high-risk groups and a potential target for chemoprevention. *Eur Urol* 35:474–478.
74. Sakr WA, Grignon DJ, Haas GP. (1998) Pathology of premalignant lesions and carcinoma of the prostate in African-American men. *Semin Urol Oncol* 16:214–220.
75. Billis A. (1996) Age and race distribution of high grade prostatic intraepitelial neoplasia: An autopsy study in Brazil (South America). *J Urological Pathol* 5:175–181.
76. Algaba F. (1999) Evolution of isolated high-grade prostate intraepithelial neoplasia in a Mediterranean patient population. *Eur Urol* 35:496–497.
77. Bostwick DG, Qian J, Frankel K. (1995) The incidence of high grade prostatic intraepithelial neoplasia in needle biopsies. *J Urol* 154:1791–1794.
78. Wills ML, Hamper UM, Partin AW, Epstein, J.I. (1997) Incidence of high-grade prostatic intraepithelial neoplasia in sextant needle biopsy specimens. *Urol* 49:367–373.
79. Orozco R, O'Dowd G, Kunnel B, Miller MC, Veltri RW. (1998) Observations on pathology trends in 62,537 prostate biopsies obtained from urology private practices in the United States. *Urol* 51:186–195.
80. Pacelli A, Bostwick DG. (1997) Clinical significance of high-grade prostatic intraepithelial neoplasia in transurethral resection specimens. *Urol* 50:355–359.
81. Gaudin PB, Sesterhenn IA, Wojno KJ, Mostofi FK, Epstein JI. (1997) Incidence and clinical significance of high-grade prostatic intraepithelial neoplasia in TURP specimens. *Urol* 49:558–563.
82. Andrews GS. (1949) Latent carcinoma of the prostate. *J Clin Path* 2:197–211.
83. Edwards CN, Steinthorsson E, Nicholson D. (1953) An autopsy study of latent prostatic cancer. *Cancer* 6:531–644.
84. Franks LM. (1954) Latent carcinoma of the prostate. *J Path Bact* 68:603–609.
85. Breslow N, Chan CW, Dhom G, Drury RAB, Franks LM, Gellei B, et al. (1977) Latent carcinoma of the prostate at autopsy seven areas. *Int J Cancer* 20:680–688.
86. Potosky AL, Miller BA, Albertsen PC, Kramer BS. (1995) The Role of Increasing Detection in the rising incidence of prostate cancer. *JAMA* 273:548–552.
87. Gilliland FD, Becker TM, Key CR, Samet JM. (1994) Contrasting trends of prostate cancer incidence and mortality in New Mexico's Hispanics, non-Hispanic whites, American Indians and blacks. *Cancer* 73:2192–2199.

88. Gilliland FD, Becker TM, Smith A, Key CR, Samet JM. (1994) Trends in prostate cancer incidence and mortality in New Mexico are consistent with an increase in effective screening. *Cancer Epidemiol Biomarker Prev* 3:105–111.
89. Reynolds, T. (1993) Prostate cancer rates climbed sharply in 1990. *JNCI* 85:947–948.
90. Jacobsen SJ, Katusic SK, Bergstralh EJ, et al. (1995) Incidence of prostate cancer diagnosis in the eras before and after serum prostate-specific antigen testing. *JAMA* 274:1445–1449.
91. Pearson JD, Carter, HB. (1994) Natural history of changes in prostate specific antigen in early stage prostate cancer. *J Urol* 152:1743–1748.
92. Stamey TA, Donaldson AN, Yemoto CE, McNeal JE, Soezen S, Gill H. (1998) Histological and clinical findings in 896 consecutive prostates treated only with radical retropubic prostatectomy: epidemiologic significance of annual changes. *J Urol* 160:2412–2417.
93. Mandelson MT, Wagner EH, Thompson RS. (1995) PSA Screening: A public health dilemma. *Annu Rev Public Health* 16:283–306.
94. Hankey BF, Feuer EJ, Clegg LX, et al. (1999) Cancer surveillance series: interpreting trends in prostate cancer—part i: evidence of the effects of screening in recent prostate cancer incidence, mortality, and survival rates. *JNCI* 91:1017–1024.
95. Stephenson RA, Stanford JL. (1997) Population-based prostate cancer trends in the United States: patterns of change in the era of prostate-specific antigen. *World J Urol* 15:331–335.
96. Catalona WJ, Smith DS, Ratliff TL, Basler JW. (1993) Detection of organ-confined prostate cancer is increased through prostate-specific antigen-based screening. *JAMA* 270:948–954.
97. Gilliland FD, Welsh DJ, Hoffman RM, Ke CR. (1995) Rapid rise and subsequent decline in prostate cancer incidence rates for New Mexico, 1989–1993. *Cancer Epidemiol Biomarkers Prev* 4:797–800.
98. Meyer F, Moore L, Bairati I, Fradet Y. (1999) Downward Trend in Prostate Cancer Mortality in Quebec and Canada. *J Urol* 161:1189–1191.
99. Merrill RM, Potosky AL, Feuer EJ. (1996) Changing trends in U.S. prostate cancer incidence rates. *JNCI* 88:1683–1685.
100. Littrup PJ, Lee F, Mettlin C. (1992) Prostate cancer screening: current trends and future implications. *CA Cancer J Clin* 42:198–211.
101. Catalona WJ, Richie JP, Ahmann FR, Hudson MA, Scardino PT, Flanigan, RC, et al. (1994) Comparison of digital rectal examination and serum prostate specific antigen in the early detection of prostate cancer: results of a multicenter clinical trial of 6,630 men. *J Urol* 151:1283–1290.
102. Smith DS, Catalona WJ. (1994) The nature of prostate cancer detected through prostate specific antigen based screening. *J Urol* 152:1732–1736.
103. Ghavamian R, Blute ML, Bergstralh EJ, Slezak J, Zincke H. (1999) Comparison of clinically nonpalpable prostate-specific antigen-detected (cT1c) versus palpable (cT2) prostate cancers in patients undergoing radical retropublic prostatectomy. *Urol* 54:105–110.
104. Luboldt HJ, Altwein JE, Bichler KH, Czaja D, Husing J, Fornara P, et al. (1999) [Early recognition of prostate carcinoma. Initial results of a prospective multicenter study in Germany. Project Group for EarlyDetection DGU-BDULaboratory diagnosis Professional Circle]. *Urologe A* 38:114–123.
105. Schroeder FH, van der Maas P, Beemsterboer P, Kruger AB, Hoedermaeker R, Rietbergen J, et al. (1998) Evaluation of the digital rectal examination as a

screening test for prostate cancer. Rotterdam Section of the European Randomized Study of Screening for Prostate Cancer. *JNCI* 90:1817–1823.
106. Littrup PJ. (1997) Future benefits and cost-effectiveness of prostate cancer
screening. *Cancer* 80:1864–1870.
107. Smith DS, Bullock AD, Catalona WJ (1997) Racial differences in operating
characteristics of prostate cancer screening tests. *J Urol* 158:1861–1865.
108. Demark-Wahnefried W, Strigo T, Catoe K, Conaway M, Brunetti M, Rimer BK,
et al. (1995) Knowledge, beliefs, and prior screening behavior among blacks and
whites reporting for prostate cancer screening. *Urol* 46:346-351.
109. Bostwick DG. (1999) What is the significance of race to prostate carcinoma.
Cancer 86:735–737.
110. Gilliland FD, Hoffman RM, Hamilton A, Albertsen P, Eley JW, Harlan L, et al.
(1999) Predicting extracapsular extension of prostate cancer in men treated with
radical prostatectomy: results from the population based prostate cancer outcomes study. *J Urol* 162:1341–1345.
111. Jhaveri FM, Klein EA, Kupelian PA, Zippe C, Levin HS (1999) Declining rates
of extracapsular extension after radical prostatectomy: evidence for continued
stage migration. *J Clin Oncol* 17:3167–3172.
112. Demers RY, Swanson GM, Weiss LK, Kau TY. (1994) Increasing incidence of
cancer of the prostate. The experience of black and white men in the Detroit
Metropolitan area. *Arch Intern Med* 154:1211–1216.
113. Mettlin C, Murphy GP, Lee F, Littrup PJ, Chesley A, Babaian R, et al. (1994)
Characteristics of prostate cancer detected in the American Cancer Society
National Prostate Cancer Detection Project. *J Urol* 152:1737–1740.
114. Catalona WJ, Smith DS, Ratliff TL, Basler JW. Detection of organ-confined
prostate cancer is increased through prostate-specific antigen-based screening.
JAMA 270:948–954.
115. Slawin KM, Ohori M, Dillioglugi LO, Scardino PT. (1995) Screening for prostate
cancer: an analysis of the early experience. *CA Cancer J Clin* 45:134–147.
116. Amling CL, Blute MI, Lerner SE, Bergstralh EJ, Bostwick DG, Zincke H.
(1998) Influence of prostate-specific antigen testing on the spectrum of patients
with prostate cancer undergoing radical prostatectomy at a large referral practice. *Mayo Clin Proc* 73:401–406.
117. Schwartz KL, Grignon DJ, Sakr WA, Wood DP Jr. (1999) Prostate cancer histologic trends in the metropolitan Detroit area, 1982 to 1996. *Urol* 53:769–774.
118. Schwartz KL, Severson RK, Gurney JG, Montie JE. (1996) Trends in the stage
specific incidence of prostate carcinoma in the Detroit Metropolitan area, 1973–
1994. *Cancer* 78:1260–1266.
119. Feneley MR. (1999) Does screening for prostate cancer identify clinically important disease? *Ann R Coll Surg Engl* 8:207–214.
120. Bassler TJ Jr, Orozco R, Bassler IC, O'Dowd GJ, Stamey TA. (1998) Most prostate cancers missed by raising the upper limit of normal prostate-specific antigen
for men in the sixties are clinically significant. *Urol* 52:1064–1069.
121. Lerner SE, Seay TM, Blute ML, Bergstalh EJ, Barrett D, Zincke H (1996)
Prostate specific antigen detected prostate cancer (clinical stage T1c): an interim
analysis. *J Urol* 155:821–826.
122. Yang XJ, Lecksell K, Potter SR, Epstein JI. (1999) Significance of small
foci of Gleason score 7 or greater prostate cancer on needle biopsy. *Urol*
54:528–532.

123. Soh S, Kattan MW, Berkman S, Wheeler TM, Scardino PT. (1997) Has there been a recent shift in the pathological features and prognosis of patients treated with radical prostatectomy? *J Urol* 157:2212–2218.
124. Merrill RM, Stephenson RA (2000) Trends in mortality in patients with prostate cancer during the era of prostate specific antigen screening. *J Urol* 163:503–510.
125. Meyer F, Moore L, Bairati I, Fradet Y (1998) Quebec prostate cancer mortality dropped in 1996. *Cancer Prev Control* 2:163–166.
126. Feng J, deGuia K, Gharibian A, Grignon D, Sakr W (2000) Changes in the frequency and volume of "index" tumors and HGPIN in radical prostatectomy specimens (RPS) in the 1990s. *Mod Path* 13:99A.

2 Natural History of Prostate Cancer

Peter C. Albertsen, MD

INTRODUCTION

Prostate cancer encompasses a wide spectrum of clinical outcomes. Some patients suffer a rapid progression of their disease: others live with their disease for many years, ultimately succumbing to competing medical hazards. Only about 30% of the patients in the Veterans Administration Cooperative Urological Research Group (VACURG) studies of prostate cancer actually died from prostate cancer *(1)*. In 1999, an estimated 179,300 American men will be diagnosed with prostate cancer and 37,000 will die from this disease *(2)*. These statistics suggest that variable outcomes are as prevalent today as they were approximately half a century ago.

The wide spectrum of clinical outcomes poses a special burden to the physician treating patients with prostate cancer. Physicians cannot easily determine whether the interventions they propose are likely to alter the natural outcome of this disease. Unlike some cancers where death is a virtual certainty in the absence of treatment, the natural history of prostate cancer is much more varied. When counseling patients with this

From: *Current Clinical Urology: Prostate Cancer Screening*
Edited by: I. M. Thompson, M. I. Resnick, and E. A. Klein
© Humana Press Inc., Totowa, NJ

disease, clinicians often follow the safest approach and recommend aggressive therapy. If the disease progresses, the physician takes solace in that he or she has done everything possible. If the disease does not progress, the physician assumes that he or she has "cured" the patient.

Unfortunately, the efficacy of different treatment strategies remains uncertain for many patients. Neither surgery nor radiation therapy has been shown to be an effective method of controlling disease among a substantial number of patients who are at the highest risk of dying from prostate cancer. The advent of testing for prostate-specific antigen (PSA) has dramatically increased our ability to detect early-stage prostate cancer and monitor the progression of this disease, but it has also increased the uncertainty concerning how best to manage men with less aggressive forms of this disease. To understand the true benefit of treatment, clinicians must have a good understanding of the natural history of prostate cancer.

The purpose of this chapter is to review the critical studies that have led to our current understanding of the natural progression of prostate cancer. Both tumor histology and tumor volume should be assessed when advising patients concerning the likely clinical outcome of this disease. Using standardized assessments of tumor histology and volume, clinicians can better estimate the relative risk posed by different prostate cancers and the relative value provided by different treatment strategies. By refining our understanding of the risks and benefits of different therapeutic approaches, patients can select a strategy appropriate to their disease that hopefully optimizes their life expectancy with a minimal compromise to their quality of life.

THE SIGNIFICANCE OF HISTOLOGY

The VACURG Studies and the Gleason Grading System

Many physicians have recognized the important relationship between histology and the clinical outcome of prostate cancer (3–4). This information, however, has only recently been incorporated into treatment decision analysis. Prior to the publication of the Gleason grading system, many pathologists found it difficult to classify prostate cancers consistently according to their malignant potential. Gleason's accumulated experience with almost 3000 tumors from the VACURG studies confirmed that prostate cancer histology was strongly correlated with the clinical behavior of this cancer and that prostate cancer histology provided information concerning outcome that was independent of clinical stage. Because of its relative simplicity, pathologists have adopted

Gleason's scoring system as the standard for assessing prostate cancer histology.

The VACURG studies were begun in 1960 as controlled, randomized, prospective comparisons of the different treatments available for prostate cancer (5). Three different protocols enrolled a total of 2911 men. Study 1 (1960–1967) compared placebo vs 5 mg of diethylstilbestrol (DES)/d following radical prostatectomy for patients with clinically localized disease. Men with regional and metastatic disease were randomized to one of four treatment groups: placebo; 5 mg of DES/d; orchiectomy alone; orchiectomy plus 5 mg DES/d. Study 2 (1967–1969) compared radical prostatectomy with no surgery for men with localized disease. Men with regional and advanced disease were randomized to one of four arms: placebo; 0.2 mg DES/d; 1 mg DES/d; 5 mg DES/d. Study 3 opened for accrual in 1969 and randomized men with localized disease to radical prostatectomy vs no surgery, while men with regional or advanced disease were randomized into four groups: 1 mg DES/d; 2.5 mg of conjugated equine estrogens (Premarin)/d; 30 mg of medroxyprogesterone acetate (Provera)/day; 30 mg of medroxyprogesterone acetate plus 1 mg DES/d.

By 1974, 2911 cases were available for follow-up clinical correlation. For each case the cause of death was determined by an evaluation committee that consisted of three participating clinicians. Original histology slides were re-evaluated by Dr. Donald Gleason and assigned a score according to his classification system. The system developed by Gleason involved an assessment of the degree of glandular differentiation viewed under low-power magnification. Originally nine independent patterns were identified, but these were combined into the classic patterns that constitute the Gleason grading system.

The VACURG assessed clinical outcomes by calculating the number of deaths per patient-year of follow-up. This statistic is calculated by dividing the number of deaths in the group under consideration by the sum of the follow-up times for all the patients (both living and dead) in that group. The follow-up time was measured from the date of admission to the study to the date of death or to the date of last known follow-up. Time was recorded in months and ranged from 0 to 14 yr/patient.

The observed incidence of the primary and secondary histology patterns was strongly correlated. Low-grade primary patterns were usually associated with low-grade secondary patterns and high-grade primary patterns were usually associated with high-grade secondary patterns. Mortality rates were strongly correlated with both the primary and secondary histology patterns, but the average histology pattern provided the strongest correlation. Accordingly, Gleason proposed summing the pattern scores to provide the best predictor of clinical outcome. This sum is now frequently called a Gleason score.

A review of the clinical outcomes of the patients involved in the VACURG study shows that grading prostate cancers by histology can separate patients into groups that experience markedly different mortality rates (Fig. 1). Patients with Gleason score 2–5 tumors had a cancer death rate of only 0.012 or 1.2 deaths/100 patient-yr. The remaining 2187 patients with Gleason scores from 6 to 10 had a cancer death rate of 0.124 deaths/patient-yr; a rate that is 10 times higher than the rate for men with low-grade disease.

The Johansson Studies

Between 1989 and 1997, Johansson and colleagues published a series of three articles that documented the natural history of untreated prostate cancer in a population-based cohort of patients diagnosed with prostate cancer in Orebro Medical Center in Sweden, a hospital with a strictly defined catchment area (6–8). No screening for prostate cancer took place during the period when this study population of 648 consecutive cases was assembled. They found relatively low 5- and 10-year mortality rates among men with clinically localized disease and challenged the use of aggressive initial treatment for all patients with early-stage prostate cancer. Their studies were criticized primarily because of issues surrounding the selection of the study cohort.

Johansson et al. utilized a prospective, population-based study design to assemble their study cohort. Between March 1977 and February 1984, all consecutive cases of clinically diagnosed prostate cancer were enrolled in the study. Diagnoses were confirmed by fine-needle aspiration biopsy of palpable prostate tumors in 542 (84%) of the 648 cases. In another 106 cases (16%), the diagnosis was made during surgery for benign prostate hyperplasia. Staging examinations included chest radiography, intravenous pyelography, bone scan, and skeletal radiography of suspicious lesions on bone scan. Digital rectal examination was also performed to determine the clinical stage of the disease. Medical information on six patients could not be located.

Of the 642 patients evaluated, 300 had disease localized to the prostate (T0–T2) and 183 patients had locally advanced disease (T3–T4) without detectable metastases (M0). Metastatic disease was found in 159 patients (25%). Of the 300 patients with localized disease, 223 received no initial treatment. Of the remaining 77 patients, 2 underwent a radical prostatectomy and 75 received some combination of external beam radiation, estrogen, estramustine, or an orchiectomy. Of the 342

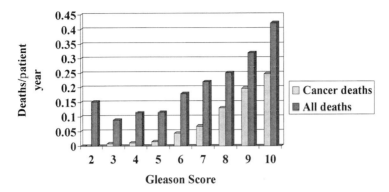

Fig. 1. Mortality rates of patients enrolled in the VACURG studies stratified by Gleason score.

patients with locally advanced disease or with metastatic disease, most were treated with hormonal therapy, predominantly with estrogen or estramustine.

All patients were followed until death or until the end of the observation period on September 1, 1994. The observation period ranged from 126 to 210 mo, the average being 168 mo (14 yr). Patients were followed at least every year and some much more frequently. Prostate cancer was recorded as the underlying cause of death, a contributory cause of death, or unrelated to the cause of death for each patient who died during the follow-up period. An autopsy was performed if the cause of death was unclear. If the treatment of the prostate cancer was related to the patient's death, (e.g., cardiovascular complications following estrogen therapy), prostate cancer was recorded as a contributory cause of death. Cause of death determinations were reviewed and compared with the classification assigned by the county tumor registrar. There was agreement in 90% of cases, and no evidence of systematic overascertainment or underascertainment of prostate cancer cause of death. The authors performed several survival analyses, including an analysis of all-cause survival and disease-specific survival. The effect of different variables on survival was determined using the Cox proportional hazards model.

At the end of the observation period, 541 (84%) of all 642 patients in the study cohort had died. Prostate cancer was considered the underlying cause of death in 201 patients (31%), whereas in 35 patients (5%), prostate cancer contributed to the cause of death. Prostate cancer accounted for more deaths among younger patients compared with older patients at the time of diagnosis. More patients with poorly differentiated tumors and/or advanced local tumors died of prostate cancer. For

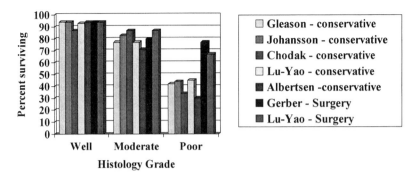

Fig. 2. Ten-year disease-specific survival estimates stratified by tumor histology derived from five studies analyzing outcomes following conservative management and two studies analyzing outcomes following radical prostatectomy.

the 300 men with localized disease at the time of diagnosis, 37 (12%) developed metastases and 33 (11%) died of their disease. Of these 300 patients, 223 received no initial therapy. Among these 223 patients, 29 (13%) developed metastases, 25 (11%) died of prostate cancer, and 4 died of prostate cancer as a contributing cause of death (Fig. 2).

A careful review of the 223 patients receiving no initial therapy reveals that 148 had well differentiated disease and 66 had moderately differentiated disease. Presumably, these cases would be classified as Gleason 2–6 tumors. Of the 148 patients with well-differentiated disease, only 9 (6%) died from prostate cancer and only 2 developed distant metastases. Results were not quite as good for men with moderately differentiated disease. Of these 66 men, 11 (17%) died from prostate cancer and 2 (1.8%) developed metastatic disease. The nine men with poorly differentiated disease fared poorly. Three patients developed local progression and six developed metastases. Five of these patients had died from prostate cancer at the time of last follow-up.

Based on their findings, Johannson et al. stated that men with well-differentiated or moderately differentiated disease have an excellent prognosis in the absence of any aggressive treatment. These findings are in agreement with those published by Gleason. Unfortunately, men with poorly differentiated prostate cancer had a high incidence of progression and death from their disease. This finding is also similar to that of Gleason. Of the 201 men who died from prostate cancer in the entire cohort of 642 men, 28 (13%) of these patients had well-differentiated prostate cancers, 101 (33%) had moderately differentiated cancers and 72 (58%) had poorly differentiated cancers. When contributory causes are considered, a total of 68% of men presenting with poorly differentiated disease and 38% of men with moderately differentiated disease died from prostate cancer. Johannson et al. concluded their study by noting that because of the favorable survival rate among the untreated patients with early-stage disease, at least 80% of these patients would be treated without survival benefit. Although this may be true for older men with well-differentiated and moderately differentiated disease, these results cannot be generalized to younger men and men with poorly differentiated cancers. The distribution of Gleason scores in contemporary series of incident cases is more heavily weighted toward moderate and poorly differentiated disease compared with the sample reported by Johannson et al.

The Chodak study

In 1994, Chodak et al. published a report concerning the results of conservative management of clinically localized prostate cancer (9). Unlike the Johannson report, this study consisted of a pooled analysis of 828 case records from 6 nonrandomized studies published during the decade preceding the report. None of the patients included in the report underwent a radical prostatectomy or received radiation therapy. Patients who had symptomatic progression or who developed metastases received hormonal therapy. The final report contained information derived from six previously reported studies (6,7,10–14). Two were conducted in the United States, two in Sweden and one each in Scotland and Israel. The final series consisted of 828 patients ranging in age from 37 to 93 yr at the time of diagnosis. The median follow-up of the study group was approx 6.5 yr.

A Cox proportional hazards regression model was initially used to determine the combined effects of the patient's age at diagnosis, tumor grade, disease stage, and the origin of the patient cohort on disease-specific survival. The risk ratio for disease progression was substantially higher for patients with poorly differentiated histology when compared with all the other risk ratios. As a result, the authors stratified patients into three categories by biopsy tumor histology for subsequent analysis. The goal of the study was to calculate conservative estimates of the effect of nonaggressive treatment on disease-specific survival, overall survival, survival among patients who did not die of prostate cancer (noncancer survival), and metastasis-free survival among men with clinically localized prostate cancer.

Disease-specific survival and metastasis-free survival for men with well-, moderately, and poorly differentiated disease were reported. Patients with poorly differentiated (grade 3) cancers had a significantly lower cancer-specific survival rate (34%) when compared with men who had well-differentiated (grade 1) or moderately (grade 2) differentiated cancers (87%). Men with moderately differentiated cancer (grade 2) had a lower disease-specific survival rate when compared with men who had well differentiated disease (grade 1), but the difference was not statistically significant (Fig. 2). The rate of progression to metastasis differed significantly among men with the three tumor grades. Men with poorly differentiated tumors were much more likely to progress to metastatic disease compared with men who were diagnosed with well-differentiated disease. These results are similar to those reported by Gleason and Johannson et al.

The authors tested for several potential biases that could have compromised their findings. They concluded that the relatively favorable outcome associated with conservative management could not be explained by the inclusion of men with shorter than average life expectancies. They also investigated the potential impact of including patients with small, focal tumors because these patients are thought to have a more favorable outcome when compared with patients with other stages of localized disease. They found that the inclusion of these cases did not affect the overall rates of disease-specific survival reported for the entire population of patients.

Based on these findings, the authors concluded that prostate cancer is a progressive disease when managed conservatively. Furthermore, the prognosis of men with poorly differentiated disease is considerably worse when compared with men with well-differentiated or moderately differentiated disease. The authors also commented that aggressive treatment of prostate cancer may result in a lower mortality from prostate cancer at 10 yr among men with well-differentiated and moderately differentiated disease, but the differences appear to be small. The relative benefit of aggressive treatment for poorly differentiated disease is less clear. These patients face a significant risk of disease progression in the absence of treatment, therefore the potential benefit of more aggressive treatment is substantially larger.

The Lu-Yao Study

In 1997, Lu-Yao and Yao published an analysis of 59,876 prostate cancer registry patients at age 50–79 years at diagnosis to ascertain overall and prostate cancer-specific survival rates among men treated with surgery, radiation, or a more conservative approach (15) Their study relied on the population-based records compiled by the Surveillance, Epidemiology and End Results (SEER) of the National Cancer Institute. Their study utilized the SEER histology classification system: grade 1 (Gleason scores 2–4), grade 2 (scores 5–7), grade 3 (scores 8–10) and grade unknown. The patients included in the study were diagnosed between January 1, 1983 and December 31, 1992. Men with other cancers were excluded from the analysis.

Using an intention to treat analysis, they found that cancer grade had a significant effect on overall survival. All patients with well-differentiated disease had similar or even better overall survival when compared with an age-matched control regardless of treatment. In contrast, patients with poorly differentiated disease had much lower overall survival than their age-matched controls in all treatment groups. The risk of dying of prostate cancer within 10 yr of diagnosis was ten times greater for men with poorly differentiated disease compared with men with well-differentiated disease. Poorly differentiated cancers had a uniformly poor outcome for men with localized disease as well as regional disease. Furthermore, the authors found that the effect of poorly differentiated disease on survival was rapid. Five years after diagnosis, patients with poorly differentiated disease managed conservatively had a relative survival of only 0.61 compared with age-matched controls and a disease-specific survival of only 63–69%.

Ten-year disease-specific survival rates for the entire cohort ranged from 45% to 94% (Fig. 2). For men with well-differentiated disease, survival rates were 94%, 90%, and 93%, respectively, for men undergoing prostatectomy, radiation therapy, and conservative management. For men with moderately differentiated disease (Gleason score 5–7), 10-yr disease-specific survival rates were 87%, 76%, and 77%, respectively. Men undergoing prostatectomy appeared to have a significant survival advantage in this group compared with men treated with radiation or managed conservatively. Men with poorly differentiated disease had the worst 10-yr disease-specific survival rates. They were 67%, 53%, and 45%, respectively, for men undergoing prostatectomy, radiation therapy and conservative management. Patients undergoing prostatectomy and radiotherapy had a higher relative and prostate-cancer-specific survival with poorly differentiated disease.

The Albertsen Study

We recently reported long-term outcomes of a competing risk analysis of 767 men diagnosed between 1971 and 1984 who were managed expectantly for clinically localized prostate cancer (16). Our study design consisted of a case series analysis of patients identified through the Connecticut tumor registry who satisfied several criteria. First, we searched for men with long-term follow-up extending 10–20 yr after diagnosis to capture the impact of prostate cancer and competing medical hazards. Second, we looked for men aged 55–74 yr at diagnosis to identify a group of men who had an average life expectancy of more than 10 yr. Third, we recovered the original histology slides of these patients to permit reanalysis using contemporary Gleason grading standards. Finally, we assembled a patient cohort sufficiently large to permit stratification by the biopsy Gleason score and age at diagnosis, factors known to be important determinants of outcome.

Long-term outcome information was obtained from the Connecticut tumor registry and the vital statistics bureau of the Department of Public Health. The mean follow-up of the patient cohort from diagnosis until death was 8.6 yr. Of the 157 patients lost to follow-up or known to be alive as of March 1, 1997, the mean follow up was 15.4 yr. Only 2 of these men were lost to follow-up before 10 yr, 76 of these men were followed for 10–14 yr and the remaining 79 were followed for 15 yr or more. Cause of death was determined by reviewing death certificates for each of the men who had died. Connecticut death certificates follow the format recommended by the World Health Assembly and contain two parts. Part I contains three lines for physicians to record the train of medical events leading directly to the patient's death. Part II contains one line for physicians to record any "other significant conditions: conditions contributing to death, but not related to cause." For this study, men were classified as dying from prostate cancer if any of the lines on Part I of the death certificate mentioned prostate cancer.

The results of our study are presented in Fig. 3. Few men (4–7%) with Gleason 2–4 tumors identified by prostate biopsy had progression leading to death from prostate cancer within 15 yr of diagnosis. A majority of the younger men are still alive, but they face the possibility of death from prostate cancer in the future. In contrast, most of the older men with Gleason 2–4 tumors identified by biopsy at diagnosis have died from competing medical hazards rather than prostate cancer.

Compared with men with well-differentiated tumors, men with Gleason 5 and 6 tumors identified by prostate biopsy experienced a somewhat higher risk of death from prostate cancer when managed expectantly (6–11% and 18–30%, respectively). Of the younger men with Gleason 5 and 6 tumors, more than half are still alive after 15 yr, whereas a majority of the older men have died from competing medical hazards.

Men with Gleason scores 7 and 8–10 tumors identified by prostate biopsy experienced a very high rate of death from prostate cancer regardless of their age at diagnosis (42–70% and 60–87%, respectively). Very few of these men of any age are still alive. Most have died from prostate cancer, except for approximately one-third of the oldest men, who died from competing medical hazards.

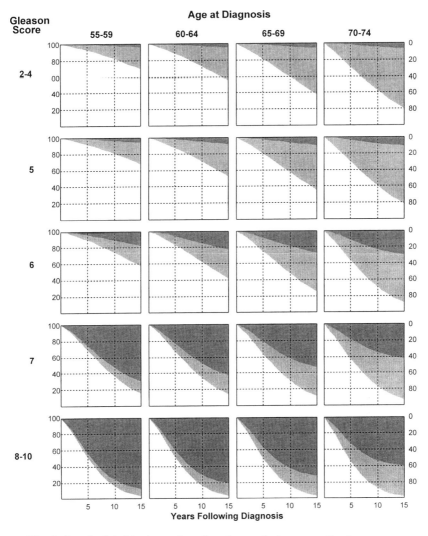

Fig. 3. Survival (white lower band) and cumulative mortality from prostate cancer (dark gray upper band) and other causes (light gray middle band) up to 15 yr after diagnosis stratified by age at diagnosis and Gleason score. The percentage of men alive can be read from the left-hand scale, and the percentage of men who have died from prostate cancer or from other causes during this interval can be read from the right-hand scale. [From Albertsen PC, Hanley JA, Gleason DF, Barry MJ (1998) Competing risk analysis of men aged 55 to 74 years at diagnosis managed conservatively for clinically localized prostate cancer. *JAMA* 280:975–980, with permission. Copyrighted 1998, American Medical Association.]

Our data are remarkably consistent with those reported by Gleason, Johansson et al., Chodak et al. and Lu-Yao et al. After 15 yr, men diagnosed with low-grade disease (Gleason score 2–4) have a small risk of dying from prostate cancer. Men with moderate-grade disease (Gleason score 5–6) have a slightly higher risk of dying from prostate cancer, whereas men with high-grade disease (Gleason score 7–10) have a substantial risk of dying from their disease when managed expectantly.

The Aus Study

In 1995, Aus et al. published an article that appeared to contradict these findings *(17)*. These investigators assembled a group of 514 Swedish men who died during the period 1988–1990. All of these men were alive at the time of diagnosis and received only noncurative therapy. Prostate cancer was diagnosed by fine-needle aspiration in 359 cases, by examination of surgical specimens in 128, by needle biopsy in 19, and by clinical findings in 14. The stage of disease was assigned retrospectively. Patients received either primary endocrine therapy (324) or deferred treatment (185). Cause of death was determined by consensus by two urologists after reviewing the medical records and the death certificates. The main outcome of the study was the cause of death among patients with disease who died during a 3 yr interval. Of the 514 patients studied, 108 (21%) had no evidence of metastatic disease, 296 (58%) had metastatic disease, and 110 (21%) had inadequate staging to determine their clinical status. Of the 301 patients without evidence of metastatic disease, 50% died of prostate cancer.

Unlike traditional population-based studies that accrue patients based on the date of their diagnosis, Aus et al. accrued patients on their date of death. By sampling only men who had died, the authors assembled a study cohort that was enriched by men who had moderately or poorly differentiated disease. The distribution of men by histology was 24%, 38%, and 35%, respectively, for men with well-differentiated, moderately and poorly differentiated cancers. In Johannson's study, this distribution was approx 33%, 48%, and 19%, respectively; in Lu-Yao's study, this distribution was 32%, 50%, and 18%, respectively; and in our study, this distribution was 33%, 56% and 10%, respectively. The 10% of patients with Gleason 8–10 tumors in our series accounted for 25% of the cancer deaths, and the 19% of men with poorly differentiated cancers in Johannson's series accounted for 36% of the cancer deaths. Because their accrual methodology yielded a significantly higher percentage of men with poorly differentiated disease, the estimates by Aus et al. of 15-yr mortality from prostate cancer are much higher than those reported by Gleason, Johansson, Chodak, Lu-Yao, and us. All five of these studies are in agreement that men with poorly differentiated prostate cancers have a high probability of dying from their disease when managed conservatively.

THE SIGNIFICANCE OF VOLUME AS ASSESSED BY SERUM PROSTATE SPECIFIC ANTIGEN

The volume of prostate cancer at the time of diagnosis is the other key variable that consistently predicts long-term clinical outcomes. Prior to the advent of testing for prostate specific antigen, clinicians relied on the digital rectal examination (DRE) and imaging studies such as the bone scan and computerized tomography (CT) to assess the extent of disease. The advent of testing for PSA has enabled clinicians to identify disease much earlier than previously imagined.

McNeal and colleagues have demonstrated that tumors less than 0.5 cc frequently occur in older men, but rarely extend beyond the confines of the prostate. Tumors greater than 3.0 cc often demonstrate seminal vesicle invasion and loss of normal histology features. Tumors that are 6.0 cc or larger are rarely curable even with aggressive management. In a large autopsy series, McNeal and colleagues showed that only tumors containing poorly differentiated histology features, specifically patterns 4 and/or 5, grow to sufficient size to metastasize *(18)*.

Stamey et al. have shown that many prostate cancers grow at a very slow rate *(19)*. Half of all prostate cancers take more than 5 yr to double in size, as compared with breast cancers, which can double in size every 3 mo. Most men over age 50 yr with prostate cancers smaller than 0.5 cc at the time of diagnosis will not live long enough for their cancers to achieve sufficient size to metastasize. Most clinicians now utilize a standard sextant biopsy technique to evaluate men who are suspected of having prostate cancer. Stamey has determined that patients with one or more cores containing more than 3 mm of tumor are likely to have a prostate volume greater than 0.5 cc *(20)*.

Although serum PSA levels are not sufficiently reliable to predict tumor burden for individual patients, serum PSA levels do correlate with tumor volume when evaluating large groups of men. In a classic analysis of over 10,000 men aged 50 yr and older participating in a screening program for prostate cancer, Catalona et al. reported that only 45% of men with a PSA score greater than 10 ng/mL had disease localized to the prostate *(21)*. Recently, Partin et al. combined information provided by serum PSA level, Gleason score, and clinical stage to generate a series of nomograms to predict local tumor extension and capsule penetration *(22)*.

The Carter Study

One of the early studies that contributed to our understanding of the natural progression of prostate cancer as measured by a rising PSA is the report by Carter et al. that evaluated longitudinal changes of PSA in men with and without prostate cancer *(23)*. They performed a case-control study utilizing men participating in the Baltimore Longitudinal Study of Aging (BLSA). Although the sample size was small, consisting of only 18 men with prostate cancer, 20 men with benign prostate hyperplasia and 16 controls, the authors suggested that the rate of change of PSA was an early clinical marker of the development of prostate cancer.

Thirty-seven men with the diagnosis of prostate cancer were identified from 1459 male participants in the BLSA. Of these patients, 18 were older than age 60 yr and had participated in the study for at least 7 yr prior to the diagnosis of cancer. Patients were classified as having local, regional or metastatic disease based on the clinical examination, prostatic acid phosphatase determination, bone scan results, and pathology reports from the treating physician's records. Sixteen subjects had no prior history of prostate disease and were selected as controls. Patients identified as controls were recruited between January 1990 and October 1990 when approximately 200 men returned for their routine visits. Serum samples available in the BLSA serum bank were tested for serum PSA. Unfortunately, serum samples were not available for all subjects for each visit.

A mixed-effects regression model was used to test the hypothesis that, after controlling for the effect of age at diagnosis, PSA values increase faster in subjects with prostate cancer compared with controls. Observed PSA levels are shown for each patient as a function of years prior to diagnosis for subjects with prostate cancer (Fig. 4). The patients with prostate cancer had significantly greater rates of change in PSA levels when compared with those patients without prostate cancer up to 10 yr before diagnosis. The graphs also demonstrate the variable progression of disease. Some patients with local or regional disease at diagnosis had an elevated serum PSA as much as 8 yr prior to diagnosis. Among patients presenting with metastatic disease, one patient had an elevated serum PSA level 16 yr prior to diagnosis. Unfortunately no information was provided concerning the Gleason score of the patients with prostate cancer who were included in the study.

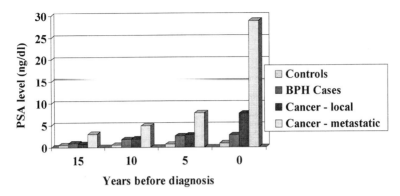

Fig. 4. Mean prostate-specific antigen levels of diagnostic groups evaluated by Carter et al. at 5-yr intervals prior to diagnosis. (Data derived from ref *23*.)

The Gann Study

In 1995, Gann and colleagues published a nested case-control study of men participating in the Physician's Health Study (PHS), an ongoing randomized trial of β-carotene that enrolled 22,071 men aged 40–84 yr in 1982 *(24)*. Their purpose was to evaluate the validity of using PSA to screen for prostate cancer. A total of 366 men diagnosed with prostate cancer were matched to three controls by age. Controls were randomly selected from the entire cohort at risk at the time of case diagnosis. Gann reviewed the medical records of each case to determine the stage at diagnosis, tumor grade, Gleason score, type of presentation (screening vs symptoms), and the PSA level just prior to treatment. If multiple tissue samples were available for evaluation, the highest Gleason score was recorded. Patients with regional or distant extension of their disease and all patients with Gleason scores of 7 or higher were classified as having aggressive cancers. Patients with pathologically determined localized disease and Gleason score 6 or less were classified as having nonaggressive cancers. The remaining patients who could not be staged pathologically and who had Gleason score 6 tumors or less were classified as having indeterminate aggressiveness. The mean age at baseline for both case patients and control patients was 62.9 yr and the mean age at prostate cancer diagnosis was 68.7 yr.

Fig. 5 presents the distributions of lead times for fatal cancers and all cancers that were detectable by the baseline PSA level at a cutoff of 4 ng/mL. On average, the diagnosis of prostate cancer was advanced 5.5 yr compared with the time of diagnosis in the pre-PSA era. This potential gain in lead-time was based on a single-screening PSA mea-

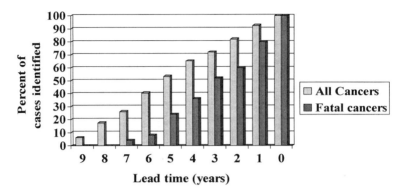

Fig. 5. Percent of tumors that theoretically could have been detected at earlier time than the actual diagnosis by prostate cancer screening using prostate specific antigen. (Data derived from ref. *24.*)

surement and most likely underestimates the potential gain achieved by periodic screening. Lead-time distributions for aggressive cancers (those with regional or distant extension of Gleason scores of 7–10) were similar to those of nonaggressive cancers (those with local extension only and a Gleason score of 6 or less).

THE HISTORY OF PROSTATE CANCER FOLLOWING DIAGNOSIS AND TREATMENT WITH RADICAL SURGERY

Determining the efficacy of therapeutic interventions for prostate cancer is notoriously difficult. Utilizing data from two case-series analyses and two population-based studies, an attempt has been made to estimate the 10-yr disease-specific survival of men diagnosed with prostate cancer in the PSA era. Because PSA testing has introduced a lead time of at least 5 yr and possibly longer, the estimates provided in Figs. 2 and 3 are likely to be conservative. Unfortunately, these estimates do not account for several known and unknown selection biases that can impact the construct of any case series. Despite these concerns, some cautious comparisons are possible if attempts are made to match patients by known risk factors such as clinical stage and Gleason score.

Gerber et al. published a multi-institutional pooled analysis of men with clinically localized prostate cancer treated by radical prostatectomy between 1970 and 1993 *(25)*. They reported excellent 10-yr disease-specific survival estimates of 94%, 80%, and 77% for men with well-differentiated (Gleason 2–4), moderately differentiated (Gleason

5–7) and poorly differentiated (Gleason 8–10) disease. Lu-Yao and Yao estimated 10-yr disease specific survival rates for men undergoing radical prostatectomy to be 94%, 87%, and 67% for men with well-differentiated, moderately differentiated and poorly differentiated disease, respectively *(14)*. A review of these data initially suggests that radical prostatectomy is most efficacious among men with well differentiated disease and least efficacious among men with poorly differentiated disease (Fig. 2).

When compared to the retrospective, population-based sample of 767 men diagnosed with localized disease in Connecticut during the same time period, we found that the 10-yr disease-specific survival for men treated expectantly was 94%, 71%, and 30% for men with well-differentiated, moderately differentiated and poorly differentiated disease *(15)*. Lu-Yao and Yao estimated the 10-yr disease specific survival for expectant management to be 94%, 77%, and 45%. These results are identical to those reported by Gerber et al. for men with well-differentiated disease, suggesting that expectant management achieves comparable results when compared with radical prostatectomy for this subset of men. Conversely, results were much worse for men with poorly differentiated disease receiving expectant management, suggesting a potentially significant advantage following surgery among men with poorly differentiated disease. These findings may be the result of selection biases, but the data suggest that expectant management is clearly not the optimal strategy for men with poorly differentiated cancers.

For men with Gleason 5–7 tumors, the group of men most frequently targeted for aggressive intervention, disease-specific survival outcomes do not appear to be dramatically different. Gerber reported a 10-yr disease-specific survival of 80% (95% confidence interval of 74–85%) following radical prostatectomy. Data from Lu-Yao and Yao estimates a 10-yr diseas-specific survival of 77% (95% confidence interval of 74–80%) and our analysis suggests a 10-yr disease-specific survival of 72% (95% confidence interval of 67–76%) for men managed expectantly. Because of the significant selection biases inherent to all three study groups and the inadequate staging of many patients managed expectantly, it is difficult to determine the relative efficacy of surgery over expectant management for this group of patients.

Lu-Yao and colleagues also addressed this question from a different perspective *(26)*. Using Medicare claims, they estimated the need for secondary cancer therapy among a group of Medicare patients diagnosed with prostate cancer during the period January 1, 1985 through December 31, 1991 and undergoing radical prostatectomy before December 31,

1992. Patients were considered to have had additional cancer therapy if they had radiation therapy, orchiectomy, and/or androgen-deprivation therapy by injection after radical prostatectomy. The interval between the initial treatment and any follow-up treatment was calculated from the date of radical prostatectomy to the first day of the follow-up cancer therapy. The study population consisted of 3494 Medicare patients, 3173 of whom underwent radical prostatectomy within 3 mo of cancer diagnosis.

A review of the surgical pathology reports suggested that less than 60% of patients whose records were included in the study had organ-confined disease. Overall, the 5-yr cumulative incidence of having any additional cancer treatment after a radical prostatectomy was 35%. For patients with organ-confined disease, the group most likely to benefit from surgery, the 5-yr cumulative incidence of the need for additional cancer therapy was 24% and ranged from 16% for men with well-differentiated disease to 42% for men with poorly differentiated disease. Men with disease extending beyond the prostate capsule at the time of surgery had a much higher probability of needing additional treatment. Approximately 68% of men with poorly differentiated disease and extracapsular extension required additional cancer treatment within 5 yr of prostatectomy. For men at the greatest risk of disease progression, more than half required additional cancer therapy within 5 yr of undergoing a radical prostatectomy. These patients clearly need more effective therapies.

SUMMARY

Prostate cancer is a complex disease with an extraordinarily variable clinical outcome. The natural history of this disease is best predicted by its histology as measured by the Gleason scoring system. Based on information provided by randomized trials, population-based studies, and case-series analyses, it appears that prostate cancer will inevitably progress to systemic disease and death if given sufficient amount of time. The competing risk analysis presented in Fig. 3 provides patients and clinicians with estimates of disease progression given a patient's age and tumor histology at the time of diagnosis. These estimates are conservative and do not incorporate the lead time introduced by PSA testing. The advent of screening for prostate cancer using serum PSA has advanced the date of diagnosis for most patients diagnosed in the contemporary era. The leadtime provided by PSA testing appears to be at least 5 yr and is similar for men with well-differentiated disease and poorly differentiated disease.

The impact of treatment on the natural history of prostate cancer is uncertain and is best assessed through randomized clinical trials.

Although case-series and population-based analyses suggest excellent outcomes for men with well-differentiated disease regardless of treatment, it is unclear how much aggressive intervention alters the natural history of this disease for men with moderately differentiated disease. Men at high risk of dying from prostate cancer are those men diagnosed with Gleason score 7–10 tumors. These men have a 10-fold increased risk of dying from prostate cancer in the absence of treatment. How much aggressive intervention alters outcomes for these men remains to be determined.

By carefully documenting clinical outcomes and precisely stratifying patients by Gleason score and tumor volume assessed using PSA measurements, clinicians and patients can obtain greater insights concerning how best to manage this complex disease. Ideally, such studies will lead to more carefully designed clinical trials. Until then, we are haunted by the words of the late Willet Whitmore who ended his manuscript on the natural history of prostate cancer with the following comment:

> *Only with better methods for defining the natural history of the particular tumor, more sophisticated means for anticipating life expectancy of the individual host, and good data on the effects of various treatments on the quality and quantity of survival in patients with appropriately stratified tumors will it be possible to inject more science into the extant art of treatment of the prostatic cancer patient and substitute an era of cold fact for the present era of heated opinion (27).*

Although written over 25 yr ago, these words summarize the continued debate concerning the appropriate management of clinically localized prostate cancer.

REFERENCES

1. The Veterans Administration Cooperative Urological Research Group. (1967) Carcinoma of the prostate: Treatment comparisons. *J Urol* 98:516.
2. Landis SH, Murray T, Bolden S, Wingo PA (1999) Cancer statistics. *CA Cancer J Clin* 1999; 49:8–31.
3. Wiederanders RE, Stuber RV, Mota C, O'Connell D, Haslam GJ. (1963) Prognostic value of grading prostatic carcinoma. *J Urol* 89:881–888.
4. Mellinger GT, Gleason D, Bailar J III (1967) The histology and prognosis of prostatic cancer. *J Urol* 97:331–337.
5. Gleason DF. (1977) Histologic grading and clinical staging of prostatic carcinoma. In: *Urologic Pathology*: The Prostate. Tannenbaum M, ed., Philadelphia: Lea &Febiger, pp. 171–198.
6. Johansson JE, Adami HO, Andersson SO, Bergstrom R, Krusemo UB, Kraaz W. (1989) Natural history of localized prostate cancer: a population based study of 223 untreated patients. *Lancet* 1:799–803.

7. Johansson JE, Adami HO, Andersson SO, Bergstrom R, Holmberg L, Krusemo UB. (1992) High 10 year survival rate in patients with early, untreated prostate cancer. *JAMA* 267:2191–2196.

8. Johansson JE, Holmberg L, Johansson S, Bergstrom R, Adami HO. (1997) Fifteen year survival in prostate cancer: a prospective, population based study in Sweden. *JAMA* 277:467–471.

9. Chodak GW, Thisted RA, Gerber GS, Johansson JE, Adolfson J, Jones G, et al. (1994) Results of conservative management of clinically localized prostate cancer. *N Engl J Med* 330:242–248.

10. Jones GW. Prospective, conservative management of localized prostate cancer. *Cancer* 1992; 70:Suppl:307–310.

11. Whitmore WF Jr, Warner JA, Thompson IM, Jr. (1991) Expectant management of localized prostate cancer. *Cancer* 67:1091–1096.

12. Adolfsson J, Carstensen J, Lowhagen T. (1992) Deferred treatment in clinically localized prostatic carcinoma. *Br J Urol* 69:183–187.

13. Goodman CM, Busuttil A, Chisholm GD (1988) Age, and size and grade of tumour predict prognosis in incidentally diagnosed carcinoma of the prostate. *Br J Urol* 62:576–580.

14. Moskovitz B, Nitecki A, Richter-Levin D. (1987) Cancer of the prostate: is there a need for aggressive treatment? *Urol Int* 42:49–52.

15. Lu-Yao GL, Yao SL. (1997) Population-based study of long-term survival in patients with clinically localised prostate cancer. *Lancet* 349:906–910.

16. Albertsen PC, Hanley JA, Gleason DF, Barry MJ. (1998) Competing risk analysis of men aged 55 to 74 years at diagnosis managed conservatively for clinically localized prostate cancer. *JAMA* 280:975–980.

17. Aus G, Hugosson J, Norlen L. (1995) Long term survival and mortality in prostate cancer treated with noncurative intent. *J Urol* 154:460–465.

18. McNeal JE, Bostwick DG, Kindrachuk RA, Redwine EA, Freiha FS, Stamey TA. (1986) Patterns of progression in prostate cancer. *Lancet* 1(8472):60–63.

19. Stamey TA, Yang N, Hay AR, McNeal JE, Freiha FS, Redwine E. (1987) Prostate specific antigen as a serum marker for adeno-carcinoma of the prostate. *N Engl J Med* 317:909–916.

20. Stamey TA, Freiha FS, McNeal JE, Redwine EA, Whittemore AS, Schmid HP. (1993) Localized prostate cancer. Relationship of tumor volume to clinical significance for treatment of prostate cancer. *Cancer* 71:933–938.

21. Catalona WJ, Smith DS, Ratliff TL, Basler JW. (1993) Detection of organ-confined prostate cancer is increased through prostate-specific antigen based testing. *JAMA* 270:948–954.

22. Partin AW, Kattan MW, Subong EN, Walsh PC, Wojno KJ, Oesterling JE, et al. (1997) Combination of prostate-specific antigen, clinical stage, and Gleason score to predict pathological stage of localized prostate cancer. A multi-institutional update. *JAMA* 277:1445–1451.

23. Carter HB, Pearson JD, Metter EJ, Brant LJ, Chan DW, Andres R, et al. (1992) Longitudinal evaluation of prostate-specific antigen levels in men with and without prostate disease. *JAMA* 267:2215–2220.

24. Gann PH, Hennekens CH, Sampfer MJ. (1995) A prospective evaluation of plasma prostate-specific antigen for detection of prostatic cancer. *JAMA* 273:289–294.

25. Gerber GS, Thisted RA, Scardino PT, Frohmuller HG, Schroeder FH, Paulson DF, et al. (1996) Results of radical prostatectomy in men with clinically localized prostate cancer. *JAMA* 276:615–619.

26. Lu-Yao GL, Potosky AL, Albertsen PC, Wasson JH, Barry MJ, Wennberg JE. (1996) Follow-up cancer treatments after radical prostatectomy: a population-based study. *J Natl Cancer Inst* 88:166–173.
27. Whitmore, WF Jr. (1973) The natural history of prostatic cancer. *Cancer* 32:1104–1112.

3 Mathematical Issues: PSA Testing

Ruth Etzioni and David F. Penson

Contents

INTRODUCTION

The discovery of prostate-specific antigen (PSA) has, no doubt, been one of the most exciting and controversial developments in the history of prostate cancer control. Simple in principle, the test presents numerous challenges in practice. From a clinical perspective, the nature of prostate cancer detected through PSA screening is unclear. An ongoing debate concerns whether these mostly localized tumors represent disease that is likely to become life-threatening if left untreated.

The challenges posed by PSA testing extend beyond the realm of clinical medicine however. From an analytic perspective, there still is no clear consensus about the appropriate definition of a PSA reference range outside of which a test may be reliably classified as abnormal. Researchers have also debated the relative merits of total PSA and other PSA-based diagnostic contenders, including PSA density, PSA velocity, and the ratio of free to total PSA. Although these alternatives have not been proven to surpass PSA, they may be informative in some settings and are often used in clinical practice.

From: *Current Clinical Urology: Prostate Cancer Screening*
Edited by: I. M. Thompson, M. I. Resnick, and E. A. Klein
© Humana Press Inc., Totowa, NJ

Table 1
Data From a Typical Diagnostic Test

	Diseased	Healthy
Test +	TP	FP
Test −	FN	TN
Totals	D	H

Note: TP: true positives; FP: false positives; TN:
true negatives; FN: false negatives; D: diseased; H:
healthy. Sensitivity is TP/D. Specificity is TN/H.

In this chapter, we review some of the major studies to date concerning the diagnostic performance of PSA as a screening test, with particular focus on methods for assessing its sensitivity, specificity, predictive value, and comparative performance relative to other screening tests for the disease. The implications of diagnostic performance for true efficacy of the test (i.e., in preventing adverse outcomes of the disease) are important but not addressed in detail herein.

We begin with a brief review of the most commonly used measures of diagnostic performance and the methods for assessing and comparing them across multiple tests. This section provides us with a vocabulary for describing the two study designs that have been used most frequently to assess the diagnostic properties of PSA, and the advantages and limitations of each. Our goal is to give the reader some tools to critically appraise studies of the diagnostic properties of PSA and other related tests. In our discussion, we assume that biopsy-detectable prostate cancer is the condition that PSA and the other diagnostic tests discussed seek to identify. This assumption is important because it implies that there exists a reliable method (i.e., prostate biopsy) for verifying whether or not an individual has the condition of interest. The methods we review for assessing diagnostic performance rely on the existence of such a gold standard.

DIAGNOSTIC MEASURES

When introducing a new diagnostic test, the primary consideration is whether the test is reliably able to detect latent disease. The *sensitivity* of a test is the likelihood that the test will identify disease that is present. Quantitatively, the proportion of disease cases gives the sensitivity whose test yields a positive result. Table 1 is a schematic of the data typically considered in diagnostic testing. The sensitivity is the ratio of the true-positive tests to the number of diseased individuals.

Sensitivity is probably the quantity most often quoted as a measure of the goodness of a diagnostic test. Certainly, a test can ultimately only be of benefit if it identifies the condition of interest so that it can be treated. However, consider a test that is always positive. This is a very sensitive test, but, clearly, not clinically useful. Such a test will certainly identify all disease cases, but it will also label as diseased all subjects that are, in fact, healthy. Thus, in measuring the usefulness of a diagnostic test, it is also important to consider the likelihood that the test will falsely declare a healthy individual to be diseased, the false-positive probability. Equivalently, one may consider the complement of the false-positive probability, or the *specificity* of the test. The specificity is the ratio of the true-negative tests to the number of healthy individuals.

Both sensitivity and specificity are critical in developing appropriate guidelines for use of a screening or diagnostic test. Low sensitivity implies that a large proportion of latent cases will remain undiagnosed with potentially adverse consequences. However, low specificity is problematic because of the costs and morbidity associated with false positive diagnoses. A number of studies have proposed PSA cutoffs on the basis of (apparently) cancer-free individuals *(1,2)*. Inasmuch as these studies attempt to identify "normal ranges", or ranges among non-diseased individuals, they are effectively considering only test specificity.

In practice, estimation of the sensitivity and specificity is straightforward so long as disease status is known for all participating subjects. If the availability of disease status information (e.g., through biopsy) depends on the test result or on the results of other tests conducted simultaneously, then estimates of sensitivity and specificity will be subject to *verification bias (3,4)*.

Table 2 illustrates the impact of verification bias in a setting in which all subjects with a positive test result are biopsied but only 20% of the subjects testing negative are biopsied. Although the true sensitivity and specificity are 80% and 90% respectively, the estimated sensitivity and specificity are 95% and 64% respectively.

Most studies of PSA as a screening test are subject to verification bias, because their protocols explicitly specify biopsy as a follow-up to a positive test, but do not recommend biopsy following a negative test. Some statistical methods have been developed to adjust results for verification bias *(4)*, but the issue is still a topic of active research. Methods available require at least some patients with negative results to be biopsied, as well as knowledge of the factors that affect the likelihood of receiving a biopsy. These may include family history of disease,

Table 2
Illustration of Verification Bias

	Diseased	Healthy
Truth: sensitivity=0.8; specificity=0.9		
Test +	80	90
Test –	20	810
Observed: sensitivity=0.95; specificity=0.64		
Test +	80	90
Test–	4	162

socioeconomic status, and the outcomes of other tests conducted at the same time as the test of interest.

As an example of a simple adjustment for verification bias *(4)*, consider the hypothetical example of Table 2. Suppose that these results are from a prospective screening study comparing PSA with digital rectal exam (DRE), with all participants receiving both tests. Then, considering all possible test results yields four possible strata: PSA positive and DRE positive (suppose this combination occurs with frequency 7%); PSA positive and DRE negative (10%); PSA negative and DRE positive (3%); and both PSA and DRE negative (80%). Additionally, suppose that all patients in the first three strata were biopsied and a random 15% of patients in the fourth stratum were biopsied. Finally, suppose that among patients biopsied within each stratum, the frequencies of disease were 50%, 45%, 10%, and 2% to the closest percentage point respectively. Then, the corrected estimate of sensitivity, from Begg and Greenes *(4)*, is given by: [(0.5) (0.7) + (0.45)(0.10)/(0.5)(0.7) + (0.45)(0.10) + (0.10)(0.03) + (0.02)(0.8)], which is equal to 0.81. However, typically, not all patients in the first three strata are biopsied, and those in the fourth stratum who receive biopsies tend to do so for highly selective reasons. The formulation of Begg and Greenes may still be used in an extended form to adjust for verification bias so long as the factors that influence individuals to undergo biopsy are known and recorded. For example, suppose that individuals with a family history of disease are known to request prostate biopsy regardless of their test results. Then, the indicator of family history together with the PSA and DRE test results can be used to define a new stratum system (with eight strata), to which the method of Begg and Greenes *(4)* can be applied.

Naturally, this approach to verification bias has limitations when test results and relevant factors are continuous variables, which cannot be dichotomized easily; methods to adjust for verification bias in such cases are a topic of active research. Finally, if the factors that influence individuals to undergo biopsy are not known, or if no screen-negatives are biopsied, then statistical methods are available to adjust for verification bias, but they require the user to make potentially unverifiable assumptions about the prevalence of disease in the various strata, e.g., Baker *(5)*. In such a case, it may be instructive to conduct a sensitivity analysis (i.e., to examine the impact of various different assumptions on the analysis). Crawford et al. used a combination of adjustment for verification bias and sensitivity analysis in their presentation of the results from Prostate Cancer Awareness Week *(6)*. For the first three strata defined earlier, they assumed that latent cancer rates among non-biopsied subjects were similar to those among biopsied test-positive subjects *within strata* defined by DRE results and categories of actual PSA level. For the last stratum, they considered assumed a range of values for disease prevalence and noted that their results were relatively robust within a reasonable range of assumptions.

When considering a test like PSA, which yields a quantitative result, a central question concerns the cutoff that defines a positive vs a negative test. One of the great debates in the case of PSA concerns the appropriate cutoff for the test and whether the cutoff should be different for younger and older men. Moving the cutoff affects both sensitivity and specificity simultaneously. A lower cutoff leads to greater sensitivity at the expense of specificity (i.e., improving the true-positive rate will also increase the false-positive rate). To understand the trade-offs between the true-positive and false-positive rates as the cutoff varies, it is convenient to plot true-positive rates against false-positive rates for different cutoff values. This display is the *receiver-operating characteristic* (ROC) curve *(7,8)*. Figure 1 shows a hypothetical ROC curve; the diagonal line is the ROC curve that would result from a test that randomly classifies individuals as diseased or nondiseased and, therefore, provides no information.

In practice, the estimation of the ROC curve may be accomplished in a number of ways using the test results for diseased and healthy individuals. The most straightforward approach is simply to vary the cutoff over a defined range and to plot the empirical true-positive rate against the empirical false-positive rate for values of the cutoff within this range. The resulting points may be connected linearly or by using a step function. So long as the sample size is sufficiently large, this will yield a reasonable approximation to the true ROC curve. However, for smaller

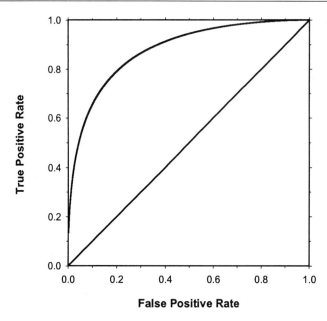

Fig. 1. Hypothetical ROC curve.

samples, the number of distinct points will be few, and connecting the dots either linearly or by a step function may not be sufficient to adequately approximate the true curve. An alternative is to assume that the test values for diseased and healthy individuals follow a known statistical distribution. The form of the assumed statistical distribution implies an expression for the ROC curve. In the past, ROC curves have commonly been based on normal distributions, however, other distributions may also be considered. In addition, methods have recently been developed for estimation of smooth ROC curves without making restrictive assumptions about the distributions of test outcomes for diseased and healthy subjects.

The area under the ROC curve (AUC) is often quoted as a summary measure of test accuracy. The AUC is an estimate of the likelihood that the test result for a randomly selected, diseased subject exceeds that for a randomly selected, healthy subject. The area under the empirical ROC curve is equivalent to the Mann–Whitney U-statistic *(19)* applied to the test outcomes for diseased and healthy subjects, which is included in most statistical software packages. When normal distributions are assumed for the test results, the area under the ROC curve is given by Φ $[(m^1-m^2)/(s^1-s^2)]$, where Φ is the standard normal distribution function,

Table 3
Illustration of How the PPV Changes
with Disease Prevalence for a Test with
Sensitivity 80% and Specificity 70%

Prevalence	PPV
0.1	0.28
0.2	0.47
0.3	0.60
0.4	0.70

m^1 and m^2 are the means for the diseased and healthy individuals, respectively, and s^1 and s^2 are the standard deviations.

A second pair of test accuracy measures used in practice are the positive and negative predictive values. The positive predictive value (PPV) is the likelihood that an individual with a positive screen is, in fact, a disease case. Quantitatively, the positive predictive value is given by the proportion of subjects with a positive test result who are found to have the disease. Similarly, the negative predictive value (NPV) is the proportion of subjects with a negative test result who are found to be free of disease. Predictive values are relevant clinically because they quantify how likely it is that the subject has the disease, given the results of the test. However, they are intrinsically dependent on the population prevalence of disease; for instance, it can be shown that

$$PPV = p*TP/p*TP + (1-p)*FP$$

where p is the prevalence, and TP and FP are the true-positive and false-positive rates, respectively, associated with the test. This explains why the positive predictive value of the PSA varies with age and it is substantially higher for older than for younger men. Table 3 illustrates how the PPV varies with disease prevalence for a test with sensitivity 80% and specificity 70%.

In practice, estimation of the positive predictive value is straightforward so long as all subjects with positive tests or a random sample thereof are evaluated for the presence of disease. If this is not the case, then bias may be present in the predictive value estimates. For instance, if a study protocol calls for all men with a PSA level above 4.0 ng/mL to be biopsied but only a subset of these subjects comply, then, if the subjects complying are a selective high-risk sample, they will bias the PPV upward.

COMPARING DIAGNOSTIC TESTS

Statistical methodology for comparing the diagnostic properties of competing tests is currently an area of active research. Most studies of PSA and alternative tests are conducted using a paired design, with each subject receiving all candidate tests. When verification bias is not an issue, comparison of sensitivities and specificities in this setting has been traditionally accomplished through the McNemar's-test *(9)*, a straightforward comparison test available in most statistical software packages. The McNemar's-test statistic is based solely on subjects with discordant results on the two tests. For the situation in which subjects testing positive on either test are biopsied, the McNemar's-test can be applied to compare sensitivities and specificities *(10)*.

Because PSA and its biomarker-based competitors are quantitative tests, comparisons of ROC curves are appropriate. Statistical formulas are available for comparing the areas under two curves. Recently, however, regression analysis methods have been developed for comparison of the curves themselves *(11)*. These methods vastly expand the practitioner's repertoire for comparing quantitative tests. They make far fewer assumptions about distributions of data values, allow for other covariates like age or ethnicity to enter into the comparison and—best of all—may be implemented using standard statistical software packages. Etzioni and colleagues *(8)* recently used ROC curve regression to compare the ROC curves for total PSA and the ratio of free to total PSA at various times prior to diagnosis. They found that whereas PSA and the ratio performed similarly at approx 8 yr prior to diagnosis, total PSA became significantly better as the time of clinical diagnosis approached.

Regression analysis methods have also been developed that allow for the comparison of sensitivities and specificities as well as for the comparison of predictive values *(12)*. The methods are more flexible than the traditional approach because they allow sensitivity, specificity, and predictive values to depend on other factors like age and ethnicity, in addition to the test itself. To compare sensitivities, the results (positive or negative) of the competing tests for disease cases are entered as the dependent variable into a regression where the independent variables consist of an indicator of which test the result is from, as well as indicators of the covariates of interest. As an example, consider comparing the sensitivity of PSA using a cutoff of 4.0 ng/mL with the test using an age-specific cutoff by Oesterling et al *(2)*. For each disease case, the binary results (positive, negative) according to the two PSA cutoffs would be recorded. This set of values would be entered as the dependent variable; the test type (fixed or age-specific cutoff) would be entered as the independent variable, together with indicators of factors like age and ethnicity that might impact sensitivity. If, for instance, it is suspected that ethnicity may affect the relative sensitivity of the two tests, then the regression could include an interaction term consisting of the product of test type and ethnicity.

MULTIPLE MARKERS

In some settings, new diagnostic tests may be developed to augment, rather than compete with, existing tests. An example of such a test is the ratio of free to total PSA (*f/t* ratio). The *f/t* ratio has been proposed for use in cases where the total PSA falls in the diagnostic gray zone, between 4 and 10 ng/mL, where specificity tends to be low. Several studies have suggested that with total PSA in this range, low values of the *f/t* ratio may be helpful in distinguishing false from true positives. Thus, the proposal is to use the *f/t* ratio in combination with total PSA as follows: PSA below 4 ng/mL, test is negative; PSA above 10 ng/mL, test is positive. PSA between 4 and 10 ng/mL, if *f/t* ratio is below some level x, the test is positive, otherwise negative.

Identification of the optimal value of x in practice is challenging *(13)*. Previous studies have used the data to identify a value for x that leads to a clinically significant improvement in specificity without a substantial loss in sensitivity. For this value of x, the reduction in sensitivity relative to the test PSA > 4.0 ng/mL is quoted, together with the reduction in the false-positive rate. For instance, Catalona et al., in a study of 63 men with benign prostatic hyperplasia (BPH) and 50 men with cancer, all of whom had prediagnostic PSA levels between 4 and 10 ng/mL, found that a *f/t* ratio cutoff of 23.4% or lower reduced false-positive rates by over 30% with a reduction in true-positive rates of only 10% *(14)*.

As the cutoff for the *f/t* ratio varies, a trade-off becomes apparent between the reductions in the true- and false-positive rates. This trade-off may be represented graphically, much like an ROC curve. Indeed, a plot of the percentage true positives remaining against the percentage false positives remaining for various values of x is technically an ROC curve, representing true- versus false-positive rates for subjects within the PSA diagnostic grey zone. A plot of this ROC curve is useful in determining the trade-offs as x varies and may ultimately be of use in selecting a value, or range, for x, below which a test may be declared positive. Studies that quote reductions in true- and false-positive rates for a single value of x are simply quoting a single point from this ROC curve; this may be suggestive but is not, by itself, sufficient to infer whether the f/t ratio provides significant diagnostic advantage in general.

STUDY DESIGNS

Two classes of study designs have been employed by researchers addressing the diagnostic properties of PSA as a screening test. *Prospective screening studies* select a group of men who are prospectively assayed for their PSA levels without knowledge of their underlying disease status. Typically, subjects with suspicious PSA levels, or with levels outside of a predetermined "normal" range, are biopsied to ascertain whether or not they have prostate cancer. PSA levels among prostate cancer cases are then compared with those among men not diagnosed with prostate cancer. *Retrospective case-control studies* are usually done in association with prior studies, which have collected and stored serum for their purposes. From these study subjects, individuals diagnosed with prostate cancer (cases) are identified and their serum that was stored prior to diagnosis is assayed for PSA. Similarly, individuals not diagnosed with prostate cancer are selected as controls, and their stored serum assayed for PSA. PSA levels for cases are compared with those for controls.

Both study designs have their merits if they are executed appropriately. Prospective studies mimic the sequence of events that occurs in practice when the test is applied to screen a population. Hence, they are able to provide information about the diagnostic performance of the test in practice. In particular, a prospective study of randomly selected individuals contains a study sample whose prevalence of the disease reflects that of the population. In principle, therefore, prospective studies are excellent sources for estimates of positive predictive values. Examples of prospective studies are those reported by Catalona et al. *(15,16)*, Mettlin et al. *(17,18)* and Brawer et al. *(19)*.

Prospective studies are subject to a host of potential biases. Many prospective studies are conducted among selected populations, including referral populations. Such studies are subject to *selection bias*, and caution should be exercised when generalizing their results to other populations.

Prospective studies are also most susceptible to *verification bias (3,4)*, which occurs when the decision to biopsy a study subject depends on test outcome and possibly on other, related factors. In addition, even though the protocols of prospective screening studies call for all subjects screening positive to be biopsied, this typically does not occur, particularly in large population-based studies that call for men testing positive to follow up with their own physicians after the test. If the subjects testing positive who decide to follow up are a selective group, estimates of positive predictive values from such may also be biased. Studies that restrict attention to compliant subjects or assume that compliant subjects constitute a random sample of subjects screening positive are particularly subject to bias in this case.

Retrospective studies are powerful in that they contain, by definition, a verified sample of disease cases with ascertainment of disease status obtained independently of the PSA levels in their banked serum. Consequently, these studies are able, in principle, to estimate test sensitivity so long as serum samples are available for cases relatively close to their time of diagnosis. Retrospective studies have been conducted by Gann et al. (20), Carter et al. (21), Whittemore et al. (22), Slate et al. (23), Pearson et al. (24), Etzioni et al. (8), and Jacobsen et al. (25). However, these studies may also be subject to serious biases, chief among them being *selection bias*. If the case group consists of men diagnosed with prostate cancer prior to the PSA era, then it is clear that such a group constitutes a selective sample of patients that is probably not representative of the pool of latent cases in the population. Sensitivity estimates from such a study may be thought of as restricted to the cases that would have become clinically apparent even in the absence of PSA. The situation is not necessarily remedied if the case group is ascertained from men diagnosed in the post-PSA era. Indeed, if the case group contains many prostate cancer cases diagnosed through PSA testing, the resulting estimates of sensitivity will be inflated, because those very cases included in the study will consist predominantly of those diagnosed through PSA testing who, by definition, have elevated PSA levels.

Controls in retrospective studies are typically selected on the basis of an absence of disease diagnosis by the time of case ascertainment, or, at best, a clinical evaluation (without prostate biopsy) that suggests individuals are healthy. Inasmuch as these controls may harbor latent disease, the control groups in such studies may misrepresent the specificity of the PSA test.

A characteristic of retrospective studies is that PSA levels are typically measured not at the time of diagnosis but at the time that serum was stored in the study database. This may be months or years before the diagnosis took place. An exception to this rule is the study of Jacobsen et al. (25); these authors used retrospective PSA data not from a serum bank, but from medical records. Cases were included in the study only if they had had a PSA test within 6 mo prior to their diagnosis.

When PSA tests are available over an interval prior to diagnosis, then it is not possible to determine test sensitivity as it is traditionally defined.

Table 4
Studies Providing Estimates of Test Sensitivity

Study	Population	Design	Sensitivity	Specificity
Gann et al. (20)	Participants in Physicians Health Study	Retrospective	73%	91%
Mettlin et al. (17)	Participants in NPCDP	Prospective	71.9%	90%
Jacobsen et al. (25)	Olmsted County 1990–1992	Retrospective	83%	85%
Catalona et al. (15)	Men biopsied for various reasons	Prospective	79%	59%

Rather, sensitivity is defined relative to an interval. Gann et al. (20), in their retrospective study, estimate 4-yr sensitivity to be 73%, which means that among men diagnosed with prostate cancer, 73% will have a positive result on a PSA test conducted within 4 yr prior to diagnosis. With the prostate cancer cases in this estimate consisting solely of men diagnosed in the pre-PSA era, the relationship between this estimate of test sensitivity and the definition of test sensitivity in a prospective setting is questionable. In particular, the interval estimate pertains to the subgroup of cases that are ultimately diagnosed with clinically apparent disease, whereas the traditional estimate pertains to the population of cases with latent disease.

To illustrate how the different designs are applied in practice, we consider estimating the sensitivity of the PSA test at a cutoff of 4.0 ng/mL. Table 4 summarizes four studies that provide estimates of test sensitivity and specificity.

The study of Gann et al. (20) was a typical, retrospective case-control study, with cases consisting of prostate cancer diagnoses occurring within 10 yr of entry into the Physicians' Health Study (PHS). At the time of entry into the PHS, participants provided a blood sample, which was retrospectively assayed for PSA. The cases upon which the sensitivity estimate is based were diagnosed within 4 yr of their entry into the PHS in 1992. The sensitivity estimate is the proportion of these cases whose serum sample showed an elevated PSA. As noted earlier, this is not interpretable as a prospective estimate of sensitivity. Controls were participants in the PHS who were age-matched to cases and who had not been diagnosed with prostate cancer prior to the date of diagnosis of their matched case. A small percentage of controls was subsequently found to have the disease, but most controls still had not been diagnosed with prostate cancer by 1992. Therefore, the specificity estimate from this study is likely to be a fairly accurate approximation to the specificity of the test when applied in the population.

The study of Mettlin et al. *(18)* reports data from the National Prostate Cancer Detection Project, which prospectively tested almost 3000 men for prostate cancer using DRE, transrectal ultrasound, and PSA. The men were tested annually over a period of 5 yr. The cases upon which the sensitivity estimate is based consisted of the 171 men with prostate cancer detected during the course of the study through any of these tests. Because of the prospective nature of the study and the lack of definitive evaluation of men with negative PSA tests, this estimate is subject to verification bias and is likely an overestimate of the sensitivity in this population.

Like the study of Gann et al. *(20)*, the Jacobsen et al. *(25)* study is a retrospective study. However, there are some key differences between the two studies. The cases in the study of Jacobsen et al. consist of all cases diagnosed in Olmsted County between 1990 and 1992 who had had a PSA test within 6 mo of their diagnosis. Therefore, unlike the study of Gann et al., the cases in this study are predominantly detected on the basis of their PSA levels. Consequently, the sensitivity estimate from this study is based on a sample of cases that are likely to have elevated PSA, therefore, it is probably an overestimate of the sensitivity.

The sensitivity and specificity estimates of Catalona et al. *(15)* are based on a cohort of men who had been biopsied for a variety of reasons, including an abnormal DRE, evidence of BPH, and elevated biomarker levels. This cohort is clearly atypical relative to the general population and is biased toward cases with elevated PSA levels, hence the relatively high estimate of sensitivity from this study. Similarly, this cohort represents a group of men with a high prevalence of benign disease, which is known to lead to elevated PSA levels. This explains the low specificity observed in this study. Thus, the study is subject to selection bias. The study is prospective in the sense that PSA (and other tests) were conducted prior to ascertaining disease status.

In conclusion, the study design is a key factor in determining the accuracy and interpretability of any measures of diagnostic performance. All the studies referenced show evidence of either selection bias or verification bias, which acts to inflate estimates of test sensitivity. We conclude that the sensitivity of the PSA test at a cutoff of 4.0 ng/mL is, at best, close to 70% on the basis of these data.

DISCUSSION

The evaluation of PSA as a screening test raises a host of mathematical issues. How should a positive test be defined? What is the optimal way to use the test in combination with other competing tests? How do the alternatives compare in terms of their diagnostic performance and, ultimately, their benefits? To address all of these issues would require an entire volume. Therefore, this chapter has focused on the most basic issues raised by the evaluation of the diagnostic performance of PSA and related tests. Many researchers have addressed this topic; the goal of the current chapter is to provide readers with a vocabulary to critically appraise this literature and with tools to address these issues.

Although statistical methodology for assessing the accuracy of diagnostic tests is less well-developed than in the area of clinical trials, for example, the field is undergoing a dramatic expansion. Certainly, the tools available are not yet standardized, but the number of methods that may be implemented through standard software packages is growing (e.g., Pepe [26]). We encourage clinicians to explore these methods and hope that this chapter will inspire dialogue between clinicians and statisticians regarding ways to best evaluate PSA and its diagnostic properties.

As noted in the Introduction, the methods presented rely on the existence of a reliable "gold standard", namely, a test or procedure that guarantees identification of the condition of interest if it is present. For this reason, we have defined the condition of interest as biopsy-detectable cancer. If the condition of interest were autopsy-detectable prostate cancer, then biopsy would misclassify some truly diseased individuals as healthy. The fact that biopsy is not perfect in identifying all men with autopsy-detectable prostate cancer would bias the estimates of accuracy of the PSA test as well as other diagnostic tests. Some methods are available to adjust for an inaccurate gold standard (27,28), but it is simpler to redefine the condition of interest as biopsy-detectable cancer, which may, in fact, be more relevant from a clinical point of view.

REFERENCES

1. DeAntoni EP, Crawford ED, Oesterling JE, Ross CA, Berger ER, McLeod DG, Staggers F, Stone NN. (1996) Age-and race specific reference ranges for prostate-specific antigen from a large community-based study. *J Urol* 48(2):234–239.
2. Oesterling JE, Jacobsen SJ, Chute CG, Guess HA, Girman CJ, Panser LA, Lieber MM. (1993) Serum prostate-specific antigen in a community-based population of healthy men. *JAMA* 270:860–864.

3. Begg CB. (1987) Biases in the assessment of diagnostic tests. *Statist Med* 6:411–423.
4. Begg CB, Greenes RA. (1983) Assessment of diagnostic tests when disease verification is subject to selection bias. *Biometrics* 39:207–215.
5. Baker SG (1995) Evaluating multiple diagnostic tests with partial verification. *Biometrics* 51(1):330–337.
6. Crawford ED, DeAntoni EP, Etzioni R, Schaefer VC, Olson RM, Ross CA, the Prostate Cancer Education Council. (1996) Serum prostate-specific antigen and digital rectal examination for the early detection of prostate cancer in a national community-based program. *Urology* 47:863–869.
7. Catalona WJ, Hudson MA, Scardino PT, Richie JP, Ahmann FR, Flanigan RC, et al. (1994) Selection of optimal prostate specific antigen (PSA) cutoffs for early detection of prostate cancer: receiver operating characteristic (ROC) curves. *J Urol* 152:2037–2042.
8. Etzioni R, Pepe M, Longton G, Hu C, Goodman G. (1999) Incorporating the time dimension in receiver operating characteristic curves: A prostate cancer case study. *Med Dec Making* 19:242–251.
9. Conover WJ. (1971) *Practical Nonparametric Statistics.* New York; Wiley.
10. Schatzkin A, Connor RJ, Taylor PR, Bunnag B. (1987) Comparing new and old screening tests when a reference procedure cannot be performed on all screenees: Example of automated cytometry for early detection of cervical cancer. *Am J Epidemiol* 125(4):672–678.
11. Pepe MS. (1998) Three approaches to regression analysis of receiver operating characteristic curves for continuous test results. *Biometrics* 54:124–135.
12. Leisenring W, Pepe MS, Longton G. (1997) A marginal regression modelling framework for evaluating medical diagnostic tests. *Statist Med* 16:1263–1281.
13. Woodrum DL, Brawer MK, Partin AW, Catalona WJ, Southwick PC. (1998) Interpretation of free Prostate Specific Antigen clinical research studies for the detection of prostate cancer. *J Urol* 159:5–12.
14. Catalona WJ, Smith DS, Wolfert RL, Wang TJ, Rittenhouse HG, Ratliff TL, Nadler RBC. (1995) Evaluation of percentage of free serum prostate-specific antigen to improve the specificity of prostate cancer screening. *JAMA* 274:1214–1220.
15. Catalona WJ, Smith DS, Ratliff TL, Dodds KM, Coplen DE, Yuan JJ, Petros JA, Andriole GL. (1991) Measurement of prostate-specific antigen in serum as a screening test for prostate cancer. *N Eng J Med* 324:1156–61.
16. Catalona WJ, Richie JP, Ahmann FR, Hudson MA, Scardino PT, Flanigan RC, et al. (1994) Comparisons of digital rectal examination and serum prostate specific antigen in the early detection of prostate cancer: results of a multicenter clinical trial of 6,630 men. *J Urol* 151:1283–90.
17. Mettlin C, Littrup PJ, Kane RA, Murphy GP, Lee F, Chesley A, Badalament R, Mostofi FK. (1994) Relative sensitivity and specificity of serum prostate specific antigen (PSA) level compared with age-referenced PSA, PSA Density, and PSA Change. *Cancer* 74(5):1615–1620.
18. Mettlin C, Murphy G, Babaian R, et al. (1996) The results of a five-year early prostate cancer detection intervention. *Cancer* 77(1):150–159.
19. Brawer MK, Chetner MP, Beatie J, Buchner DM, Vessella RL, Lange PH. (1992) Screening for prostatic carcinoma with prostate specific antigen. *J Urol* 147:841–845.
20. Gann PH, Hennekens CH, Stampfer MJ. (1995) A prospective evaluation of plasma prostate-specific antigen for detection of prostate cancer. *JAMA* 273:289–294.

21. Carter HB, Morrell CH, Pearson JD, Brant LJ, et al. (1992) Estimation of prostatic growth using serial prostate-specific antigen measurements in men with and without prostate disease. *Cancer Res* 52:3323–3328.
22. Whittemore AS, Lele C, Friedman GD, Stamey T, Vogelman JH, Orentreich N. (1995) Prostate-Specific Antigen as predictor of prostate cancer in black men and white men. *J Nat Cancer Inst* 87(5):354–360.
23. Slate EH, Clark LC. (1999)Using PSA to detect prostate cancer onset: An application of Bayesian retrospective and prospective changepoint identification. In: Case Studies in Bayesian Statistics IV. Gatsonis C, Carlin B, Carriquiry A, Gelman A, Kass R, Verdinelli I, West M, eds. Springer-Verlag, New York, pp. 511–534.
24. Pearson JD, Luderer AA, Metter J, Partin AW, Chan DW, Fozard JL, Carter HB. (1996) Longitudinal analysis of serial measurements of free and total PSA among men with and without prostatic cancer. *Urology* 48(6A):4–9.
25. Jacobsen SJ, Bergstralh EJ, Guess HA, Katusic SK, Klee GG, Oesterling JE, Lieber MM. (1996) Predictive properties of serum prostate-specific antigen testing in a community-based setting. *Arch Int Med* 156:2462–2468.
26. Pepe MS. (2000) An interpretation for the ROC curve and inference using GLM procedures. *Biometrics* 56:352–359.
27. Baker SG. (1991) Evaluating a new test using a reference test with estimated sensitivity and specificity. *Commun Statist Theory Methods* 20:2739–2752.
28. Walter S, Irwig L. (1988) Estimation of test error rates, disease prevalence, and relative risk from misclassified data: a review. *J Clin Epidemiol* 41:923–937.

4   Evidence of Benefit of Screening in Other Cancers

Ismail Jatoi, MD, PhD, FACS

CONTENTS

INTRODUCTION
SCREENING FOR CANCERS
CONCLUSIONS
REFERENCES

INTRODUCTION

Cancer screening has been studied extensively in recent years. There is now considerable evidence to suggest that screening for cervical, colorectal, and breast cancers can effectively reduce mortality. Thus, screening may eventually play a significant role in reducing cancer mortality throughout the world. However, we must also consider the impact of screening on the quality of life. After all, cancer screening targets large, asymptomatic populations, and its impact on the quality of life is therefore of paramount concern. Breast cancer screening, in particular, has been the subject of intense investigation and controversy in recent years. In this review, I shall discuss the progress made in our understanding of cancer screening, with particular emphasis on what we have learned about breast cancer screening.

*The opinions or assertions contained herein are the private views of the authors and are not to be construed as reflecting the views of the Departments of the Army, Air Force or Defense.

From: *Current Clinical Urology: Prostate Cancer Screening*
Edited by: I. M. Thompson, M. I. Resnick, and E. A. Klein
© Humana Press Inc., Totowa, NJ

Over the last 35 yr, numerous studies were undertaken to determine the efficacy of cancer screening: case-control, retrospective, and prospective studies. However, we cannot accept the results of these studies at face value. Before discussing the merits of cancer screening, we must consider three biases pertinent to many of these studies: lead time, length, and selection.

Lead-Time Bias

Screening advances the time of cancer diagnosis. *Survival* refers to the interval of time between diagnosis of cancer and death. Thus, patients with screen-detected cancers will have better survival rates than those with clinically detected cancers, even if screening does nothing to delay the time of death. *Lead-time bias* refers to the interval of time between the diagnosis of cancer by screening and by usual clinical detection. Lead-time bias may lead one to think that screening prolongs life when, in fact, it simply extends the period over which the cancer is observed. Comparing survival between screen-detected and clinically detected cancers is therefore meaningless. Rather, we must determine whether screening reduces the cancer-specific mortality. The lung cancer screening trials undertaken in the 1970s provide a good example of lead-time bias *(1)*. Those trials showed improved survival in the screen-detected cases but no reduction in lung cancer mortality. Those early studies on lung cancer screening suggested that lung cancer screening simply moved the time of diagnosis backward but had no real impact on the length of life.

Length Bias

The slower-growing cancers exist for a longer period in the preclinical phase and are more likely to be detected by screening. In contrast, the more aggressive cancers exist for a shorter period in the preclinical phase and are more likely to be detected clinically in the intervals between screening sessions. This phenomenon is termed *length bias* and further complicates any comparisons between screen-detected and clinically detected cancers. Klemi et al. compared the biology of breast cancers detected by screening with those detected clinically *(2)*. The authors compared several biological properties in the two groups, including histology, differentiation, tumor necrosis, mitotic counts, estrogen and progesterone receptors, DNA-ploidy, and S-phase fraction. Overall, the breast cancers detected by screening had a more favorable tumor biology. This study suggests that screening tends to detect the biologically indolent, slow-growing cancers. In the absence of screening, many of these cancers might never have been diagnosed during the lifetime of the patient.

Selection Bias

Individuals who are health conscious are more likely to volunteer for screening. Such individuals would be expected to have a lower mortality from all causes (they may, for example, also eat well and exercise regularly). Thus, any comparisons between volunteers and nonvolunteer controls might be subject to a *selection bias*. The effect of selection bias has been shown in several studies. In one notable study from the United Kingdom, the authors studied women in a district where breast cancer screening was available (screening district) and those from another district where screening was not available (control district) *(3)*. The authors found that breast cancer mortality was higher among the nonvolunteers of the screening district, when compared to the women in the control district. This study demonstrates the potential confounding effect of selection bias and the problem of comparing volunteers with non-volunteer controls.

SCREENING FOR CANCERS

How do we account for the above discussed biases? The best way is to undertake large, randomized controlled trials with cancer-specific mortality as the end point. Such trials compare cancer-specific mortality between screened and unscreened populations. These trials account for selection bias because individuals are randomized to either undergo periodic screening or usual care (no screening). Other studies (retrospective, case control, and nonrandomized prospective) fail to account for the biases discussed above and are not reliable in determining the efficacy of a cancer screening method. Randomized controlled trials have improved our understanding of cancer screening and have provided important insights into the natural history of cancer. Interest in cancer screening has focused on several cancers with a high prevalence (Table 1). These are discussed below.

Cervical Cancer

Screening for cervical cancer is undertaken by a method developed by Papanicolaou over 50 yr ago *(4)*. This technique involves the cytological examination of cervical scrapes that are smeared onto slides and stained by the Papanicolou method (Pap smear). World War II delayed the implementation of the Pap smear as a screening method for cervical cancer. However, in the 1960s, organized screening programs were

Table 1
Cancers Where Screening is Effective

Cancer	Screening Method	Evidence
Cervical	Pap smear	National mortality data
Colorectal	Fecal occult blood testing (FOBT)	Randomized controlled trials
Breast	Mammography	Randomized controlled trails

initiated in all the Nordic countries, with the exception of Norway *(5)*. By the mid-1970s, very significant reductions in cervical cancer mortality were observed in the Nordic countries (except Norway). In Britain, organized cervical cancer screening programs were initiated in the 1980s, and reductions in mortality have become apparent in recent years *(6)*. In other countries, cervical cancer screening programs have been less well-organized, and effects on mortality are therefore less clear.

Lung Cancer

Four randomized controlled trials were undertaken in the 1970s to examine the efficacy of lung cancer screening in high-risk individuals *(1)*. The Memorial Sloan-Kettering and Johns Hopkins trials examined the value of screening with sputum cytology *(7,8)*. The Mayo Clinic and Czech trials studied the impact of screening with both sputum cytology and chest radiography *(9,10)*. In all four trials, screening for lung cancer was found to have no impact on mortality. However, the design of these four trials has been criticized recently *(1)*. The Memorial Sloan-Kettering and Johns Hopkins trials did not examine the value of chest radiography. In the Czech trial, the study group underwent screening with chest radiography and sputum cytology twice a year for 3 yr. Yet, in the subsequent 6 yr of follow-up, both the screened group and the study group had annual chest radiographs, and this might have diluted out the possible benefit of screening. Although the Mayo Clinic trial is perceived as the definitive, negative trial, there were several flaws in this study as well. The trial was underpowered and could only detect a 50% reduction in mortality. Additionally, 50% of the controls underwent annual chest radiography, and this might have diluted out the benefit of screening in the study group. Finally, the compliance rate in the study group was only 75%.

Now, some investigators have argued that screening for lung cancer merits additional investigation. Recently, the Early Lung Cancer Action Project (ELCAP) evaluated the potential role of annual helical low-dose computed-tomography (CT) scanning as a screening modality (11). Low-dose CT improved the detection of lung cancer at an early and potentially more curable stage. Additional studies are planned to further evaluate its effectiveness as a screening modality.

Colorectal Cancer

Screening for colorectal cancer by means of fecal occult blood testing (FOBT) has been studied in three randomized controlled trials involving over 250,000 participants *(12)*. These trials were undertaken in the United States, the United Kingdom, and Denmark. The US trial, undertaken at the University of Minnesota, involved about 47,000 men and women aged between 50 and 80 yr *(13)*. In that study, individuals were screened annually with Hemoccult slides, mostly rehydrated. After 13 yr of follow-up, a 33% reduction in mortality from colorectal cancer was reported in the screened group. The UK and Danish trials showed statistically significant reductions in mortality in the screened group of 15% and 18%, respectively *(14,15)*. However, individuals in these studies were screened every 2 yr by FOBT, without rehydration. Thus, evidence from clinical trials indicates that screening with FOBT can significantly reduce mortality from colorectal cancer.

Breast Cancer

More is known about breast cancer screening than screening for any other type of cancer. There have been eight randomized controlled studies that have examined the impact of mammographic screening on breast cancer mortality *(16)*. These are the Health Insurance Plan (HIP), Swedish Two County, Gothenburg, Stockholm, Malmo, Edinburg, Canadian National Breast Screening Study I (NBSS I), and the NBSS II. In total, nearly 500,000 women were enrolled in these eight trials, and 175,000 of these women were below the age of 50 at the start of the trials. During the last 15 yr, two large randomized controlled trials have also examined the impact of screening with breast self-examination (BSE) on breast cancer mortality *(17,18)*. These trials were undertaken in St. Petersburg (formerly Lenningrad), Russia and Shanghai, China and recruited 120,310 and 267,040 women, respectively.

The results of each of the eight mammographic screening trials have been reported. In addition, several overviews (meta-analyses) incorporating the results of the mammographic screening trials have been published *(19,20)*. Overall, the results of the mammographic screening trials indicate that, for women aged 50 or over at entry, a significant reduction in breast cancer mortality of around 25% is evident after 7–9 years of follow-up *(20)*. For women below age 50 at entry, a significant reduction in breast cancer mortality of only 18% is observed, but only after 12 yr of follow-up *(20)*.

Why should age determine the effectiveness of mammographic screening? Age 50, of course, corresponds approximately to the time of menopause, which has an enormous impact on the epidemiology and biology of breast cancer *(21)*. There is, for example, a steep rise in breast cancer incidence until about age 50, followed by a less rapid increase thereafter *(22)*. In addition, obesity is associated with a lower risk of premenopausal but higher risk of postmenopausal breast cancer *(23)*. Also, premenopausal women have a lower percentage of estrogen receptor positive tumors than do postmenopausal women, making hormonal therapy (tamoxifen) more effective in older women *(24)*. Thus, the results of the mammographic screening trials are consistent with other studies showing differences in the epidemiology and biology of premenopausal and postmenopausal breast cancer.

Thus, one might speculate that menopause influences the efficacy of mammographic screening, and there are several possible ways that this might occur. As screening advances the time of diagnosis and allows for the early initiation of therapy, one might speculate that early therapy is of greater benefit in postmenopausal than premenopausal women. Alternatively, cancers in premenopausal women may grow more rapidly than those in postmenopausal women. As a result, many cancers in the premenopausal age group may escape detection by biennial mammographic screens. Indeed, there is evidence that the incidence of interval cancers (diagnosed between screening sessions) is greater in premenopausal than postmenopausal women *(25)*. If this is the case, then reducing the intervals between screening sessions in premenopausal women (from 2 yr to 1 yr) may improve the effectiveness of mammographic screening in younger women. Finally, some suggest that the sensitivity of mammography is less in premenopausal than postmenopausal women, making it a less effective screening test in younger women *(21)*. This is often attributed to an increased density of the breasts in younger women, but the issue remains controversial.

There are other factors (besides menopause) that might explain the difference in results between screening younger and older women. Breast cancer is much less common in younger women, with 75% of all breast cancers occurring in women over age 50 *(26)*. Thus, much larger numbers of women might be needed to detect a statistically significant benefit from screening younger women during the early years of follow-up. Kopans estimates that, for a screening trial to have an 80% power to demonstrate a 25% mortality reduction with statistical significance during the early years of follow-up, 500,000 women below age 50 would be required *(27)*. However, all the trials to date have included only 175,000 women below age 50 at entry *(28)*. Yet, if such large numbers of women are indeed required to demonstrate a significant benefit from screening younger women, then, in absolute terms, the benefit must be very small.

It is important to remember that the mammographic screening trials took several years to complete. Thus, many women who were below age 50 at entry into these trials continued to undergo mammographic screening beyond the age of 50. Several authors now suggest that the delayed benefit of screening women below age 50 at entry might actually be derived from screening these women when they are over the age of 50. To address this possibility, de Koning et al. used a computer simulation model known as MISCAN (Mirosimulation Screening Analysis) and studied the results from the Swedish randomized trials (Two-County, Gothenburg, Stockholm, Malmo) in their analysis *(29)*. The MISCAN model suggests that, for the Swedish trials, about 70% of the 10% observed reduction in breast cancer mortality for women who were between the ages of 40 and 49 at the start of the screening trials was indeed the result of screening these women after they passed the age of 50. This hypothesis will be further tested in a large, randomized prospective trial that has been initiated in the United Kingdom *(30)*. In this trial, women will be aged 40–41 at entry. A study group of 65,000 women will be offered mammographic screening at the first visit and annually thereafter for seven or eight rounds, and a control group of 135,000 women will be offered the usual care with no screening. Upon reaching the age of 50, both groups will be offered regular mammographic screening. Thus, this study is designed to address the impact of mammographic screening specifically for women between the ages of 40 and 49. Women in this study will be followed for 14–15 yr. The trial has been designed with 80% power to detect a mortality reduction of 20%, assuming that 70% of the women accept the offer to undergo mammographic screening.

Screening with BSE is widely promoted as a means of reducing breast cancer mortality. However, there is little evidence to support its efficacy. There have only been two randomized prospective trials that have examined the effectiveness of screening with BSE *(17,18)*. A trial was initiated in St. Petersburg, Russia between the years 1985 and 1990 under the auspices of the World Health Organization (WHO) *(17)*. That trial recruited 120,310 women, with half randomized to receive BSE training and the other half receiving usual care. A report published in 1992 indicated no significant difference in the number of breast cancers detected between the two groups (190 cases in the BSE group and 190 in the control group) *(17)*. In addition, there were no significant differences between the two groups with respect to size of the tumors, incidence of lymph node metastasis, or mortality. The effectiveness of screening with BSE was also studied in a clinical trial initiated in Shanghai, China between the years 1989 and 1991 *(18)*. In that trial, 267,040 women were randomly assigned on the basis of work sites (520 textile factories) to receive either intensive BSE instruction (study group) or instruction on the prevention of low-back pain (control group). After 5 yr of follow-up, there was more than a two-fold increase in number of breast biopsies in the BSE group in comparison to the control group. However, the number of breast cancer cases and breast cancer mortality were nearly identical in the two groups.

Physical examination (PE) using trained personnel is yet another method of screening for breast cancer. Unfortunately, there are as yet no randomized prospective trials that have evaluated the efficacy of screening by PE alone. However, four of the eight mammographic screening trials also included PE as a screening modality: HIP, Edinburgh, and the CNBSS I and II *(31–34)*. The HIP trial compared screening with mammography and PE to no screening *(31)*. Ultimately, 45% of the cancers in the screened group of the HIP trial were detected by PE alone, 33% by mammography alone, and 22% by mammography and PE. Thus, 67% of the screen-detected cancers were detectable by PE, suggesting that this alone might have contributed to much of the 30% reduction in breast cancer mortality observed in the screened group. In the CNBSS II trial, women aged 50–59 were randomized to undergo either annual screening with mammography and PE (study group) or annual PE alone (control group) *(34)*. After 7 yr of follow-up, there was no significant difference in breast cancer mortality between the two groups. One might interpret these results to mean that screening by mammography contributes nothing to mortality reduction above and beyond the benefit of screening by PE alone. In the Edinburgh trial, women aged 45–64 were randomized to undergo screening with mammography and PE or no screening *(32)*. This trial showed a nonsignificant 18% reduction in breast cancer mortality in the study group after 10 yr of follow-up, and 74% of the cancers in that group were detectable by PE. Finally, the CNBSS I study randomized women aged 40–49 to screening with mammography and PE or no screening *(33)*. The results of the CNBSS I were consistent with other studies showing no benefit to screening women below age 50 during the first 7–10 yr of follow-up. However, 59% of the cancers in the study group were detectable by PE. The results of these various studies suggest that screening by PE alone may reduce breast cancer mortality, at considerably less cost than screening with mammography.

In view of these findings, a randomized controlled trial addressing the impact of screening by PE will be initiated in Mumbai, India under the direction of Dr. Indraneel Mittra *(28)*. This trial will enroll 70,000 women, equally divided between study and control groups. The study group will be taught BSE and receive annual breast cancer screening for 5 yr with PE using trained personnel; the control group will receive usual care. Women enrolled in this study will be followed for 5 yr.

Mittra has long argued that it is not necessary to detect cancers as early as possible, but only as early as needed to produce an improvement in outcome. Although the cancers detected by PE are generally larger than those detected by mammography, this does not necessarily mean that PE is a less effective screening modality. Mammographic screening detects many occult cancers (both invasive and noninvasive) that, in the absence of screening, might never become symptomatic or pose a threat to a woman's life. This *overdiagnosis* of cancer can adversely affect quality of life, as discussed later. In contrast, screening by PE detects early symptomatic cancers. Thus, the overdiagnosis of breast cancer is of less concern in women who undergo screening by PE.

In contrast to most medical interventions that target symptomatic individuals, cancer screening targets large, asymptomatic populations. The studies cited earlier suggest that, where screening is effective, the benefit is not as great as one might have expected. Therefore, the impact of screening on quality of life is of considerable concern. There are three adverse effects of screening that merit particular attention: lead time, false positives, and overdiagnosis (Table 2). These are discussed in the following sections.

LEAD TIME

Screening advances the time of diagnosis. However, finding cancers *early* does not necessarily reduce mortality. For example, in the lung cancer screening trials, early detection had no impact on lung cancer mortality *(1)*. In the breast cancer screening trials, screening reduced breast cancer mortality by only about 25% in postmenopausal women *(28)*. Thus, for most women, the early detection of breast cancer did not favorably alter the natural history of the disease. As a result of screening, most women simply found out *early* that they had breast cancer, but derived no tangible gain from this advanced notice. This *lead-time effect* of screening often results in unnecessary anxiety, financial hardships, and other adverse effects on quality of life.

FALSE POSITIVES

False positives are those cases reported as suspicious or malignant by screening that, on subsequent evaluation, prove to be benign. For mam-

Table 2
Cancer Screening's Adverse Effects on Quality of Life

Adverse Effect	Consequences
Lead time	Some patients might be given advanced notice of a cancer diagnosis with no tangible gain.
False positive	Leads to further costly, invasive tests (such as biopsies).
Overdiagnosis	Falsely labeling someone as a "cancer patient"; this has adverse financial/emotional consequences.

mographic screening, the false-positive rates in the United States are much higher than in Europe. This is generally attributed to the fear of litigation in the United States and, hence, a greater unwillingness of American radiologists to commit themselves to a benign diagnosis. Indeed, in the American Breast Cancer Detection and Demonstration Project (BCDDP), the positive predictive value of mammographic screening was only 10%, meaning that nine women had a false-positive result on screening for every cancer found *(35)*. In contrast, the positive predictive value of mammographic screening in European centers generally ranges from 30% to 60% *(36)*.

A recent study in the United States found that after 10 screening mammograms, a woman has about a 49% cumulative risk of a false positive result *(37)*. For women between the ages of 40 and 49, that risk is about 56%, whereas for women aged 50–79 it is about 47%. False-positive mammograms result in unnecessary breast biopsies (surgery), anxiety, and increase in health care expenditures.

OVERDIAGNOSIS

Since the advent of mammographic screening, the incidence of breast cancer (both *in situ* and invasive) has increased dramatically *(38)*. This suggests that many screen-detected cancers might never have been clinically detected during the lifetime of a woman. Peeters and colleagues define *overdiagnosis* as a *histologically established diagnosis of intraductal or invasive cancer that would never have developed into a clinically manifest tumor during the patients normal life expectancy if no screening examination had been carried out (39)*.

To understand how screening results in the overdiagnosis of invasive cancer, consider the case of a 75-yr-old woman with severe carotid occlusive disease who undergoes routine mammographic screening. Let us assume that an occult (nonpalpable) invasive breast cancer is discovered, and, as a result of that diagnosis, the patient is treated with surgery, systemic therapy, and radiotherapy. Let us also assume that our hypothetical patient dies of a stroke 1 yr later. Mammographic screening generally advances the time of breast cancer diagnosis by 2–4 yr *(16)*. Had our patient not undergone mammographic screening, she probably would have died of a stroke, never knowing that she had breast cancer. Therefore, this case illustrates the effect of screening mammography in *overdiagnosing* invasive cancer. Thus, one might speculate that mammographic screening is at least partly responsible for the increased incidence of invasive breast cancer reported in the United States.

However, the term *overdiagnosis* is more often applied to the diagnosis of noninvasive (*in situ*) cancers by mammographic screening. Ductal carcinoma *in situ* (DCIS) is rarely detectable by physical examination of the breast and is usually detected by mammographic screening *(40)*. DCIS accounted for 7% of new breast cancers diagnosed in the United States in 1985; today, it accounts for more than 14% of breast cancers and for about 30% of those discovered mammographically *(41,42)*.

It is generally assumed that DCIS is a preinvasive breast cancer that, if left untreated, invariably leads to invasive cancer. This assumption is based on two observations: DCIS is often found adjacent to invasive breast cancer and, with simple excision of DCIS, recurrences can occur, and these recurrences are often invasive cancer *(43)*. However, there is now considerable evidence to suggest that not all cases of DCIS progress to invasive cancer. Nielsen et al. reported the results of 110 medicolegal autopsies undertaken at the Fredricksburg Hospital in Copenhagen *(44)*. In their series, DCIS was found in 15% of cases, a prevalence four to five times greater than the number of clinically overt cancers expected to develop over a 20-yr period. This study suggests that occult DCIS is not uncommon in younger women. Additionally, in autopsies of women with a history of invasive breast cancer, Alpers and Wellings found that 48% had occult DCIS in the contralateral breast *(45)*. Yet, only 2–11% of women with breast cancer develop contralateral breast cancer in their lifetime *(46)*.

There are also retrospective studies that suggest that not all cases of DCIS progress to invasive cancer. Rosen et al. and Page et al. retrospectively reviewed benign biopsy findings and found a number of instances where DCIS was overlooked by the original pathologist *(47,48)*. Thus, these patients received no treatment for DCIS other than a diagnostic biopsy. In the series reported by Rosen et al., 30 patients with DCIS were identified, and after an average follow-up of 18 yr, only 8 patients developed clinically detectable breast cancer. In the series by Page et al., 28 women with DCIS were identified, and clinically apparent breast cancer developed in only 7 of these patients after 15 yr of follow-up.

Taken together, the autopsy studies and the retrospective studies cited suggest that only about one out of every four cases of DCIS progresses to a clinically manifest cancer during the lifetime of a patient. Thus, most cases of DCIS, if left untreated, would have no impact on mortality. However, with the advent of mammographic screening, large numbers of women are being diagnosed with DCIS. These women are falsely labeled as *cancer patients* and face difficulties obtaining life insurance, health insurance, loans, and even employment *(49)*. Clearly, the overdiagnosis of breast cancer has adversely affected the quality of life for many women. This adverse effect of screening has received very little attention in the medical literature and the lay press. The effects of screening on quality of life should be addressed and we must take necessary steps to reduce overdiagnosing asymptomatic women as *breast cancer patients.*

CONCLUSION

Clearly, screening does find cancers *early*. However, the early detection of cancer is not a sufficient basis for recommending screening. We must first determine whether the early detection of cancer (by screening) can effectively reduce mortality. Randomized controlled trials have provided important information on the effects of screening on mortality. These trials suggest that, for some cancers, screening does reduce mortality. However, the impact of screening on mortality is generally less than one might have expected.

It is absolutely essential that we also consider the impact of screening on quality of life. Screening targets large, asymptomatic populations. For many, screening may adversely affect quality of life. Therefore, we should inform our patients about the potential risks and benefits of screening.

REFERENCES

1. Smith IE. (1999) Screening for lung cancer: time to think positive. *Lancet* 354:86.
2. Klemi PJ, Joensuu H, Toikkanen S, et al. (1992) Aggressiveness of breast cancers found with and without screening. *Br Med J* 304:467–469.
3. Moss SM, Summerley ME, Thomas BJ, et al. (1992) A case-control evaluation of the effect of breast cancer screening in the United Kingdom trial of early detection of breast cancer. *J Epidemiol Comm Health* 46:362–364.
4. Kline TS. (1997) The Papanicolaou smear. A brief historical perspective and where we are today. *Arch Pathol Lab Med* 121(3):205–209.

5. Laara E, Day NE, Hakama M. (1987) Trends in mortality from cervical cancer in the Nordic countries: association with organized screening programmes. *Lancet* 1:1247–1249.
6. Sasieni P, Cuzick J, Farmery E. (1995) Accelerated decline in cervical cancer mortality in England and Wales. *Lancet* 346:1566–1567.
7. Melamed MR, Flchinger DJ, Zaman MB, et al. (1984) Screening for lung cancer: results of the Memorial Sloan Kettering study in New York. *Chest* 86:44–53.
8. Tockman MS. (1986) Survival and mortality from lung cancer in a screened population: the Johns Hopkins Study. *Chest* 89:324–25S.
9. Fontana RS, Sanderson DR, Woolner LB, et al. (1986) Lung cancer screening: the Mayo program. *J Occup Med* 28:746–750.
10. Kubik A, Parkin DM, Khlat M, et al. (1990) Lack of benefit from semi-annual screening for cancer of the lung: follow-up report of a randomized controlled trial on a population of high-risk males in Czechoslovakia. *Int J Cancer* 45:26–33.
11. Henschke CI, McCauley DI, Yankelevitz DF, et al. (1999) Early lung cancer action project: overall design and findings from baseline screening. *Lancet* 354(9173):99–105.
12. Levin B. (1999) Colorectal cancer screening: sifting through the evidence. *J Natl Cancer Inst* 91(5):399–400.
13. Mandel JS, Church TR, Ederer F, Bond JH. (1999) Colorectal cancer mortality: effectiveness of biennial screening for fecal occult blood. *J Natl Cancer Inst* 91:434–437.
14. Hardcastle JD, Chamberlain JO, Robinson MH, et al. (1996) Randomized controlled trial of faecal-occult-blood screening for colorectal cancer. *Lancet* 348:1472–1477.
15. Kronborg O, Fenger C, Olsen J, et al. (1996) Randomized study of screening for colorectal cancer with faecal-occult blood test. *Lancet* 348:1461–1471.
16. Jatoi I, Baum M. (1993) American and European recommendations for screening mammography in younger women: a cultural divide? *Br Med J* 307:1481–1483.
17. Semiglazov VF, Moiseyenko VM, Bavli JL, et al. (1992) The role of breast self-examination in early breast cancer detection (results of the 5-year USSR/WHO randomized study in Leningrad). *Eur J Epidemiol* 8(4):498–502.
18. Thomas DB, Gao DL, Self SG, et al. (1997) Randomized trial of breast self-examination in Shanghai: methodology and preliminary results. *J Natl Cancer Inst* 89:355–365.
19. Kerlikowske K, Grady D, Rubin SM, et al. (1995) Efficacy of screening mammography. A meta-analysis. *JAMA* 273:149–154.
20. Hendrick RE, Smith RA, Rutledge JH, Smart CR. (1997) Benefit of screening mammography in women aged 40-49: a new meta-analysis of randomized controlled trials. *Monogr Natl Cancer Inst* 22:87–92.
21. Elwood JM, Cox B, Richardson AK. (1993) The effectiveness of breast cancer screening by mammography in younger women. *Online J Curr Clin Trial* 25 Feb 1993 (Doc No. 32).
22. Clemmensen J. (1948) Carcinoma of the breast. Results from statistical research. *Br J Radiol* 21:583.
23. Willett W. (1990) Nutritional Epidemiology. New York: Oxford University Press.
24. Henderson IC. (1992) Biologic variations of tumors. *Cancer* 69:1888–1895.
25. Tabar L, Faberberg G, Day NE, Holmberg L. (1987) What is the optimum interval between mammographic screening examinations? An analysis based on the latest results of the Swedish two-county breast cancer screening trial. *Br J Cancer* 55:547–551.

26. Landis SH, Murray T, Bolden S, Wingo PA. (1998) Cancer Statistics, 1998. *CA Cancer J Clin* 48: 6–29.
27. Kopans DB. (1994) Screening for breast cancer and mortality reduction among women 40–49 years of age. *Cancer* 74:311–322.
28. Jatoi I. (1999) Breast cancer screening. *Am J Surg* 177(6):518–524.
29. deKonig HJ, Boer R, Warmerdam PG, et al. (1995) Quantitative interpretations of age-specific mortality reductions from the Swedish breast cancer screening trials. *J Natl Cancer Inst* 87:1217–1223.
30. Editorial. (1991) Breast cancer screening in women under 50. *Lancet* 337:1575–1576.
31. Shapiro S, Venet W, Strax P, et al. (1988) Periodic screening for breast cancer. In: *The Health Insurance Plan Project and Its Sequelae, 1963–1986.* Baltimore, MD: Johns Hopkins University Press.
32. Alexander FE. (1997) The Edinburgh randomized trial of breast cancer screening. *Monogr Natl Cancer Inst* 22:31–35.
33. Miller AB, Baines CJ, To T, Wall C. (1992) Canadian National Breast Screening Study I. Breast cancer detection and death rates among women aged 40 to 49 years. *Can Med Assoc J* 147:1459–1476.
34. Miller AB, Baines CJ, To T, Wall C. (1992) Canadian National Breast Screening Study II. Breast cancer detection and death rates among women aged 50 to 59 years. *Can Med Assoc J* 147:1477–1488.
35. Baker LH. (1982) Breast cancer detection demonstration project: 5-year summary report. *CA Cancer J Clin* 42:1–35.
36. Reidy J, Hoskins O. (1988) Controversy over mammography screening. *Br Med J* 297:932–933.
37. Elmore JG, Barton MB, Moceri VM, et al. (1998) Ten-year risk of false positive screening mammograms and clinical breast examinations. *N Engl J Med* 338:1089–1096.
38. Jatoi I, Baum M. (1995) Mammographically detected ductal carcinoma in situ: are we overdiagnosing breast cancer? *Surgery* 118: 118–120.
39. Peeters PHM, Verbeek ALM, Straatman H, et al. (1989) Evaluation of overdiagnosis of breast cancer in screening with mammography: results of the Nijmegen programme. *Int J Epidemiol* 18:295–299.
40. Hwang ES, Esserman LJ. (1990) Management of ductal carcinoma in situ. *Surg Clin North Amer* 79(5): 1007–1030.
41. Bland KI, Menck HR, Scott-Conner CE, et al. (1998) The National Cancer Data Base 10-year survey of breast carcinoma treatment at hospitals in the United States. *Cancer* 83: 1262–1273.
42. Ernster VL, Barclay J, Kerlikowske K, et al. (1996) Incidence of treatment for ductal carcinoma in situ of the breast. *JAMA* 275:913–918.
43. Van Dongen JA, Fentiman IS, Harris JR, et al. (1989) In-situ breast cancer: the EORTC consensus meeting. *Lancet* 2:25–27.
44. Nielsen M, Thomsen JL, Primdahl S, et al. (1987) Breast cancer and atypia among young and middle aged women: a study of 110 medicolegal autopsies. *Br J Cancer* 56:814–819.
45. Alpers CE, Wellings SR. (1985) The prevalence of carcinoma in situ in normal and cancer-associated breasts. *Hum Pathol* 16:796–807.
46. Chen Y, Thompson W, Semenciw R, Mao Y. (1999) Epidemiology of contralateral breast cancer. *Cancer Epidemiol Biomarkers Prev* 8(10): 855–61.
47. Rosen PR, Braun DW Jr, Kinne DW. (1980) The clinical significance of pre-invasive breast carcinoma. *Cancer* 46:919–925.

48. Page DL, Dupont WD, Rogers LW, Landenberger M. (1982) Intraductal carcinoma of the breast: followup after biopsy only. *Cancer* 49:751–758.
49. Berkman BJ, Sampson SE. (1993) Psychosocial effects of cancer economics on patients and their families. *Cancer* 72:2846–2849.

5

The Role of Prostate Specific Antigen and Its Variants in Prostate Cancer Screening

Faiyaaz M. Jhaveri, MD,
Michael K. Brawer, MD,
and Eric A. Klein, MD

INTRODUCTION

Prostate-specific antigen (PSA) is the most important marker for the detection and management of prostate cancer. PSA-based screening has been responsible for a profound downward stage migration in newly diagnosed prostate cancer compared to those detected in the pre-PSA era *(1)*. This has been the result of the increased lead time for prostate cancer diagnosis that has resulted in the identification of prostate cancer earlier in the natural history of the disease *(2)*. In addition, we have recently shown that rates of extracapsular extension in radical prostatectomy specimens have continued to decrease during the PSA era independent of preoperative serum PSA levels, T stage, and histological grade *(3)*.

From: *Current Clinical Urology: Prostate Cancer Screening*
Edited by: I. M. Thompson, M. I. Resnick, and E. A. Klein
© Humana Press Inc., Totowa, NJ

Despite impressive initial results in early detection and screening studies, PSA is not a perfect tumor marker. Although the sensitivity remains high at approx. 75% for elevation above 4.0 ng/mL, specificity remains low at only about 25%. Therefore, efforts are ongoing to improve test specifity and to thus avoid unnecessary biopsies. These efforts have resulted in the use of PSA density, PSA velocity, age-specific PSA cutoffs, and the measurement of the different molecular forms of PSA in the systemic circulation. After a discussion of the history of PSAs application to early detection and screening, each of these parameters will be addressed.

HISTORY OF PSA SCREENING

After the recognition of the PSA protein initially in the seminal plasma and, subsequently, in the serum by researchers at the Roswell Park Cancer Institute *(4)*, many investigators questioned whether PSA should be used for the early detection or screening for prostate cancer *(5,6)*. Early investigations suggested that PSA would be of limited value for screening. Because many men with benign prostatic hyperplasia (BPH) had a PSA elevation and as virtually every man undergoing screening for prostate cancer has some histological evidence of BPH, the PSA test was felt to be nonspecific and useless in a diagnostic setting.

Evidence from two early studies questioned this conclusion. Cooner et al. *(7)* performed ultrasound-guided biopsies on patients with an abnormality on transrectal ultrasound. Brawer et al. *(8)* biopsied men with an abnormality on digital rectal examination (DRE). In both studies, PSA was measured prior to histological analysis, but not used as an indication for biopsy. Both studies independently showed that a man had a 50% chance of having prostate cancer with a PSA level greater than 4.0 ng/mL. These independent studies indicated that prostate cancer could be associated with an elevated PSA level.

Furthermore, in men having simple prostatectomy for presumed BPH, a detailed histological analysis of all resected or enucleated tissue revealed that 50% of those men with incidental carcinoma, acute inflammation, or prostatic intraepithelial neoplasia had serum PSA levels greater than 4.0 ng/mL *(9)*. However, less than 4% of the men with BPH with or without chronic inflammation had PSA levels above this threshold. These observations suggested a mechanism underlying this elevation of the PSA level that was related to specific disease processes not noted in the older series.

Table 1
Confirmatory Investigations of Prostate Cancer
Correlation with PSA Level Greater than 4.0 ng/mL

Investigators	Year	No. of biopsies	Population	PPV[a]
Bazinet et al. (12)	1994	565	Referral	37
Brawer et al. (10)	1992	105	Screening	31
Catalona et al. (11)	1991	112	Screening	33
Catalona et al. (13)	1994	1,325	Screening	37
Cooner et al. (14)	1990	436	Referral	35
Rommel et al. (15)	1994	2,020	Referral	41

[a]PPV = positive predictive value.

PSA for Early Detection of Prostate Cancer

On the pathological basis that PSA had some specificity as a marker for prostate cancer, two investigations using PSA as a diagnostic test in a screening population were initiated. In both studies, men were recruited through media announcements and offered a free PSA test. Brawer et al. *(10)* showed that of the 1249 men evaluated, the detection rate was 2.6% and the positive biopsy yield was 31% if the PSA was greater than 4.0 ng/mL. A 4.6% detection rate would have been realized had all men undergone a biopsy. Similarly, Catalona et al. *(11)* evaluated 1653 men and found a 2.2% observed detection rate and a 33% positive biopsy yield. Several other investigations have demonstrated similar results in positive predictive values (PPV) (Table 1) *(10–15)*.

Drawbacks of PSA Screening

Despite the observations that PSA can be used as an indicator for prostate cancer, it is not an ideal marker. Assay variability has created substantial problems with the interpretation of PSA concentrations. Serum PSA concentrations have been found to vary in identical samples by a factor of 2 *(16)*. The clinician interpreting PSA concentrations must have detailed information on the assay-specific reference range and must be aware of the assay method used.

The primary pitfall of PSA screening is the risk of false-positive results. For this reason, considerable efforts have been made to increase the *specificity* of PSA in detecting prostate cancer. Because of the slow growing nature of prostate cancer, and the high likelihood of multiple PSA tests over a man's lifetime, the concern regarding false-negative results may be less as annual testing may detect the tumor at a curable stage. However, false-positive test results are financially and emotionally costly with as many as three-quarters of men undergoing unnecessary biopsies. Because enhancing the specificity does so at the expense of sensitivity, the goal is to maintain acceptable sensitivity, a level that must be 95% or higher.

ENHANCING PSA SPECIFICITY

To improve the performance of PSA for the detection of prostate cancer, investigators have evaluated PSA velocity, PSA density, age-specific PSA cutoffs, and molecular forms of PSA such as free/ total PSA ratio or complexed PSA (cPSA).

PSA Velocity

The rate of increase of PSA or PSA velocity has been evaluated as a method to improve PSA sensitivity. In men with advanced prostate cancer, the rate of rise is significantly greater than in men with benign disease or in healthy men of the general population (17).
Carter and collegues, in the Baltimore longitudinal study of aging (18), were the first to demonstrate this concept by showing that patients who had an increase in PSA of greater than 0.75 ng/mL per year had a higher risk of carcinoma. Using archival serum, and PSA determinations separated by a minimum of 7 yr, they demonstrated sensitivities of 75% and specificities of greater than 90% using this cutoff of PSA velocity.

The Seattle group has not been able to reproduce these results using relatively short-term PSA determinations over 1- and 2-yr intervals (19). PSA velocity did not stratify those men with or without cancer in this series. One explanation of this discrepancy is the wide biological variation and assay variability as documented by Nixon and collegues (20). They found that a 25% increase in PSA was required to ensure that the change was the result of an actual change in prostatic disease. For free PSA, an even greater change of 36% was required. Similar conclusions were reached by Catalona et al. (21), who found that PSA velocity was no more useful than PSA alone at relatively short periods of follow-up. Carter et al. (22) subsequently found that with a minimum of three consecutive measurements over a 2-yr time period, PSA velocity was most predictive in those men that had a PSA greater than 4.0 ng/mL.

PSA Density

Prostate-specific antigen density PSAD density is calculated by dividing the serum PSA by the volume of the prostate gland. This calculation takes into account the concept that benign prostatic tissue results in incremental elevations in PSA proportional to the volume of prostatic epithelium. These elements largely arise from the transition zone, which enlarges from the development of BPH.

Several studies have found that PSA density is useful for enhancing PSA specificity *(23–26)*. Littrup et al. *(25)* observed that 16–55% of negative biopsies could be avoided with only a 4–25% loss in the sensitivity if a PSA density of 0.12 was used. Bagma et al. *(26)* also demonstrated a significant reduction of negative biopsies with only 11% of cancers missed. However, several other studies were not able to reproduce these results of improved specificity of PSA density over serum PSA alone *(27–29)*.

Several factors could explain the discrepancy of these results. The biopsy sampling error may cause a larger proportion of cancer to be missed in larger glands *(30)*. It is interesting to note that in the review of the studies that support PSA density, the glands that biopsied positive for cancer were smaller than those with benign findings. However, in the series by Brawer et al. *(31)*, there was no difference in the prostate sizes. Letran et al. have demonstrated that there was a decrease in the cancer detection rate in glands greater than about 55 g *(31)*. However, ultrasound measurement error, differing histological makeup of the cohort being biopsied, and PSA assay variability all could also contribute to these findings *(23,30,33)*.

Because the transition zone is the main area of the prostate that increases in size as a result of BPH and thus causes a decrease in PSA specificity, investigators have attempted to correct for the transition-zone volume to further enhance PSA specificity. Djavan et al. *(34)* and Maeda et al. *(35)* demonstrated that using transition-zone PSA density (PSA TZD) enhances the specificity of PSA. However, Lin et al. *(36)* were unable to reproduce these results. PSA alone was found to have similar specificities when compared to PSAD and PSA TZD, and no benefit was seen in the measurement and calculation of these indexes. A possible explanation for these differing results may be related to the difficulty of accurately measuring the transition-zone volume with ultrasound. Not only is transrectal ultrasound (TRUS) costly but it is also an uncomfortable test for men to undergo. Some utility may be obtained in men being evaluated for a possible repeat biopsy, where the measurements of these volumes may alter a plan for a repeat biopsy.

Age-Adjusted PSA

It is well-known that PSA increases with advancing age *(5)*. By adjusting the PSA cutoffs based on the age of the patient, some investigators have found that PSA performance can be improved *(30)*.

Oesterling et al. suggested that to provide greater sensitivity in the younger man and to decrease the number of unnecessary biopsies in the older man it would be better to use a lower PSA cutoff in the former and higher cutoff in the latter *(37)*. They found that a man younger than 50 yr old should have a PSA cutoff of 2.5 ng/mL, whereas the cutoff for a man in his seventies is 6.5 ng/mL. Contrary to these results, Borer and collegues *(38)* raised serious concerns regarding this adjustment, finding that the majority of carcinomas that would be missed in men 60–79 yr old had characteristics of a life-threatening malignancy.

What is the optimal PSA cutoff? This remains controversial as seen by a Swedish screening study by Aus using a lower PSA cutoff *(39)*. The author observed that with a PSA of 3.0 – 4.0 ng/mL, 13.2% of men (n = 32/243) were found to have cancer. This represented an additional 23% of all cancers detected. Etzioni et al. *(40)* compared PSA with a cutoff of 4.0 ng/mL to age-specific PSA from a screening study in Seattle. The detection rate of age-specific PSA ranges was significantly less even though the positive predictive value was greater. Using estimates of US life expectancy and modeling for life years gained, they found with age adjustment that a reduction in life years gained would result even though the potential for detecting younger men with cancer would be greater (Table 2). It was recommended that a cutoff of 4.0 ng/mL would be more appropriate than using the age-specific cutoffs.

PSA Molecular Forms: Free Versus Complexed PSA

Efforts to analyze PSA have resulted in the discovery of several forms of this protein in the bloodstream. Molecular forms complexed to protease inhibitors exist in serum, as opposed to the free form in the ejaculate *(41,42)*. The two most prevalent complexes in the serum are α-1-antichymotrypsin (ACT) and α-2-macroglobulin (AMG). When PSA is complexed to AMG in the serum, all the epitopes are sterically hindered, preventing detection by currently available assays. In addition, this form of complexed PSA is found in very low quantities in vivo. In contrast, PSA complexed to ACT is more common in the serum, and two epitopes remain unhindered and available for detection by immunoassays.

Free PSA and Free-to-Total PSA Ratio

Stenmen et al. demonstrated that free PSA exists in higher proportion in men without prostate cancer compared to those with the disease *(42)*. Christensson et al. discovered that they could enhance the specificity of free PSA by showing that the ratio of free-to-total PSA was decreased in men with cancer *(43)*. Luderer et al. showed that in the

Table 2
Age-Specific PSA Reference Range vs Cutoff of 4.0 ng/mL

	Age-specific PSA level[a]	PSA 4.0 ng/mL
Positive predictive value	42%	37%
Cancer detection rate	3.8%	5.7%
Life saved (yr)	757	1091

Source, Ref. *40.*
[a]Cutoffs from Oesterling et al. *(37)*

diagnostic gray zone of PSA between 4.0 and 10.0 ng/mL, the total PSA did not differ between men with and without prostate carcinoma *(44)*. However, the ratio of free-to-total PSA was significantly lower in men with cancer.

The most definitive study on the performance of free-to-total PSA was recently reported by Catalona et al *(45)*. In this multicenter trial involving seven institutions, the Hybritech free and total PSA assays were evaluated in men with total PSA levels between 4.0 and 10.0 ng/mL and negative DREs. Of the 773 men evaluated, 379 (49%) were found to have cancer. The total PSA was found to be higher in men with cancer, and the free-to-total PSA ratio was found to be lower in this group. When using free-to-total PSA cutoffs of less than 25%, the sensitivity of detecting cancer was 95% and the specificity was enhanced by 20%. Therefore, for missing cancer in 5%, 1 out of 5 biopsies could be avoided if this cutoff was used. Depending on the percent of free-to-total PSA, the probability of detecting cancer can vary widely (Table 3) *(45)*.

Although free-to-total PSA improves the specificity of prostate cancer detection, two main issues regarding its clinical use must be addressed. First, the analytical problems of measuring free and total PSA by different manufacturers of assays and the preanalytical handling and storage of sera can cause widely variable results. Second, the target population of men that free-to-total PSA values would be most useful in, remains to be defined.

Owing to the molecular structure and, in part, to protease activity in the sample, levels of free PSA may decrease during sample storage *(46)*. Furthermore, the PSA–ACT complex may also decompose and increase the amount of free PSA levels in the sample *(47)*. This dissociation rate, however, is insignificant under optimal storage conditions *(48)*. Therefore, preanalytical handling instructions must be standardized and enforced.

Differences between assay manufacturers may result in differing serum PSA levels in the same patient's sera *(49,50)*. These differences

Table 3
Percent Free-to-Total PSA and Probability
of Cancer Detection in Men with PSA 4–10 ng/mL
and Benign Prostate DRE

Percent free-to-total PSA	Probability of cancer
0–10%	56%
10–15%	28%
15–20%	20%
20–25%	16%
>25%	8%

Source: Ref. 45.

are compounded when two analytes are measured to obtain the free-to-total PSA ratio (51). For example, for free-to-total PSA cutoffs to give a 95% sensitivity, the Dianon free PSA to Hybritech total PSA ratio gives a specificity of only 19% (cutoff 34%), significantly lower than the Hybritech free PSA to Hybritech total PSA ratio of 38% (cutoff 22%). Therefore, clinicians should be aware of the assays that their laboratories are using, and the performance of each free-to-total PSA assay in their patient population should be defined prior to its clinical use.

Another important concern is when a clinician should use free-to-total PSA ratio. Should it be used only on men with PSA in the diagnostic gray zone of PSA 4–10 ng/mL? Another possibility is its use in men with PSA less than 4.0 ng/mL, where approximately 25% of cancers are detected. Recently, Djavan et al. (52) compared free-to-total PSA with standard PSA assays in men with serum PSA 2.5–4.0 ng/mL in a referral population. They found that in a cohort of 273 men, free-to-total PSA and transition-zone PSA density was the most powerful predictors of prostate cancer. With a 95% sensitivity and a free-to-total PSA cutoff of 41%, the specificity was 29.3% and would result in the lowest number of unnecessary biopsies compared to all the other PSA-related parameters.

Another potential use of free-to-total PSA is in the evaluation of men after a previously negative biopsy. Malignancy can be detected in 20–30% of men on repeat biopsy, and, recently, Letran et al. (53) showed that free-to-total PSA can help identify men that harbor cancer despite an initial negative biopsy.

Complexed PSA

Even though it has been recognized that PSA complexed to α-1-antichymotrypsin (PSA–ACT complex or cPSA) is the form that occurs to a greater extent in men with prostate cancer *(42)*, because of technical problems it has been difficult to measure and is not commercially available *(43)*. Recently, the Bayer Corporation has developed an immunoassay that is specific for cPSA *(54)*.

Brawer et al. *(55)* performed a study using the Bayer Immuno 1 cPSA Assay on archival sera obtained from 300 men, 75 of whom had biopsy-proven prostate cancer. At cutoffs yielding 95% sensitivity, specificities for total PSA, free-to-total PSA, and cPSA alone were 21.8%, 15.6%, and 26.7%, respectively. Complexed PSA alone performed better than the other parameters and obviated the need for a second analyte determination. These results have been recently confirmed by Maeda et al. *(56)* using cPSA assays manufactured by Chugai Pharmaceutical, Japan. They found cPSA to be more specific than total and free-to-total PSA in their cohort of 137 men with PSA levels of 4.0–10.0 ng/mL. Such findings suggest that using the single analyte of cPSA may lead to significant economic savings and reduction of patient discomfort by reducing the number of unnecessary biopsies without sacrificing sensitivity of detecting prostate cancer.

SUMMARY

Undoubtedly, PSA has had a profound impact on the detection and management of men with prostate cancer, and its role in screening is well established. Its main drawback is the limited specificity at high sensitivities. Free-to-total PSA, complexed PSA, and the various volume indexes have been used to help enhance PSA specificity in attempts to decrease the number of unnecessary biopsies. Interpreting these and new markers that are being identified in the individual patient is the challenge that clinicians face when screening for this most common human malignancy.

REFERENCES

1. Catalona WJ, Smith DS, Ratliff TL, et al. (1993) Detection of organ-confined prostate cancer is increased through prostate-specific antigen based screening. *JAMA* 270:948.
2. Carter HB, Pearson JD, Metter JE, et al. (1992) Longitudinal evaluation of prostate specific antigen levels in men with and without prostate disease. *JAMA* 267:2215–2220.
3. Jhaveri FM, Klein EA, Kupelian PA, et al. (1999) Declining rates of extracapsular extension in radical prostatectomy: evidence for continued stage migration. *J Clin Oncol* 17:3167–3172.
4. Wang MC, Valenzuela LA, Murphy GP, Chu TM. (1979) Purification of a human prostate antigen. *Invest Urol* 17:159–163.

5. Stamey TA, Yang N, Hay AR, et al. (1987) Prostate-specific antigen as serum marker for adenocarcinoma of the prostate. *N Engl J Med* 317:909–916.
6. Ercole CJ, Lange PH, Mathisen M, et al. (1987) Prostate specific antigen and prostatic acid phosphatase in the monitoring and staging of patients with prostatic cancer. *J Urol* 138:1181–1184.
7. Cooner WH, Eggers CW, Lichtenstein P. (1987) Prostate cancer: New hope for early diagnosis. *Alabama Med* 56:13.
8. Brawer MK, Lange PH. (1989) PSA in the screening, staging and follow up of early-stage prostate cancer: A review of recent developments. *World J Urol* 7: 7–11.
9. Brawer MK, Rennels MA, Nagle RB, et al. (1989) Serum prostate specific antigen and prostate pathology in men having simple prostatectomy. *Am J Clin Pathol* 92: 760–764.
10. Brawer MK, Chetner MP, Beatie J, et al. (1992) Screening for prostate carcinoma with prostate specific antigen. *J Urol* 147: 841–845.
11. Catalona WJ, Smith DS, Ratliff TL, et al. (1991) Measurement of PSA in serum as a screening test for prostate cancer. *N Engl J Med* 324: 1156–1161.
12. Bazinet M, Meshref AW, Trudel C, et al. (1994) Prospective evaluation of prostate specific antigen density and systematic biopsies for early detection of prostatic carcinoma. *Urology* 43:4–51.
13. Catalona WJ, Richie JP, Ahmann FR, et al. (1994) Comparison of digital rectal examination and serum prostate specific antigen in the early detection of prostate cancer: Results of a multicenter clinical trial of 6,630 men. *J Urol* 151: 1283–1290.
14. Cooner WH, Mosley BR, Rutherford CL Jr, et al. (1990) Prostate cancer detection in a clinical urological practice by ultrasonography, digital rectal examination and prostate specific antigen. *J Urol* 143: 1146–1154.
15. Rommel FM, Agusta VE, Breslin JA, et al. (1994) The use of prostate specific antigen and prostate specific antigen density in the diagnosis of prostate cancer in a community based urology practice. *J Urol* 151:88–93.
16. Semjonow A, Brandt B, Oberpenning F, Roth S, Hertie L. (1996) Discordance of assay methods creates pitfalls for the interpretation of prostate-specific antigen values. *Prostate* 7:3–16.
17. Williford WO, Lepor H, Dixon CM, et al. (1996) Serum PSA levels after 52 weeks of therapy with finasteride, terazosin, combination and placebo: results of the VA cooperative study #359. *J Urol* 155: (Suppl) 533A
18. Carter HB, Morrell CH, Pearson JD, et al. (1992) Estimation of prostatic growth using serial prostate specific antigen measurements in men with and without prostate disease. *Cancer* 52:3323–3328.
19. Porter JR, Hayward R, Brawer MK. (1994) The significance of short-term PSA change in men undergoing ultrasound guided prostate biospy. *J Urol* 151(Suppl.) :264 (abstract 293).
20. Nixon RG, Wener MH, Smith KM, et al. (1997) Biological variation of prostate specific antigen levels in serum: An evaluation of day-to-day physiological fluctuations in a well-defined cohort of 24 patients. *J Urol* 157:2183–2190.
21. Catalona WJ, Smith DS, Ratliff TL. (1993) Value of measurement of the rate of change of serum PSA levels in prostate cancer screening. *J. Urol* 150 (Suppl.):300 (abstract 1502).
22. Carter HB, Pearson JD, Chan DW, Guess HA, Walsh PC. (1991) Prostate-specific antigen variability in men without prostate cancer: effect of sampling interval on prostate-specific antigen velocity. *Urology* 45: 591.

23. Benson MC, Whang IS Pantuck A, et al. (1992) Prostate-specific antigen density: a means of distinguishing benign prostatic hypertrophy and prostate cancer. *J Urol* 147: 815–816.
24. Rommel FM, Augusta VE, Breslin JA, et al. (1994) The use of PSA and PSAD in the diagnosis of prostate cancer in a community based urology practice J Urol 151:88–93.
25. Littrup PJ, Kane RA, Mettlin CJ, et al. (1994) Cost-effective prostate cancer detection: reduction of low-yield biopsies. *Cancer* 74(12):3146–3158.
26. Bagma CH, Kranse R, Blijenberg BG, Schroder FH. (1995) The value of screening tests in the detection of prostate cancer. Part I: Results of a retrospective evaluation of 1726 men. *Urology* 46(6): 773–778.
27. Ellis WJ, Aramburu EAG, Chen GL, Preston SD, Brawer MK. (1993) The inability of PSA density to enhance the predictive value of PSA in the diagnosis of prostate carcinoma. *J Urol* 149:415A.
28. Mettlin C, Littrup PJ, Kane RA, et al. (1994) Relative sensitivity and specificity of serum PSA level compared with age-referenced PSA, PSA density and PSA change. *Cancer* 74: 1615–1620.
29. Ohori M, Dunn JK, Scardino PT. (1995) Is prostate-specfic antigen density more useful than prostate-specific antigen levels in the diagnosis of prostate cancer? *Urology* 46: 666–671.
30. Brawer MK. (1995) How to use prostate-specific antigen in the early detection or screening for prostatic carcinoma. *CA Cancer J Clin* 45: 148–164.
31. Brawer Mk, Aramburu EAG, Chen GL, Preston SD, Ellis WJ. (1993) The inability of PSA index to enhance the predictive value of PSA in the diagnosis of prostate carcinoma. *J Urol* 150: 369–373.
32. Letran J, Meyer G, Loberiza F, Brawer M. (1998) The effect of prostate volume on the yield of needle biopsy. *J Urol* 160(5): 1718–1721.
33. Wener MH, Daum PR, Brawer MK. (1995) Variation in measurement of PSA: The importance of method and lot variability. *Clin Chem* 41(12) 1730–1737.
34. Djavan B, Zlotta AR, Byttebier G, et al. (1998) Prostate specific antigen density of the transition zone for the early detection of prostate cancer. *J Urol* 160: 411–419.
35. Maeda H, Ishitoya S, Maekawa S, et al. (1997) Prostate specific antigen density of the transition zone in the detection of prostate cancer. *J Urol* :158(4):58A.
36. Lin DW, Gold MH, Ransom S, Ellis WJ, Brawer MK. (1998) Transition zone PSA density: Lack of utility in prediction of prostatic carcinoma. *J Urol* 160:77–82.
37. Oesterling JE, Jacobson SJ, Chute CG, et al.(1993) Serum prostate specific antigen in a community-based population of healthy men: establishment of age-specific reference ranges. *JAMA* 270: 860–864.
38. Borer JG, Serman J, Solomon MC, et al. (1996) Age-specific reference ranges for prostate-specific antigen and digital rectal examination may not safely eliminate further diagnostic procedures. *Urol J* 155: 48A.
39. Aus G. Screening for Prostate Cancer in Sweden. Eighth International Prostate Cancer Update. Feb 1998
40. Ezioni R, Shen Y, Petteway JC, Brawer MK. (1996) Age-specific PSA: a reassessment. *Prostate* 7: 70–77.
41. Christensson A, Laurell CB, Lilja H. (1990) Enzymatic activity of prostate-specific antigen and its reaction with extracellular serine proteinase inhibitors. *Eur J Biochem* 194:755.
42. Stenman U, Leinonen J, Alfthan H, Rannikko S, Tuhkanen K, Althan O. (1991) A complex between PSA and a 1-antichymotrypsin is the major form of PSA in

serum of patients with prostatic cancer: assay of the complex improves clinical sensitivity for cancer. *Cancer Research* 51:222.

43. Christensson A, Bjork T, Nilsson O, et al. (1993) Serum prostate-specific antigen complexed to alpha-1 antichymotrypsin as an indicator of prostate cancer. *J Urol* 150(1): 100–105.

44. Luderer AA, Chen Y, Thiel R, et al. (1995) Measurement of the proportion of free-to-total PSA improves diagnostic performance of PSA in the diagnostic gray zone of total PSA. *Urology* 46(2): 187–194.

45. Catalona WJ, Partin AW, Slawin KM, et al. (1998) Use of the percentage of free prostate specific antigen to enhance the differentiation of prostate cancer from benign prostatic disease: a prospective multicenter clinical trial. *JAMA* 279:1542–1547.

46. Piironen T, Pettersson K, Suonpaa M, et al. (1996) In vitro stability of free prostate-specific antigen (PSA) and prostate-specific antigen (PSA) complexed to alpha-1-antichymotrypsin in blood samples. *Urology* 48(6A): 81–87.

47. Stenman UH, Hakama M, Knekt P, Aromaa A, Teppo L, Leinonen J. (1994) Serum concentrations of prostate-specific antigen and its complex with alpha-1-antichymotrypsin before the diagnosis of prostate cancer. Lancet 344: 1594–1598.

48. Pettersson K, Piironen T, Seppala M, et al. (1995) Free and complexed prostate-specific antigen (PSA): In vitro stability, epitope map, and development of immunoflurometric assays for specific and sensitive detection of free PSA and PSA-alpha-1-antichymotrypsin complex. *Clin Chem* 41: 1480–1488.

49. Brawer MK, Daum P, Petteway JC, Wener MH. (1995) Assay variability in serum prostate specific antigen determination. *Prostate* 26:1-6.

50. Brawer MK, Bankson DD, Haver VM, Petteway JC. (1997) Comparison of three commercial PSA assay: results of restandardization of the Ciba Corning method. *Prostate* 30: 269–273.

51. Nixon RG, Meyer GE, Blasé AB, et al. (1998) Comparison of 3 investigational assays for the free form of prostate specific antigen. *J Urol* 160:420–425.

52. Djavan B, Zlotta A, Kratzik C, et al. (1999) PSA, PSA density, PSA density of transition zone, free/total PSA ratio, and PSA velocity for early detection of prostate cancer in men with serum PSA 2.5 to 4.0 ng/mL. *Urology* 54: 517–522.

53. Letran JL, Blasé AB, Meyer GE, Brawer MK. (1998) Repeat ultrasound-guided prostate needle biopsy: the utility of free-to-total PSA ratio in predicting those men with or without prostatic carcinoma. *J Urol* 160(2):426–429.

54. Allard WJ, Zhou Z, Yeung KK, et al. (1998) Novel immunoassay for the measurement of complexed prostate-specific antigen in serum. *Clin Chem* 44:1216–1223.

55. Brawer MK, Meyer G, Letan J, et al. (1998) Measurement of complexed PSA improves specificity for early detection of prostate cancer. *Urology* 52: 372–378.

56. Maeda H, Arai Y, Aoki Y, et al. (1999) Complexed prostate-specific antigen and its volume indexes in the detection of prostate cancer. *Urology* 54: 225–228.

6 The Digital Rectal Examination in Prostate Cancer Screening

Joseph Basler, PhD, MD

Contents

INTRODUCTION

Digital rectal examination (DRE) remained the primary means of diagnosis of prostate cancer until the popularization of the prostate-specific-antigen (PSA) in the late 1980s and early 1990s. This part of the physical examination still constitutes the cornerstone of clinical staging of prostate cancer but remains quite subjective and subject to wide interobserver variability. This chapter will discuss the method of obtaining accurate information from the DRE and its utility in the early detection of prostate cancer.

TECHNIQUE

Positioning of the patient is crucial to allowing adequate access to the rectum, especially when the patient is obese. The preferred positions are the "squatting" position (bent over at the waist, knees bent and leaning slightly forward), the lateral decubitus position (lying on the right or left side with the knees tucked into the chest for maximal hip flexion), or lithotomy (lying on the back with the hips flexed upward and the knees bent). The choice of right or left lateral decubitus depends on the "hand-

From: *Current Clinical Urology: Prostate Cancer Screening*
Edited by: I. M. Thompson, M. I. Resnick, and E. A. Klein
© Humana Press Inc., Totowa, NJ

edness" of the examiner: A right-handed examiner will approach the patient in the right lateral decubitus position from his anterior side and the patient in the left lateral decubitus position from the posterior side. Lithotomy is generally reserved for examination under anesthesia or debilitated patients who are unable to roll onto their sides.

Size estimation is one of the more variable aspects of the process and depends heavily on the physician's experience with other imaging modalities such as transrectal ultrasound (TRUS) and computed tomography (CT) scans and surgical experience with the prostate (transurethral resection of prostate [TURP], simple or radical prostatectomy). Terminology that utilizes such nondescript phrases such as 1+, 2+, and so forth, are of little value and should be avoided. The more the physician has been able to compare his or her subjective results with a measurable standard or actual sizing of the examined gland, the more accurate will be subsequent estimates of size. For those not routinely dealing with modalities that allow more precise measurements, a simple method of estimating size follows. Begin by measuring the width and length of the examining finger in centimeters. This will allow a general calculation of the posterior surface area of the gland as the exam proceeds. The lubricated, gloved examining finger is introduced atraumatically per rectum and extended toward the base of the prostate in the midline. This usually allows a fairly accurate estimate of the sagittal length when correlated with the known length of the finger to the creases. Next, the finger is moved laterally to the sulcus on either side. Starting from one lateral edge, the finger is sequentially placed medially until the central urethral furrow is encountered. The numbers of finger widths on either side are added to obtain the total transverse diameter. Anteroposterior (AP) measurements are not possible, but a reasonable estimate is that the AP diameter is approx. 0.75 times the transverse diameter. Together, the sagittal × transverse × AP measurement will provide a good "ballpark" estimate of the prostate size in cubic centameters.

Further information to be gained from the DRE must include a description of the character of the tissue with respect to the known pathologic conditions that can affect the prostate. In general, several conditions can be entertained resulting from the information gained at DRE: "normal," benign prostatic hypertrophy (BPH), prostatitis, prostatic abscess, prostatic calculi, and prostate cancer. The *normal* examination includes a symmetric prostate with a consistency of the relaxed adductor pollicis brevis musculature of the thenar eminence of the hand. *Benign prostatic hypertrophy* has a similar consistency but may be palpably lobular. Size also plays a part in this diagnosis because BPH implies some degree of enlargement. Prostatitis, if acute is exquisitely tender to the touch and the consistency varies from normal to "boggy" (similar to a marshmallow). Chronic prostatitis may vary in consistency from normal to firm and will often mimic the induration of prostate cancer. *Prostatic abscesses*, when palpable again are exquisitely tender and fluctuant. *Prostatic calculi* are discrete, smooth nodules that are stony hard and, if multiple, can often be felt to grind over one another. The distinction between a calculus and cancer is occasionally difficult to make. *Prostatic cancer* can vary in consistency from "normal" to stony hard. Typically, the suspicious areas felt on screening examinations are *"indurated"*, having the consistency similar to a callus, or *"hard"*, palpably similar in texture to a bony prominence (e.g., knuckle).

Needless to say, there can be considerable variation in the interpretation of the DRE. The findings within the same prostate on the same day by two different examiners are often divergent *(1)*. The level of experience of the examiner also plays an important role and should be taken into account when considering setting up large-scale prostate-cancer-screening events. If relatively inexperienced physicians will be performing the DREs, a training session with readily available rubber prostate models may be an appropriate prescreening step for the examiners.

OBJECTIVE ASSESSMENT OF DRE FINDINGS
Correlation with TRUS

Following the discovery of an abnormal area in the prostate on DRE, an imaging assessment of the area in question is usually done, most commonly with TRUS. Magnetic resonance imaging may also be helpful, but the expense involved is usually prohibitive, especially in the screening setting. In general, it is wise to have the initial examiner (urologist) perform the TRUS in conjunction with a repeat rectal examination so that the area in question can be adequately assessed. Large series, in which the examiner and ultrasonographer may be different and have a different interpretation of "abnormal" on DRE, report poor correlation between ultrasound-directed biopsies and DRE findings *(2)*.

Correlation with PSA

As might be expected from the higher incidences of cancer with higher PSAs and patient age, the positive predictive value (PPV) of a suspicious DRE increases with PSA and age *(3)*. In large screening studies, 18–25% of prostate cancers were detected solely by DRE, whereas about 40–45% were detected solely by PSA *(4)*. Two recent studies define the utility of DRE for cancer detection in patients whose PSA is <4.0 ng/mL. In the first, Carvalhal et al *(5)*, describe their experience with 2703 men having a suspicious DRE and a PSA <4.0 ng/mL. This group represented about 12% of a large volunteer screening group. Of these, 70% agreed to recommendations for biopsy and underwent quadrant or sextant ultrasound-directed biopsies. In the group undergoing biopsies, the overall PPV of suspicious DRE was 13% [244/1905] for Caucasian men and 26% [14/53] for African-Americans). Table 1 shows the PPV of suspicious DRE broken down by PSA intervals. In general, the higher the PSA, the more likely the DRE will accurately predict cancer. The second study, Eastham et al. *(6)*, reported on the findings for 700 men with suspicious DRE and a PSA <4.0 ng/ml. The percentage of African-Americans was higher for this group (36% vs 2.9% in the Carvalhal study), but the cancer detection rate was the same for both ethnic groups. The overall detection rate was less (9% vs 13%) and the PPV was lower for each interval but still increased with PSA (Table 1). The trend of increasing PPV for suspicious DRE continues with PSAs above 4.0 ng/mL as well.

Correlation with Biopsy

The discrepancy between the suspicious area on DRE and biopsy-proven cancer is exemplified in the study by Flanigan et al. *(2)*. This large, multicenter study examined the correlation of DRE and biopsy results by quadrants of the prostate. The suspicious DRE was predictive of cancer in the same quadrant only 11% of the time, but it missed 74% of cancers detected on quadrant biopsies. Even when crediting the positive biopsies found away from areas of palpable induration, the positive predictive value of DRE for cancer was only 39%. Optenberg and Thompson *(7)* reviewed eight DRE-based screening studies and noted an average 6.5% abnormal DRE in the screened population, a 1.2% overall cancer detection rate, and an average 18% PPV for the suspicious DRE. Other studies put the figure for PPV from 6% to 39% *(8)*.

Stages and Grades of Cancers Detected by DRE

The correlation of results regarding staging and grading of tumors discovered through DRE must be interpreted in the context of the discovery. Traditional means of detecting prostate cancer include annual physical examinations and assessment of obstructive or irritative voiding symptoms and/or other symptoms of advanced disease (bone pain, fatigue, weight loss, etc.). In this setting, the cancers detected primarily as a result of obvious disease on DRE are locally advanced or metastatic about 60% of the time. However, in the setting of screening asymptom-

Table 1
PPV of a Suspicious Rectal Examination
as a Function of Various PSA Ranges

PSA (ng/ml)	PPV of Suspicious DRE		
	Carvalhal et al, 1999	Eastham et al, 1999*	Catalona et al, 1994
0.0–1.0	5%	2.8%	
1.0–2.5	14%	10.5%	
2.5–4.0	30%	22%	—
4.0–10.0	—		40.8%
>10.0	—		69.1%

*These data are a compilation of data provided in this paper for smaller PSA intervals.

atic men greater than 50 yr of age, the proportion of locally advanced or metastatic cancers drops to about 30% *(9)*. The cancers detected only by DRE in men with a PSA <4.0 ng/mL (Hybritech) tend to be lower grade and stage as may be expected from the lower correlative PSAs. However, within the 0.0 to 4.0 ng/mL PSA range, both the pathologic stage and Gleason score vary directly with PSA *(10)*. PSA is a better predictor of grade and ultimate pathologic stage in the >4.0-ng/mL range as well.

CONCLUSIONS

The DRE remains an important part of the screening armamentarium for prostate cancer, especially for men whose PSA is less than 4.0 ng/mL. Significant numbers of men with predominantly moderately differentiated carcinoma are detectable in this group through DRE. Because current screening efforts utilizing DRE and PSA >4.0 ng/mL still result in some cancers being detected at advanced stages, other efforts are underway to further expand the detection of potentially curable cancers in the group of men with lower PSAs and normal DREs *(10)*. Although it is possible that PSA derivatives such as the free-to-total ratio may eventually be found to be a reasonable replacement, the data presently available suggest that DRE remain a part of the overall design of screening efforts.

REFERENCES

1. Smith DS, Catalona WJ, (1995)Inter-examiner variability of digital rectal examination in detecting prostate cancer. Urology 45(1):70–74.

2. Flanigan RC, Catalona WJ, Richie JP, Ahmann FR, Hudson MA, Scardino PT, et al. (1994) Accuracy of digital rectal examination and transrectal ultrasonography in localizing prostate cancer. J Urol 152(5 Pt 1):1506–1509.

3. Richie JP, Catalona WJ, Ahmann FR, Hudson MA, Scardino PT, Flanigan RC, et al. (1993) Effect of patient age on early detection of prostate cancer with serum prostate-specific antigen and digital rectal examination. Urology 42(4):365–374.

4. Catalona WJ, Richie JP, Ahmann FR, et al. (1994) Comparison of digital rectal examinationand serum prostate specific antigen in the early detection of prostate cancer: results of a multicenter clinical trial of 6630 men. J Urol 151: 1283–290.

5. Carvalhal GF, Smith DS, Mager DE, Ramos C, Catalona WJ. (1999) Digital rectal examination for detecting prostate cancer at prostate specific antigen levels of 4 ng/ml or less. J Urol 161: 835–839.

6. Eastham JA, May R, Robertson JL, Sartor O, Kattan MW. (1999) Development of a nomogram that predicts the probability of a positive biopsy in men with an abnormal digital rectal examination and a prostate specific antigen between 0 and 4 ng/ml. Urology 54(4): 709–713.

7. Optemberg, SA, Thompson IM. (1990) Economics of screening for carcinoma of the prostate. Urol Clin North Am 17(4):719.

8. Gerber GS, Chodak GW. (1990) Digital rectal examination in the early detection of prostate cancer. Urol Clin North Am 17(4): 739–744.

9. Catalona WJ, Smith DS, Ratliff TL, Basler JW. (1993) Detection of organ-confined prostate cancer is increased through PSA-based screening. JAMA 270: 948–954.

10. Catalona WJ, Partin AW, Finlay, JA, Chan, DW, Rittenhouse HG, Wolfert RL, Woodrum DL. (1999) Use of percentage of free prostate-specific antigen to identify men at high risk of prostate cancer when PSA levels are 2.51 to 4 ng/ml and digital rectal examination is not suspicious for prostate cancer: an alternative model. Urology 54: 220–224.

7 Philosophical Reflections on PSA Screening
What Should We Now Think and Do?

Paul H. Lange

Without getting entangled in arcane philosophical discussions, it is safe to say that all action ultimately comes from ideas (hopefully articulated as hypotheses) that in science (including clinical medicine) must be verifiable (or more accurately falsifiable). Yet, this goal is not always possible in fact or in time so that instead (or during the interim) clinicians constantly face a variety of conundrums, constantly say "we don't know, but.....", and continually hear (now under increased pressures for interview efficiency), "yes, doctor but what would you do?" We euphemistically place these situations under the rubric of "the art of medicine", and call up the phenomenon of "common sense" to rescue us, knowing full well that, as Oliver Wendall Holmes said, "Certitude is not the test of certainty. We have been cock-sure of many things that were not so" *(1)*. Yet usually they are true and this remains an anchor of medicine by those practicing physicians who cannot afford the luxury of operational nihilism.

Like many who are labeled "experts" in prostate cancer, I have struggled with the problem of prostate-specific antigen (PSA) screening and what I should think and do for my patients, and for audiences both lay and professional. There are three reasons why my reflections may be of more value than some:

1. Very early on, I was involved in discovering the clinical value of PSA and participating in one of the earliest PSA screening trials.*(2–4)* The explosion in the application of PSA-based early diagnosis and the consequent dramatic increase in the number of men given localized therapies has been (and continues to be) surprising and concerning.

From: *Current Clinical Urology: Prostate Cancer Screening*
Edited by: I. M. Thompson, M. I. Resnick, and E. A. Klein
© Humana Press Inc., Totowa, NJ

2. Unfortunately I seem to be one of the few "experts" who actually had prostate cancer. Because of my early PSA work, I had been following my PSA for more than 15 yr and had a biopsy when it hit 3.5, which was positive, and, subsequently, I had a radical prostatectomy. I am almost certainly cured and have all my important functions intact. Although for me this experience was relatively easy, I have come to appreciate the issues of PSA screening and therapies for apparently localized prostate cancer with greater insight.

3. Over 5 yr ago, I wrote a mainly philosophical piece about screening titled "Future Studies in Localized Prostate Cancer: What Should We Think? What Should We Do?"*(5)* In light of what has occurred to me and in the field subsequently, it seems prudent to revisit this effort again.

Of the many ideas in that article, *(5)* the one that is still most relevant is the reintroduction of the concept of viewing prostate cancer allegorically as:

Three animals in a box in a garden. (Fig. 1) All the animals grow to a certain size before they have the capacity to escape and ruin the garden, but obviously at different rates. The turtles grow slowly and take a long time to reach a size where they are capable of crawling out of the box. Only occasionally do they do so and then only after much time. The rabbits grow much faster and earlier reach the critical escape size (which could be the same size as a turtles), and hop out easier but not always. The birds grow the fastest and quickly reach a size (again as large as the turtles or birds) where they can and almost always do fly out and ruin the garden.

This allegory has been used frequently to conceptualize the issues surrounding screening. Some of these issues include how to detect and avoid treating the turtles and is this being done in the modern era? What is the natural history of the birds of prostate cancer? Are they "capturable" by PSA screening approaches and are they now being captured?

It seems to me that there are a variety of irrefutable facts about prostate cancer screening that have accumulated over the yr. First, the approach is very contentious. Early on, a variety of groups, whose charge is preventive medicine strategies, analyzed what data were available and concluded that the evidence did not recommend PSA screening or early diagnosis approaches. Soon thereafter, it was generally acknowledged that these recommendations were based on series where the diagnosis was predominantly made by digital rectal exam (DRE) and that this approach in the PSA era was

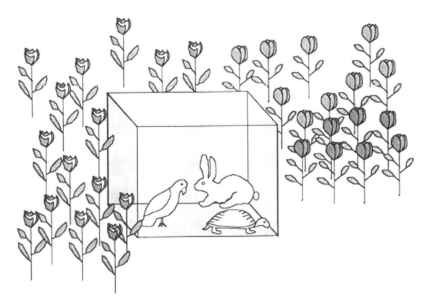

Fig. 1. Illustration of the turtle, rabbit, and bird allegory (from ref. 5– reprinted by permission)

very inadequate. Based on more modern PSA-influenced data, these same groups upgraded their estimation of the quality of the evidence and equivocated a little on the recommendations that were, nonetheless, still against screening or early diagnosis. Other groups such as the American Urological Association and the American Cancer Society issued strong statements supporting early diagnosis, especially in men who are over age 50 who have an estimated life expectancy >10 yr *(6–8)*. Randomized studies which purport to test the efficacy of PSA screening are under way *(5,9)*. However, prostate cancer support groups are confused and impatient and have applied forceful political and marketing pressures that have left many (especially primary care) physicians and health maintenance organizations in difficult positions.

A second fact is that the issue of screening is difficult operationally to separate from early diagnosis. To believe that a man >50 yr old with a 10 yr life expectancy who comes to a urologist for something other than his prostate should be urged to have a PSA and DRE, and at the same time remain silent about whether all such men should have the test, is a difficult position to hold in the practical arena.

Similarly, it is difficult to separate the issue of screening from that of the appropriate therapy for apparently localized prostate cancer (again in a man with greater than 10 yr expectancies). Although there are a variety of studies under way attempting to resolve this issue (e.g., expectant therapy vs. radical prostatectomy or radiation therapy) *(9),* the studies will take many yr to mature and, arguably, are flawed. However, in the meantime, we can confidently make a variety of statements:

1. To at least the 10-yr mark, results with expectant therapy, particularly in Sweden, seem to yield results that on first analysis seem comparable to more aggressive strategies. In my earlier essay, I postulated that this could be true not because localized prostate cancer as a whole is best treated expectedly, but because of the particular philosophical approach to prostate cancer in Sweden. This idea was stated as follows:

   Most physicians in Sweden are taught to believe that prostate cancer (localized or not) may not be treated until symptomatic. Human nature would dictate that in such a society, digital rectal exam would not be done readily, the exams would be performed without much attention to the subtleties of prostate induration, and biopsies, even if accomplished by an easy method, would be done reluctantly. When the prostate cancers in this society were discovered (albeit reluctantly), they would be discovered late. If this were done for a significant period and then the men who were diagnosed and found to only have localized prostate cancer analyzed, they would have certain inevitable characteristics which would be different from comparable patients from another society such as the United States where early diagnosis is advocated: 1) the men would be older (and in Sweden these men are) and 2) the grade of the tumors in these men would be lower (and in Sweden they are). Also, the society as a whole would have several different characteristics: 1) the death rate from prostate cancer would be greater (and in Sweden it is); and, 2) the stage of onset of prostate cancer would be weighed more to the higher stages (and in Sweden it may well be so).... (Thus, in societies such as Sweden which have conservative views toward prostate cancer diagnosis and screening), they will diagnose prostate cancer "reluctantly" and, therefore, "late," and they will have in their localized prostate cancer group a disproportionate accumulation of "turtles." Thus, the Swedish data may teach us more about the behavior of turtles, but as a realistic paradigm of localized prostate cancer, it may be an aberration. *(5)*

   Indeed, subsequently, several analyses suggested that the watch-and-wait strategy for serious albeit local disease (e.g., high-grade cancer) is not as good as aggressive approaches *(10).* Also, further long-term analysis of the Swedish watch-and-wait series suggest undesirable death rates *(11)* (e.g., even turtles, if watched long enough, escape and kill).

2. Radical prostatectomy and radiation therapy approaches are getting better with acceptable outcomes, especially in centers with high expertise. Moreover, both approaches have good survival and PSA outcomes, which promise to get better with earlier diagnosis, the use of earlier hormone ablation strategies *(12)*, and/or other adjuvant therapies *(13)*. The appropriate randomized studies comparing radiation therapy and radical prostatectomy "head to head" are under way or being planned.

Another irrefutable fact is that, especially in the PSA era, there is much experiential data to suggest that the natural history of prostate cancer is especially conducive to PSA screening. For example, it is almost inconceivable to believe that the "birds" of prostate cancer are not for the most part "capturable." Clinical observation shows that prostate cancer is not like lung cancer, where it is common to see a small lung cancer and significant metastasis or a patient with a normal chest X-ray one year and incurable cancer the next. Even in breast cancer, where screening with mammography has, for the most part been proven and certainly accepted, every clinician sees women who have a normal mammogram one year and cancer the next, which, by pathological parameters (and by subsequent follow-up), is not curable. Yet, I would maintain that in prostate cancer it is exceedingly rare to observe men who have been correctly serially followed who have obviously incurable cancer as their eventual diagnosis. The "birds" of prostate cancer are exceedingly capturable, more like cervical or colon cancer than lung or even breast cancer.

Of course, an ancillary concern is that modern aggressive diagnostic and therapeutic strategies are treating too many "turtles." It is undoubtedly true that we are treating some turtles unnecessarily, but "too many" currently seems improbable. For example, in several surgical series, the prevalence of "insignificant" cancer (variably defined as cancers <0.2 cm^3, low grade, organ confined, etc.) has been determined. Although it could be argued that some of these cancers could be "early birds", by their very growth rate, many more turtles would be in this group than birds. (A counterargument and currently irrefutable argument is that insignificant cancer is too narrowly defined.) Nonetheless, these series show that only a minority (5–15%) are "insignificant"*(14–16)*. Thus, taken together, it now seems that the caveats of length and lead-time biases are not very operational in prostate cancer; that is, we are not picking up too many turtles and missing too many of the birds because they are already gone; and/or among the early cancers that we are detecting, there are not too many birds that cannot be cured.

A final irrefutable fact is that the experience so far with aggressive diagnosis and therapy is encouraging. For example, the cancer incidence, which initially increased at an alarming rate, is decreasing and the lifetime risk may rest at little more than what was earlier realized over a man's lifetime using DRE-based approaches *(17)*. Thus, although we may be picking up cancer earlier, we are picking up mostly the cancers that previously became manifest clinically, albeit now at an earlier stage. Also (and I attest to this personally), the work up (e.g., a biopsy) and the anxiety surrounding the detection of an elevated PSA is manageable in most cases and the PPV of 15–20% that exists in men with mildly elevated PSAs, although discouraging to some preventive medicine experts, is threatening enough for most people to want to know. Most important, PSA diagnostic approaches are picking up many more prostate cancers apparently early (predominantly T1C) and over 90% of the pathologies on radical prostatectomies done on men diagnosed by serial PSAs is very localized, that is, organ-confined or only exhibiting focally positive margins or capsular extension *(18)*. These "favorable" pathologies are cured at a high frequency and/or at least take more than 10 yr to manifest metastasis *(19)*. Finally, the death rate from prostate cancer is decreasing, and although it may be too early to attribute this to PSA screening (and even if it is so, it still could be the result of lead time bias), these trends are going the right way *(17)*.

In summary, there seems to me to be a variety of irrefutable observations in the PSA era about prostate cancer that favor an aggressive approach to diagnosis and therapy for local disease. These are as follows: 1) no one has definitive proof as to their value and the appropriate studies are under way but will take many years; (2) PSA-based diagnostic strategies detect much more prostate cancer, which mostly appears significant; (3) the theoretical natural history of prostate cancer favors an optimistic view toward the value of early detection, (4) the current consequences of this approach regarding incidence, pathology, morbidities, and death rates are trending in a favorable direction. Indeed, so far, there does not seem to be a consequence of this approach that would not be expected based on the hypothesis that early diagnosis and aggressive therapy in men with more than 10 yr life expectancies is an appropriate strategy.

So what should we now think and do? I believe that for physicians that manage patients with early prostate cancer, a neutral position is almost untenable. Urology clinics are full of patients who have serious, albeit seemingly curable, cancers that would never have been detected for years using DRE alone, and urologists have the impression that the only patients with advanced disease that they now see are those who did not or could not (e.g., <55 yr old) have the recommended yearly prostate cancer screening. With that experience, reinforced almost daily, I believe it is morally, ethically, and rationally almost inevitable that such physicians would conclude that for men with appropriate life-spans, an aggressive approach to prostate cancer diagnosis and treatment is in their best interest. Thus, urologists should aggressively promote that position while acknowledging that physicians with preventive medicine agendas can hold contrary views in good conscience. One of my patients is a physician, a professor here at my medical school, and a preventive medicine expert. Nonetheless, he was diagnosed with prostate cancer, albeit somewhat late. He has become an even greater expert on the issues surrounding early prostate cancer diagnosis and treatment, is now "a true believer" in aggressive strategies, and has said it best: "The absence of proof is no excuse for the absence of common sense." Although this has always been true, today with the increasing influence of managed care organizations, it is most important to remind those of us for which prostate cancer has been our heritage and our daily concern, that the welfare of the patient must be our predominant if not exclusive agenda.

REFERENCES

1. Boorstin DJ. (1998) *The Seekers,* New YorkRandom House, p. 223.
2. Ercole C, Lange PH, Mathisen M, et al. (1987) Prostatic specific antigen and prostatic acid phosphatase in the monitoring and staging of patients with prostatic cancer. *J Urol* 138:1181–1184.
3. Brawer MK, Chetner M, Beatie J, Buchner D, Vessella RL, Lange PH. (1992) Screening for prostatic carcinoma with prostate-specific antigen. *J Urol* 147:841–845.
4. Brawer MK, Beatie J, Wener MH, Vessella RL, Preston SD, Lange PH. (1993) Screening for prostatic carcinoma with prostate specific antigen:results of the second year. *J Urol* 150:106–109.
5. Lange PH. (1994) Future studies in localized prostate cancer. What should we think? What should we do? *J Urol* 152:193–198.
6. Kramer B, Gohagan J, Prorok P. (1996) Clinical oncology update: Prostate cancer: is screening for prostate cancer the current gold standard?—"No." *Eur J Urol* 33:348–353.
7. Collins M, Barry M. (1996) Controversies in prostate cancer screening: analogies to the early lung cancer screening debate. *JAMA* 276:1976–1979.
8. Pauker S. (1997) Contentious screening decisions? Does the choice matter? *N Engl J Med* 336:1243–1244.
9. Wilt T, Brawer M. (1997) The Prostate Cancer Intervention versus Observation Trial. *Oncology* 11:1133–1143.
10. Albertsen PC, Fryback DG, Storer BE, Kolon TF, Fine J. (1995) Long-term survival among men with conservatively treated localized prostate cancer. *JAMA* 274:626–631.
11. Aus G, Hugosson J, Norlen L. (1995) Long-term survival and mortality in prostate cancer treated with noncurative intent. *J Urol* 154:460–465.
12. Messing EM, Manola J, Sarosdy M, Wilding G, Crawford ED, Trump D. (1999) Immediate hormonal therapy compared with observation after radical prostatec-

tomy and pelvic lymphadenectomy in men with node-positive prostate cancer. *N Engl J Med* 341(24):1781–1788.

13. Cadeddu J, Partin A, DeWeese T, Walsh P. (1997) Long-term results of radiation therapy for prostate cancer recurrence following radical prostatectomy. *J Urol* 159:173–178.

14. Epstein J. (1996) Can insignificant prostate cancer be predicted preoperatively in men with stage T1 disease? *Sem in Urol Oncol* 14:165–173.

15. Humphrey P, Keetch D, Smith D, Shepherd D, Catalona W. (1997) Prospective characterization of pathological features of prostatic carcinomas detected via serum prostate specific antigen based screening. *J Urol* 155:816–820.

16. Dugan JA, Bostwick DG, Myers RP, Qian J, Bergstralh EF, Oesterling JE. (1996) The definition and preoperative prediction of clinically insignificant prostate cancer. *JAMA* 275:288–294.

17. Stephenson R, Stanford J. (1997) Population-based prostate cancer trends in the United States: patterns of change in the era of prostate-specific antigen. *World J Urol* 15:331–335.

18. Ramos C, Casrvalhal G, Smith D, Mager D, Catalona W. (1999) Clinical and pathological characteristics, and recurrence rates of stage T1C versus T2A or T2B prostate cancer. *J Urol* 161:1525–1529.

19. Pound C, Partin A, Eisenberg M, Chan D, Pearson J, Walsh P. (1999) Natural history of progression after PSA elevation following radical prostatectomy. *JAMA* 281:1591–1597.

8 Imaging in Prostate Cancer Screening

Aaron Sulman, MD
and Martin I. Resnick, MD

Contents

INTRODUCTION

Because of the immense number of men affected by prostate cancer, it is imperative to develop a system of adequate screening and staging in order deliver proper treatment while not unnecessarily exhausting expensive health care resources. Recently, much progress has been made regarding the appropriate use and applicability of multiple modalities. Improving the methods used to detect and stage the local extent of prostate cancer will help identify the patients who are most likely to benefit from curative therapy *(1)*. Clinical understaging is frequent with today's current diagnostic practices, which, for example, result in 30–70% understaging of clinical stage T2 disease *(2)*. Improved imaging can help obtain more adequate staging and consequently, help in

From: *Current Clinical Urology: Prostate Cancer Screening*
Edited by: I. M. Thompson, M. I. Resnick, and E. A. Klein
© Humana Press Inc., Totowa, NJ

selecting more appropriate therapies. Among others, these imaging modalities include ultrasound, computed tomography, magnetic resonance imaging, and nuclear medical imaging techniques.

ULTRASOUND

Gray scale ultrasound can be used to stage and monitor established prostate cancers but its use for screening and early detection is less well-defined *(3)*. Ultrasonic imaging can be accomplished with a transabdominal, perineal, transurethral or transrectal scanning approach. The close proximity of the prostate to the rectum and good patient acceptance allows transrectal ultrasound (TRUS) to consistently obtain the best image quality *(4)*.

Ultrasonography can be used to identify prostate cancer directly through several characteristics to be discussed and can be used to image cancer indirectly by demonstrating various changes within the prostate. In a normal prostate, patterns and landmarks are present, including the fat plane between the base of the prostate and seminal vesicles, the presence of the ejaculatory ducts, and the echo boundary noted between the transition and peripheral zones (Fig. 1). The presence of prostate cancer can obscure these findings. Another abnormal finding suspicious for tumor extension is the presence of hypoechoic areas within the seminal vesicles. Large-volume cancers can also cause an increased anterior-to-posterior diameter and a lack of compressibility of the prostate gland with the transrectal probe *(1)*.

Ultrasonic characteristics of tumors have themselves been reported to range from hypoechoic to isoechoic to hyperechoic (Fig. 2a,b). Shinohara et al. in 1989 found the echogenicity to be related to how poorly differentiated the tumors were, with the most poorly differentiated tumors being more hypoechoic *(3)*. Others have described high-grade tumors having an isoechoic or even hyperechoic appearance. It is possible for large tumors to appear isoechoic after they have replaced all normal surrounding tissue, thereby eliminating the reference for normal ultrasound appearance. Although rare, hyperechogenicity in prostate cancer is usually associated with high-grade ductal carcinomas, which contain comedo-type tumor nests, central necrosis, and dystrophic calcifications *(5)*. More malignant tumors tend to be less echogenic because the normal glandular structure is destroyed and replaced with a "packed mass of cells containing smaller glands," which, in turn, contain fewer sonographically detectable interfaces *(3)*. Others, however, argue that ultrasound may be an ineffective screening technique because hypoechoic lesions can also be artifactual because of the similar appearance of cystic dilatation, post-inflammatory atrophy, and benign prostatic hyperplasia (BPH) *(6)*. Ultrasonography,

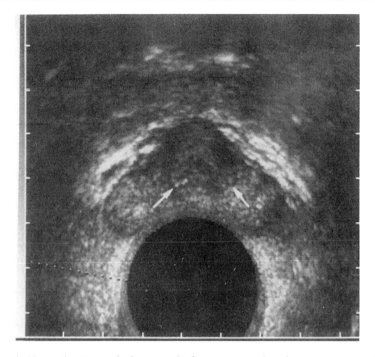

Fig. 1. Normal trasrectal ultrasound of a prostate taken in a transverse plane with a 7.5-MHz probe. Note the hypoechoic transition zone compared to the isoechoic peripheral zone. (From Fornage BD [1998] *Ultrasound of the Prostate*. New York: Wiley, p. 32.)

when used for screening, has been reported to double the prostate cancer detection rate when compared with digital rectal examination (DRE) alone *(7,8).* Tumors detected by transrectal ultrasonography (TRUS) are clinically important because they tend to be larger (more than 4.4 mm), palpable, and of higher grade *(3).* Cooner et al. found the smallest detectable tumor size to be 0.1 cm³ in volume, although ultrasound tends to underestimate the cancer diameter by 4.8 mm *(7).* Rifkin et al. noted ultrasonography to be 49% and 63% accurate in staging confined and advanced prostate cancer, and Carter et al. in 1989 noted TRUS to have a sensitivity of 52% and a specificity of 68% using pathologic evaluation of radical prostatectomy specimens as the gold standard *(9,10).* One reason for the low level of accuracy is ultrasound's inability to image microscopic local or advanced disease. Another possible cause of inaccuracies may be artifacts caused by hemorrhage or inflammation resulting from earlier biopsies *(10).*

TRUS was found by Ellis et al. to be helpful in predicting cancer when combined with prostate-specific antigen (PSA) but as a single test,

A

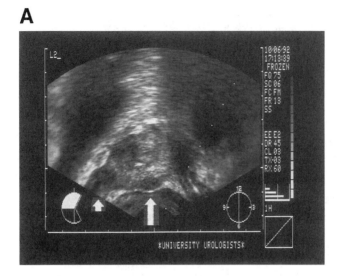

B

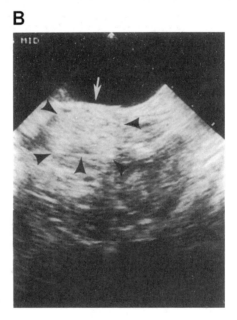

Fig. 2. (A) Transrectal ultrasound (sagittal view) showing an irregular hypoechoic region in the peripheral zone (long arrow), which was proven by biopsy to be carcinoma. Also, note normal seminal vesicle (short arrow). (Courtesy of MI Resnick, MD, Department of Urology, University Hospitals of Cleveland.) **(B)** Transrectal ultrasound showing a large hypoechoic mass with capsular bulging (white arrow) which was proven by biopsy to be carcinoma. (From Dunnich NR, McCallum RW, and Sandler CM [1991] *Textbook of Uroradiology*. Baltimore, MD: Williams and Wilkins, p. 386.)

it was noted to be inferior to PSA. TRUS can be highly operator dependent, with interpretation depending on the expertise of the user *(4,11)*. In spite of this, it remains an important tool to ensure accurate guidance of prostate biopsies within the appropriate sector of the gland *(11)*. In addition, it can be helpful in facilitating repeat biopsies in patients with a negative biopsy despite suspicious clinical and ultrasonographic findings. Although repeat biopsies may be positive, ultrasonic abnormalities are due half of the time the result of benign processes, including BPH, prostatitis, or prostatic calculi *(12)*. TRUS-negative cancers were noted by Ferguson et al. to not differ significantly from TRUS-positive tumors when comparing tumor volume, Gleason score, focality, DNA ploidy status, pathologic stage, or predominant location of the tumor *(5)*. Hypoechoic sectors, however, have been found to be more than twice as likely to contain malignancy on biopsy than are isoechoic sectors *(11)*.

The positive predictive value of a hypoechoic area in association with the combination of an abnormal DRE and an elevated PSA level was noted by Cooner et al. to be as high as 61.8%. These authors only performed TRUS in patients aged 50–64 yr if there was an abnormal DRE or PSA and, in addition, they chose to do a screening TRUS in all patients age 65 and older *(7)*. Rifkin and Choi found 20% of peripherally oriented hypoechoic prostatic lesions to be malignant although smaller cancers were often noted to be isoechoic and were poorly visualized *(13)*. The sensitivity and specificity of TRUS for detecting early-stage prostate cancer is decreased by the echogenic variability of malignant and benign tissue and because of the high false-positive and false-negative rate, Ferguson et al. suggest that, as a result, TRUS may not have utility for clinical staging of PSA-detected, nonpalpable prostate cancer *(5)*.

Regarding selection of ultrasound probes, 7.0- and 7.5-MHz probes provide excellent images of the peripheral zone, and 5.0- or 6.0-MHz probes allow more precise visualization of the transition zone in large prostates *(14)*.

An unfortunate limitation of ultrasound is that no method of imaging "that depends on gross architectural changes is likely to have a high degree of accuracy in detecting microscopic extension of extracapsular tumor frequently observed in radical prostatectomy specimens" *(1)*. Ultrasonography is also very operator dependent, although it has been used to detect tumor presence in the neurovascular bundle and in the seminal vesicle when not palpable on DRE *(1,12,15)*. There is, however, a high false-positive rate for seminal vesicle involvement *(15)*. Werner-Wasik et al. noted that in patients with a positive prostate biopsy,

TRUS abnormalities correlated with the side of the gland with the positive biopsy in a minority of patients (24%). Another study by Spencer et al., found that positive biopsies were obtained in 32 of 177 (18.1%) of patients with four-quadrant prostate biopsies despite no focal findings of a hypoechoic lesion *(17)*. The decision to biopsy and the location to biopsy thus should rarely be based on TRUS findings alone *(16)*.

COLOR DOPPLER ULTRASONOGRAPHY

Color Doppler Imaging (CDI) can be used to view the peripheral and central areas of the prostate and permits an assessment of gland symmetry. The basis of color flow doppler lies in the fact that blood flow is usually elevated in malignancy and prostatitis, and it is low in normal prostatic tissue. Angiographically, this is the result of variation in the caliber of vessels, loss of regular vessel distribution, intratumoral pooling, early venous drainage, and parenchymal staining *(18)*. Microvascular density has been shown to predict radical prostatectomy findings *(19)*, with prostatic carcinoma demonstrating an increased capillary density when compared with benign prostate tissue *(20)*. Color Doppler findings, which differentiate cancer from other regions, are based on the concept that in order for tumors to progress, they require the recruitment of native vessels, expansion or dilation of preexisting vessels, or the formation of new vessels (tumor angiogenesis). A stepwise increase in angiogenesis has been observed as one progresses toward the center of the prostate tumor *(21)*. Unfortunately color Doppler studies have not been accepted for screening because of the overlap between benign and malignant disease, as color flow can be detected in regions of prostatitis (primarily acute), prostatic intraepithelial neoplasia (PIN), and benign prostatic hyperplasia. In one study, patients who had increased flow within the tumor were 4.55 times more likely to have seminal vesicle invasion than patients with no detected flow within the tumor. Increased flow was also significantly associated with relapse *(21)*. Ismail et al. attempted to correlate color-coded flow detected with CDI with pathologic features in whole-mount radical prostatectomy specimens and calculated the sensitivity and positive predictive value (PPV) of CDI in the diagnosis of cancer to be 35% and 87.5% *(21)*. The PPV of ultrasound rises with increasing PSA levels and with increased palpability and size of the lesion and thus color Doppler ultrasonography may have the potential to better delineate lesions that are hard to visualize with gray scale imaging *(22)*. Kelly et al. found that color Doppler ultrasonography, although improving the PPV of transrectal ultrasonography (from 0.53 to 0.77), did not improve the sensitivity over TRUS alone in diagnosing prostate cancer *(18)*.

CDI is more accurate for staging posterior cancers than for cancers located in the anterior portion of the prostate *(1)*. The most accurately imaged area is the midportion of the posterior prostate and the least accurately imaged area is the anterior midportion of the gland. Accuracy in detection of extracapsular extension improves with increasing tumor volume *(1)* and the accuracy of detecting local extension varies from 60% to 100% and is quite operator dependent *(23)*.

CDI can also be used to complement gray-scale sonography. It allows real-time visualization of blood flow in conventional gray-scale, two-dimensional images (Fig. 3a,b) *(4)*. In a study by Laviopierre et al. 75% of cancers were correctly shown on gray-scale imaging but 16% were seen only on CDI. Nine percent were missed by both modalities and detected on sextant biopsy *(24)*. These authors also noted that in 18% of cases where gray-scale sonography findings were interpreted as normal, CDI correctly visualized a tumor. However, they also noted that in 18% of cases where color Doppler sonography findings were normal, cancer was visualized by gray-scale sonography. These data showed that both modalities can be used together to find lesions that would otherwise be missed, and neither one is necessarily more useful than the other. They also noted that although this method may prevent excessive biopsies and may help target lesions, TRUS is not sufficiently sensitive to allow the elimination of random sextant biopsies *(24)*. Other authors have found low sensitivity and specificity of TRUS that could lead to an increase of unnecessary biopsies *(4)*.

An advance that may enhance the performance of CDI is the use of microbubble contrast *(4)*. Microbubbles increase the Doppler signal with a linear relationship between the bubble concentration and signal intensity. Aarnink et al. suggested using contrast agents to enhance color Doppler signals and using CDI to grade tumors noninvasively by correlating abnormal areas on color Doppler with histopathology. Patients in subgroups with different vascularization patterns might therefore be graded with this technique *(4)*. Recently, Bogers at al. described using contrast enhanced color power doppler three-dimensional angiography and diagnosed suspicious lesions primarily through vascular asymmetry. Contrast enhancement was noted to improve sensitivity from 31% to 85% *(25)*.

Okihara et al. in 1997 investigated ultrasonic power Doppler imaging which has the advantage of a three-fold to four-fold increase in blood flow sensitivity compared with that of CDI *(26)*. The authors compared the localization and the vascularity of blood flow within the prostates of patients with prostate cancer with those of BPH and observed hypervascular lesions in all cases with prostate cancer compared to only 4%

A

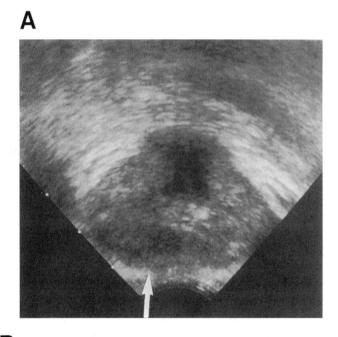

B

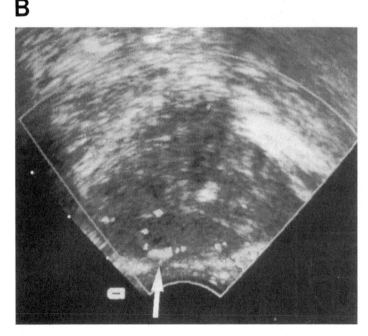

Fig. 3. (A) Gray-scale ultrasound showing subtle peripheral hypoechoic lesion.
(B) Color Doppler ultrasound of same lesion revealing increased vascularity.
This lesion was proven by biopsy to be carcinoma. (From ref. *24*)

of those with BPH. Findings in all of the prostate cancer patients were "characterized with disorderly tangles and numerous sharp kinks" *(26)*. Hypoechoic lesions were noted with this technique in 49% of BPH and 44% of prostate cancer patients *(26)*. Hypoechoic areas are malignant in 17–57% of patients *(4)*. With regard to hypervascularity, symmetry is important in differentiating BPH from prostate cancer *(26)*.

A relatively new concept is the use of computerized interpretation of ultrasound images that may reveal information imperceptible to the human eye *(4)*. This is done by creating a binary decision tree through the correlation of texture parameters of puncture images with the corresponding histology of the resected tissue. The image is then color coded with the probability of malignancy. This serves as a guide for prostate biopsy. In a study of patients scheduled for radical prostatectomy, 75% diagnostic accuracy was achieved in discriminating benign from malignant structures *(4)*.

Although it may not be the most efficient screening tool, ultrasonography can also be helpful in ruling out extraprostatic extension and to evaluate response to hormonal therapy *(12)*. It also remains a more accurate means of biopsy guidance than digital guidance for lesions that are either nonpalpable or subtly palpable *(13)*. Ultrasonography is also useful after completion of biopsies to rule out a hematoma and to compress the region of bleeding to prevent further hematoma expansion *(14)*. In addition, as noted by Rifkin and Choi, ultrasound may have a place in prostatic screening when one looks at the fact that the 21.3% malignancy rate they noted in prostatic lesions was similar to that seen in solid breast lesions detected by mammography which is an accepted modality for malignancy screening *(13)*. CDI may help identify patients at risk for progression and those with less aggressive tumors who are likely to benefit from watchful waiting (21). At the current time, PSA combined with DRE is the most sensitive and cost-effective approach and ultrasound's primary role is in guiding the biopsy needle.

COMPUTED TOMOGRAPHY

Computed Tomography (CT) has been used most commonly for staging the primary tumor and for ruling out lymph node involvement. As of 1996, 35% of men with newly diagnosed adenocarcinoma of the prostate underwent staging CTs and the vast majority showed no CT evidence of cancer spread *(27)*. Carlisle found that CT was not able to differentiate normal prostates from those with stage T1 or T2 tumors. CT was similarly unable to identify palpable nodules but was able to detect stage T3 tumors by showing extension of a mass beyond the prostate, often in the region of the seminal vesicles (Fig. 4a,b). CT was also able to image bone metastases in 60% of patients with positive bone scans. However, the authors found that CT would have understaged 23% of cancers. A limitation of CT for imaging nodal involvement is its inability to image microscopic involvement *(28)*. Huncharek and Muscat suggested that PSA may be useful in determining which patients require CT scans as they noted no patient with a normal PSA had a positive CT scan and 80% of patients with positive CTs had PSA levels greater than 20 ng/mL. Seventy-five percent of CTs and their associated costs could be avoided by only imaging patients with PSA levels greater than 20 ng/mL *(27)*.

Weaknesses of CT scanning include its inability to image low-volume or microscopic disease and to differentiate benign from malignant disease within the prostate. Additionally, the apex and seminal vesicles are poorly visualized. Biopsy artifact can also obscure tissue planes and adversely affect findings *(15)*.

With regard to detection of nodal involvement, CT's threshold for detecting lymph node involvement is 1–1.5 cm, a less than desirable threshold, as most patients with lymphadenopathy currently present with a small volume of metastatic disease (i.e., nodes smaller than 1 cm, including those with only microscopic involvement). The 95th percentile values for normal lymph node sizes of internal iliac, obturator, common iliac, and external iliac nodes are 7 mm, 8 mm, 9 mm, and 10 mm, respectively. Also, CT is unable to distinguish inflammatory lymphadenopathy from neoplastic involvement. Therefore, CT is best employed only for patients at high risk for metastasis *(15)*. Lee et al. noted negative CT scans in all 244 patients with PSAs of 15 ng/mL or less, Gleason scores of 2–7, and clinical stage T2b or less and therefore recommended staging CT scans only in patients with higher Gleason scores, PSAs, and clinical stages than those listed *(29)*.

In a retrospective analysis of the patterns of the practice of requests for imaging in patients with prostate cancer, clinicians were found to obtain a higher number of CT scans in patients with a PSA of 20 ng/mL or greater and with stage T3 or T4 tumors *(30)*. In a study of 861 men with newly diagnosed prostate cancer, only 13 (1.5%) were noted to have nodal disease on CT scan, all of whom had a PSA greater than 20 ng/mL *(31)*. The authors suggest obtaining staging CTs "only when serum PSA, biopsy Gleason score and clinical tumor stage are suggestive of systemic disease" and potentially only in patients for whom a staging pelvic lymph node dissection is planned *(30)*. Currently, CT, as well as other modalities, are used much more often than what has historically been recommended *(32)*.

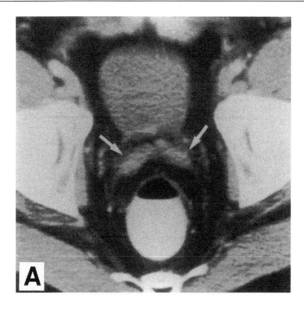

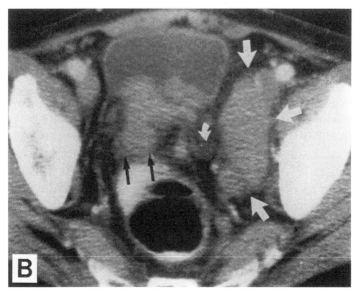

Fig. 4. (A) Pelvic CT showing seminal vesicles. **(B)** CT of pelvis showing asymmetry of seminal vesicles with prostatic carcinoma infiltration of right seminal vesicle (black arrows) compared to the normal left seminal vesicle (small white arrow) and distortion of the proper angle between the seminal vesicles and bladder. Also, note significant left external iliac lymphaden-opathy (large white arrows) and tumor infiltration of the bladder base. (From Pollack HM [1990] Clinical Urography. Philadelphia: WB Saunders, p. 1393.)

MAGNETIC RESONANCE IMAGING

Magnetic resonance imaging (MRI) has been studied extensively for use in prostate cancer screening and staging. Prostate cancer is imaged with both T1-weighted and T2-weighted images. T1-weighted images evaluate lymphadenopathy by maximizing "contrast between fat and solid organs or viscera," and T2-weighted images are used to image the prostate by providing "the maximal contrast between tumor and normal muscular tissue" (15). The neurovascular bundle (NVB) is seen on T1-weighted images when the low-signal nerves and vessels of the NVB are outlined by the high-signal periprostatic fat. It can be seen in a similar manner on T2-weighted images (Fig. 5). Normal seminal vesicles can be seen on T2-weighted images with high-signal-intensity fluid in the lumen and low-signal intensity walls (2).

On MRI, prostate cancer is usually indistinguishable from surrounding normal glandular prostatic tissue on T1-weighted images because of its intermediate signal intensity. On occasion however, carcinoma has a mildly hyperintense appearance when compared to the normal peripheral zone. Postbiopsy hemorrhage is hyperintense on T1-weighted images (2). T2-weighted images, in contrast, allow recognition of most nodules of adenocarcinoma of the prostate as these areas are low in signal intensity and are similar to muscle signal intensity (Fig. 6). In the peripheral zone, T2-weighted images show a high tissue contrast between prostate cancer and normal tissue (2,33). On T2-weighted images, most types of prostate carcinoma usually appear as low-signal intensity except for mucinous adenocarcinoma which produces high signal intensity (15,23). The central gland is more difficult to image as this region has a lower signal intensity. BPH in the transition zone is also difficult to distinguish from prostate cancer, as it has a similar signal intensity to that of prostate cancer. Nevertheless, most cancers can be imaged, as approximately 70% arise in the peripheral zone (2,34).

As with other modalities, MRI could prove to be helpful if extraprostatic extension could be detected (15). MRI's staging accuracy in prostate cancer has been reported to be as high as 75–80% (2). Sandhu et al. showed a 1-cm or more peripheral zone defect with a low-signal ill-defined border to have a 100% sensitivity and a 54% specificity for extracapsular spread. The authors found that any node over 1.5 cm was likely to be malignant. Nevertheless, for the diagnosis of nodal involvement, MRI has yet to be shown to be an improvement over CT (23). One occasional benefit of MRI is that it can be used to detect bone marrow involvement (15).

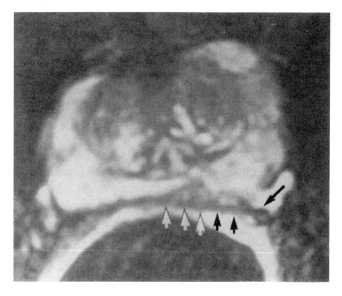

Fig. 5. Endorectal coil MRI T2-weighted image showing obliteration of rectoprostatic angle (short arrows) and asymmetry of the left neurovascular bundle (long arrow) because of prostatic carcinoma with extracapsular extension. (From Yu KK, Hricak H, Alagappan R et al. [1997] Detection of extracapsular extension of prostate carcinoma with endorectal and phased-array coil MR imaging: multivariate feature analysis. *Radiology* 202:669.)

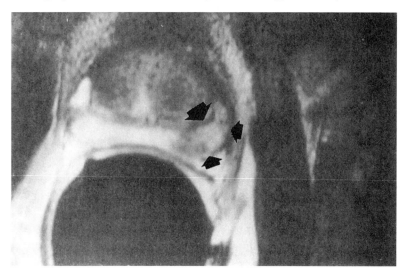

Fig. 6. T2-Weighted image using endorectal surface coil MRI demonstrates left peripheral zone lesion grossly confined to the prostatic capsule (arrow). (From Chelsky MJ, Schnall MD, Seidmon EJ et al. [1993] Use of endorectal surface coil magnetic resonance imaging for local staging of prostate cancer. *J Urol* 150:392.)

Several recent advances have improved MRI visualization of prostate cancer. Resolution has improved with the use of endorectal and pelvic phased-array coils (15). An endorectal coil consists of a small surface coil mounted on the inner surface of a balloon and an array coil consists of a set of four surface coils. Two are located anterior to the pelvis and two are located posterior to the pelvis, each with its own receiver (2,35). Glucagon is often administered before imaging to decrease artifacts caused by rectal contractions (36,37). The endorectal coil facilitates differentiation of the peripheral zone from the central gland and permits imaging of the normal prostatic urethra, the verumotanum, and portions of the ejaculatory ducts. MRI also images the capsule as a thin low-signal-intensity band that defines the posterior and lateral margins of the prostate (2). Hricak et al. (38) found integrated endorectal pelvic phased-array coils to be superior to pelvic phased-array coils for evaluating local prostatic cancer. Manzone et al. (37) found sensitivity and specificity of endorectal MRI findings of definite extracapsular disease to be 23.5% and 93.9%, respectively. They noted that although the sensitivity is low, MRI may be helpful in deciding which neurovascular bundles need to be excised and in identifying which patients are unlikely to benefit from surgery.

Among recent improvements in prostatic MRI, fat suppression techniques have been shown to improve images from pelvic body coils by reducing artifact and enhancing soft-tissue contrast. Fast spin echo imaging decreases imaging time, decreases motion artifact, and increases contrast between tissues (15,36,39).

Numerous authors describe the improved accuracy of detection of endorectal MRI. Husband and colleagues found better visualization of the anterior gland and the neurovascular bundle with the pelvic phased array coil as opposed to the endorectal MRI coil. They do, however, suggest that endorectal coils may provide superior imaging of tumor spread into the seminal vesicles and may improve imaging of early capsular penetration (40).

Postbiopsy hemorrhage can decrease the accuracy of endorectal MRI by overestimating tumor extent and by suggesting extracapsular extension. This occurs particularly when MRI is performed within 21 days following prostate biopsy. Kaji et al. (41) found that MR spectroscopic imaging significantly enhanced the ability to detect prostate cancer and to estimate its extent when postbiopsy changes interfere with interpretation using MR imaging alone. On spectroscopy, cancer is diagnosed based on the (cholene + creatine)/citrate peak area ratio. Prostate cancer is diagnosed when one or more voxels has a ratio of more than three standard deviations above the normal value. The authors noted that in the presence of hemorrhage, tumor detection improved from 52% with MR imaging alone to 75% when using combined examinations. With the combined modalities, they reported a sensitivity and specificity of 88% and 66% *(41)*.

In a multivariate analysis comparing endorectal MRI evidence of extracapsular extension to clinical staging, serum PSA values, and Gleason score, MRI was shown to be the single best predictor of tumor extent at time of radical prostatectomy. D'amico et al. *(42)* found endorectal coil MRI to have a sensitivity, specificity, and accuracy of 65%, 100%, and 84% in patients with clinical stages T1 and T2 disease, a PSA of 10–20 ng/mL, Gleason score of 7 or less, and at least 50% positive biopsy specimens on sextant biopsy. They noted that the use of the endorectal MRI for this specific population as a means of patient selection for radical prostatectomy could increase the pathologic organ confinement rate from 32% to 61% and could decrease the number of patients with extracapsular extension or seminal vesicle invasion from 35% to 18%. Importantly, with these criteria, no patients would be excluded from radical prostatectomy based on a false-positive study. As might be expected, this technique may be useful in identifying patients at high risk for postoperative PSA failure *(42)*. Like other modalities, MRI is limited by its inability to image microscopic seminal vesicle invasion or capsular penetration *(36)*.

Magnetic resonance imaging can be hampered by several factors. Radiation and hormonal therapy can compromise prostate and seminal vesicle images by obscuring the distinction between tumor and normal muscle tissue. Postbiopsy hemorrhage can hamper staging by either mimicking or masking the tumor and by decreasing the signal on T2-weighted images. In addition to hemorrhage, biopsies can alter findings by causing edema, granulation, inflammation of periprostatic fat, and irregularity, thickening, and bulging of the prostatic capsule *(2,15)*. A wait 3 weeks after prostate a biopsy before MRI has been suggested *(2)*. BPH can be confused with a tumor nodule by producing a low-signal-intensity bulge *(15)*. Also, prostatic MRI has been noted to have high interobserver variability, with accuracy, sensitivity, and specificity all dependent on the experience of the reader *(15,36,39,43,44)*. Manyak and Javitt noted that MRI was not significantly better than CT for use in evaluation of nodal involvement. In a review of data from four different series, they found MRI to have a sensitivity and specificity of 42% and 98%, respectively *(15)*. Confounding structures and processes that, like prostate cancer, are low intensity on T2-weighted images and decrease specificity include smooth-muscle hyperplasia and fibromuscular hyperplasia as well as atypical adenomatous hyperplasia, prostatitis and granulomatous prostatitis, infarcts, radiation and hormonal therapy and areas of hemorrhage postbiopsy *(2)*. Central gland tumor, infiltrative tumor growth, and measurement of tumor volume are difficult to image with adequate specificity *(2,35)*. However, gadolinium-enhanced MRI may improve assessment of volume and multifocality of the tumor as well as central gland involvement *(2)*.

In stage T3 disease, "large or gross extracapsular tumor is readily identified on [T1-weighted or T2-weighted fast-spin echo endorectal coil MRI] as low-signal-intensity tumor replacing the high-signal periprostatic fat" *(2)*. Findings that may indicate "early or minimal extra-capsular tumor" are "smooth or irregular bulging of the prostate contour adjacent to a low-signal area, low-signal capsular thickening, low-signal stranding in the periprostatic fat, capsular retraction, asymmetry of the NVB, obscuration of the periprostatic veins, 12 mm or more of low-signal intensity abutting the capsule or large tumors …abutting the capsule" *(2,45)*. Yu et al. *(43)* found that the most predictive characteristics of extracapsular extension were obliteration of the rectoprostatic angle and asymmetry of the neurovascular bundle with a sensitivity and specificity of 38% and 95%, respectively. Schnall et al. noted 82% accuracy in dif-ferentiating stage T2 from stage T3 prostate cancer and noted endorectal coil images improved prostate cancer staging accuracy by 16% when compared to body coil images *(46)*. Seminal vesical involvement is noted on T2-weighted imaging by "low-signal-intensity tumor filling the [seminal vesicle] tubules or low-signal-intensity thickening or nodularity of the walls of the [seminal vesicle] tubules" *(2)*. Ikonen et al. reported a sensitivity and specificity of 59% and 84%, respectively, for seminal vesicle invasion detection *(44)*. Bladder and rectal invasion can also be imaged on T2-weighted imaging *(2)*.

Detection of metastatic disease includes imaging of the lymph nodes. MRI cannot distinguish benign from metastatic disease by signal inten-sity and has the same sensitivity as CT for the detection of lymph node metastases when using node-size criteria. T1-weighted body coil images can also be used to detect lumbar spine and pelvic bony metastases and, although sensitive, the specificity for this indication is low *(2)*.

Several studies have correlated pathology with endorectal MRI. D'Amico et al showed a 100% biochemical failure rate in patients noted to have extracapsular extension or seminal vesicle invasion on endorectal MRI when accompanied by at least 50% positive biopsies *(42)*. Endorectal coil MRI was found to improve the detection of semi-nal vesicle invasion and extracapsular extension (accuracies of 97% and 64%) in patients with a PSA greater than 10-20ng/ml and a Gleason score of 57 *(48,49)*. False-positive findings limit MRI effectiveness, particularly with nonpalpable tumors *(50)*. Werner-Wasik et al., in a study of patients with nonpalpable prostate carcinoma, showed that although MRI abnormalities correlated better than TRUS with biopsy results (39% vs 24%), it was helpful for differentiating patients with nonpalpable stage T1C cancers from other higher stages *(16)*. Criteria that help improve sensitivity of anterior tumor detection include the presence of homogeneous, low-signal-intensity, and ground glass-like areas *(44)*.

One final indication of MRI is for the localization cancer in patients with repeatedly negative biopsy findings despite high PSA values *(44)*.

ANTIBODY NUCLEAR SCANS

Monoclonal antibody nuclear scans are promising developments for the imaging/staging of regional and distant prostate cancer *(15)*. In 1984, Vihko et al. *(57)* radiolabeled human prostate-specific acid phosphatase polyclonal antibodies raised in rabbits and used the antibodies to detect distant prostatic carcinoma metastasis, verifying these lesions on plain radiographs. Two other studies found prostatic acid phosphatase monoclonal antibodies to have utility in locating lymph node metastases with a sensitivity and specificity of 100% and 83% *(52,53)*.

Prostate-specific membrane antigen (PSMA) is a 100 kDa type II integral membrane glycoprotein that is expressed to a greater degree in prostate adenocarcinoma than in normal prostate tissue. PSMA can also be detected in peripheral blood using reverse-transcriptase-polymerase chanin reaction (RT-PCR) techniques *(15,54,55)*. This antigen was localized by Troyer et al. "at the cytoplasmic face of the plasma membrane… and within and surrounding the outer mitochondrial membrane" *(56)*. It is overexpressed in poorly differentiated and metastatic prostate carcinomas and appears to be upregulated after hormone-ablation therapy *(56)*. The degree of PSMA upregulation correlates roughly with the Gleason score of the tumor *(57)*. It is recognized by the monoclonal antibody, 7E11-C5.3, first described by Holoszewicz in 1987 and binds to it intracellularly *(55,56)*. When conjugated with indium-111, increased signal intensity is seen in foci of metastatic disease.

The ProstaScint Scan (ProstaScint; Cytogen Corporation, Inc., Princeton, NJ) is performed by injecting the patient with the monoclonal antibody-bound isotope and then performing planar and cross-sectional single-photon-emission computerized tomography (SPECT) images after the injection and then 3–5 d later (Figs. 7a,b, 8) *(15)*. Its sensitivity and specificity (91.4% and 92.0%, respectively) are highest, with a prostate/muscle count ratio of greater than 3.0 correlating to a positive

A

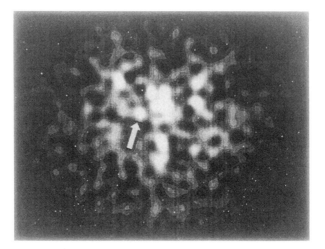

B

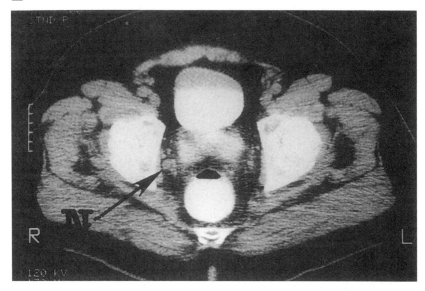

Fig. 7. (A) Prostascint scan showing an 8 mm metastatic obturator node (arrow). **(B)** CT scan of the identical region verifies the location of this node, which was proven to be metastatic prostate carcinoma on CT-guided needle biopsy. (Courtesy of D.B. Sodee, MD, Department of Radiology, Division of Nuclear Medicine, Unversity Hospitals of Cleveland.)

biopsy and less than 3.0 correlating to a negative biopsy, Acute prostatitis is a source of false positive results *(57)*.

In a study of 64 patients with proven pelvic lymph node metastases, the ProstaScint Scan had a sensitivity of 63% compared to 4% for CT and 15% for MRI. For patients with a PSA of less than 40 ng/mL and a Gleason score of less than 7, it has a negative predictive value of greater than 90%. The positive predictive value is greater than 80%, for patients having a PSA greater than 40 ng/mL and a Gleason score greater than or equal to 7 *(15)*. Babian et al. noted the scan's accuracy, sensitivity, and specificity to be 76%, 44%, and 86%, respectively and noted the nodal size detection threshold to be 5 mm *(58,59)*. For detecting extraprostatic disease, Hinkle et al. found the sensitivity and specificity to be 75% and 86%, respectively *(60)*. The CYT-356 antibody used by these authors appears to have a high affinity for detecting hormone resistant prostate cancer and thus could be a useful adjunct for the managment of advanced disease *(58)*. ProstaScint Scans are helpful in excluding nodal disease in high-risk patients prior to deciding on definitive therapy *(59)*.

BONE SCAN

The bone scan is the staging procedure of choice to assess bone involvement of prostate cancer (Fig. 9) *(61)*. It has a greater sensitivity for axial skeletal metastases than clinical evaluation, serum alkaline phosphatase levels, and skeletal radiographs. Schaffer, in a group of patients with positive bone scans, found that 43% denied bone pain, 39% had a normal prostatic acid phosphatase (PAP), 23% had a normal serum alkaline phosphatase, and 10–50% had skeletal radiographs that did not show metastases *(62)*. Bone scans are best reserved for patients with a PSA > 10 ng/mL, a Gleason score of 8–10, or an elevated serum alkaline phosphatase. The bone scan is a highly sensitive imaging modality but suffers from poor specificity. Equivocal findings should be correlated with bone radiographs of the areas in question *(15)*. Positive bone scan findings, however, often preceding X-ray detection by 3–6 mo as plain film radiographs *(61)* only reveal disease after the loss of a considerable degree of bone mass.

False-negative results can be a result of diffuse high activity throughout the skeleton (e.g., diffuse metastases, Paget's disease—the so-called "super scans") *(15)*. False-positive results can be caused by healing fractures and inflammatory conditions, including infections and arthritis *(62)*. Levran et al., in a review of 861 patients, found no positive bone scans in patients with a PSA <20 ng/mL and therefore recommended bone scans only in patients with PSA value >20 ng/mL *(31)*.

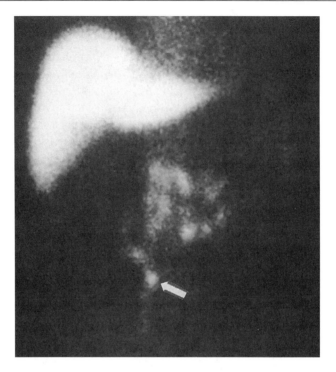

Fig. 8. Prostascint scan showing periarotic lymph node (arrow). Other areas of increased uptake represent liver and small bowel (not metastatic). (Courtesy of D.B. Sodee, MD, Department of Radiology, Division of Nuclear Medicine, Unversity Hospitals of Cleveland.)

POSITRON EMISSION TOMOGRAPHY

Positron emission tomography (PET) is an imaging modality in which the patient receives an intravenous injection of a radiotracer that accumulates in a specific tissue, then takes advantage of a specific related biochemical or physiological property. Following injection and tissue incorporation, a positron then travels a short distance through the tissue until colliding with an electron. The collision results in the destruction of both the positron and electron and the generation of two photons. These photons, traveling in opposite directions, are then detected by photon imagers and the images are reconstructed mathematically (Fig. 10) *(63)*. Recently, Hara et al. *(64)* described using PET imaging to detect early prostate cancer bone (marrow) metastases using carbon-11-choline as a radiotracer, which they noted to have a higher level of uptake in normal prostate and prostate cancer than in other pelvic organs. The authors found PET to be more sensitive for detecting bone metasta-

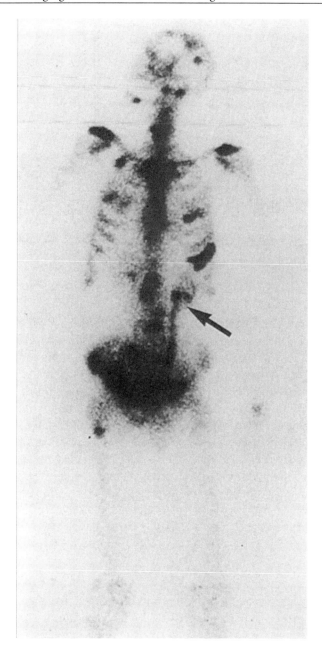

Fig. 9. Bone scan showing multiple osseous metastases as evidenced by asymmetric regions of increased radioisotope uptake. Arrow points to obstructed right kidney. (From Amis SE and Newhouse JH [1991] *Essentials of Uroradiology.* Boston: Little Brown and Company, p. 330.)

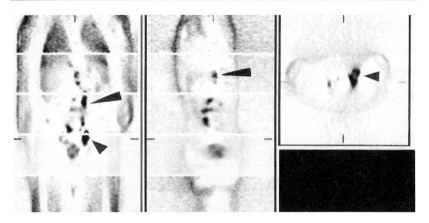

Fig. 10. PET scan with increased regions of radioisotope uptake showing evidence of prostate carcinoma metastases in periaortic (long arrows) and pelvic (short arrows) lymph nodes. (Courtesy of P.F. Faulhauber, MD, Depart-

sis than bone scintigraphy *(64)*. Carlin et al. found a 100% correlation between PET scan results and histology on subsequent lymphadenectomy *(65)*. PET scanning uses a similar amount of radiation as CT and allows the physician to obtain a volumetric set of data that can be reconstructed into tomographic images that can be displayed in a transaxial, coronal, or sagittal tomographic plane *(63)*. Hoh and colleagues *(63)* used PET with the radiotracer 18-flouro-2-deoxyglucose (FDG) and noted that it may be useful and more sensitive than CT for patients with a high PSA or high PSA velocity in the detection of lymph node metastases. A problem with PET is caused by urinary and bowel excretion of radiotracers. This phenomenon can interfere with imaging because these artifacts can be confused with lymph node metastasis. Filling the bladder with saline can reduce the likelihood of excessive pelvic artifact *(63,65)*.

MECHANICAL IMAGING

A recent innovative modality for prostate cancer screening under investigation is mechanical imaging. This technique analyzes tissues according to their viscoelastic properties. Evaluation of tissue hardness, or shear elastic modulus, is used to characterize the tissue and to identify suspicious lesions. Niemczyk et al. *(66)* imaged prostatectomy specimens and found prostate cancer in all lesions that were located with mechanical imaging. In one case, a nonpalpable tumor was detected with this technique. A prototype transrectal probe using this technique is currently being tested *(67)*. A possible advantage of this technique would be to provide better examination consistency than screening with rectal examinations by nonurologists, an examination known to have a great deal of variability in sensitivity and specificity. It may also prove helpful in guiding prostate biopsies *(66)*.

CONCLUSION

There are currently a multitude of prostate imaging modalities that have applications for screening and staging of prostate cancer. It is important that clinicians are aware of the specific benefits offered by each one and to only request those studies that provide reliable information.

REFERENCES

1. Smith JA, Scardino PT, Resnick MI, et al. (1999) Transrectal ultrasound versus digital rectal examination for the staging of carcinoma of the prostate: Results of a prospective, multi-institutional trial. *J Urol* 157:902–906.
2. Barton NM, Seidman EJ. (1995) Endorectal coil magnetic resonance imaging of prostate cancer. *Semin Urol* 8(2):113–121.
3. Shinohara K, Wheeler TM, Scardino P. (1989) The appearance of prostate cancer on transrectal ultrasonography: correlation of imaging and pathological examinations. *J Urol* 142:76–82.
4. Aarnink RG, Beerlage HP, De La Rosette JJ, et al. (1998) Transrectal ultrasound of the prostate: Innovations and future applications. *J Urol* 159:1568–1579.
5. Ferguson JK, Bostwick DG, Suman V, et al. (1995) Prostate-specific antigen detected prostate cancer: pathological characteristics of ultrasound visible versus ultrasound invisible tumors. *Euro Urol* 27:8–12.
6. Terris MK, McNeal JE and Stamey TA. (1992) Transrectal ultrasound imaging and ultrasound guided prostate biopsies in the detection of residual carcinoma in clinical stage a carcinoma of the prostate. *J Urol* 147:864–869.
7. Cooner WH, Mosley BR, Rutherford CL, et al. (1990) Prostate cancer detection in a clinical urological practice by ultrasonography, digital rectal examination and prostate specific antigen. *J Urol* 143:1146–1152.
8. Lee F, Littrup PJ, Torp-Pedersen ST, et al. (1988) Prostate cancer: Comparison of transrectal us and digital rectal examination for screening. *Radiology* 168(2):389–394.
9. Carter HB, Hamper UM, Sheth S et al. (1989) Evaluation of transrectal ultrasound in the early detection of prostate cancer. *J Urol* 142:1008–1010.
10. Rifkin MW, Zerhouni EA, Gatsonis CA et al. (1990) Comparison of magnetic resonance imaging and ultrasonography in staging early prostate cancer. Results of a multi-institutional cooperative trial. *N Engl J Med* 323: 621–626.
11. Ellis WJ, Chetner MP, Preston SD, et al. (1994) Diagnosis of prostatic carcinoma: the yield of serum prostate specific antigen, digital rectal examination and transrectal ultrasonography. *J Urol* 152:1520–1525.
12. Resnick MI, Willard JW, Boyce WH. (1980) Transrectal ultrasonography in the evaluation of patients with prostatic carcinoma. *J Urol* 124:482–484.
13. Rifkin MD, Choi H. (1988) Implications of small, peripheral hypoechoic lesions in endorectal US of the prostate. *Radiology* 166:619–622.
14. Beerlage HP, de Reijke TM, de la Rosette JJ. (1998) Considerations regarding prostate biopsies. *Euro Urol* 34:303–312.

15. Manyak MJ, Javitt MC. (1998) The role of computerized tomography, magnetic resonance imaging, bone scan, and monoclonal antibody nuclear scan for prognosis prediction in prostate cancer. *Semin Urol Oncol* 16(3):145–152.
16. Werner-Wasik M, Wittington R, Malkowicz SB, et al. (1997) Prostate imaging may not be necessary in nonpalpable carcinoma of the prostate. *Urology* 50:385–389.
17. Spencer JA, Alexander AA, Gomella L, et al. (1994) Ultrasound-guided four quadrant biopsy of the prostate: efficacy in the diagnosis of isoechoic cancer. *Clin Radiol* 49:711–714.
18. Kelly IM, Lees, WR, Rickards D, (1993) Prostate cancer and the role of color Doppler US. *Radiology* 189:153–156.
19. Brawer MK, (1996) Quantitative Microvessel Density. A Staging and prognostic marker for human prostatic carcinoma. *Cancer* 78(2):345–349.
20. Bigler SA, Deering RE, Brawer MK. (1993) Comparison of microscopic vascularity in benign and malignant prostate tissue. *Hum Pathol* 24(2):220–226.
21. Ismail M, Petersen RO, Alexander AA, et al. (1997) Color Doppler imaging in predicting the biologic behavior of prostate cancer: Correlation with disease-free survival. *Urology* 50(6):906–912.
22. Rifkin MD, Sudakoff GS, Alexander AA. (1993) Prostate: techniques, results, and potential applications of color Doppler US scanning. *Radiology* 186:509–513.
23. Sandhu SS, Kaisary AV. (1997) Localized carcinoma of the prostate: a paradigm of uncertainty. *Postgrad Med* J 73:691–696.
24. Lavoipierre AM, Snow RM, Frydenberg M, et al. (1998) Prostate cancer: role of color Doppler imaging in transrectal sonography. *Am JRoentgenol* 171:205–210.
25. Bogers HA, Sedelaar JPM, Beerlage HP, et al. (1999) Contrast-enhanced three-dimensional power Doppler angiography of the human prostate: correlation with biopsy outcome. *Urology* (54):97–104.
26. Okihara K, Kojima M, Naya Y, et al. (1997) Ultrasonic power Doppler imaging for prostatic cancer: a preliminary report. *Tohoku J. Exp. Med.* 182:277–281.
27. Huncharek M, Muscat J (1996) Serum prostate-specific antigen as a predictor of staging abdominal/pelvic computed tomography in newly diagnosed prostate cancer. *Abdominal Imaging* 21:364–367.
28. Morgan CL, Phil M, Calkins RF, et al. (1981) Computed tomography in the evaluation, staging, and therapy of carcinoma of the bladder and prostate. *Radiology* 140:751–761.
29. Lee N, Newhouse JH, Olsson CA, et al. (1999) Which patients with newly diagnosed prostate cancer need a computed tomography scan of the abdomen and pelvis? An analysis based on 588 patients. *Urology* 54(3):490–494.
30. Kindrick AV, Grossfeld GD, Stier DM, et al. (1998) Use of imaging tests for staging newly diagnosed prostate cancer: trends from the CaPsure Database. *J Urol* 160:2102–2106.
31. Levran Z, Gonzalez JA, Diokno AC, et al. (1995) Are pelvic computed tomography, bone scan and pelvic lymphadenectomy necessary in the staging of prostatic cancer? *Br J Urol* 75:778–781.
32. Plawker MW, Fleisher JM, Vapnek, et al. (1997) Current trends in prostate cancer diagnosis and staging among United States urologists. *J Urol* 158:1853–1858.
33. Carrol CL, Sommer EG, McNeal JE, et al. (1987) The abnormal prostate: MR imaging at 1.5 t with histopathologic correlation. *Radiology* 163:521–525.
34. Torp–Pedersen ST, Lee F. (1989) Transrectal biopsy of the prostate guided by transrectal ultrasound. *Urol Clin North Am* 16(4):703–712.

35. Schnall MD, Lenkinski RE, Pollack HM, et al. (1989) Prostate: MR Imaging with an endorectal surface coil. *Radiology* 172:570–574.

36. Quinn, SF, Franzini DA, Demlow TA, et al. (1994) MR Imaging of prostate cancer with an endorectal surface coil technique: correlation with whole-mount specimens. *Radiology* 190:323–327.

37. Manzone TA, Malkowicz B, Tomaszewski JE, et al. (1998) Use of Endorectal MR imaging to predict prostate carcinoma recurrence after radical prostatectomy. *Radiology* 209.537–542.

38. Hricak H, White S, Vigneron D, et al. (1994) Carcinoma of the prostate gland: MR imaging with pelvic phased-array coils versus integrated endorectal-pelvic phased-array coils. *Radiology* 193:703–709.

39. Tempany CM, Zhou X, Zerhouni EA, et al. (1994) Staging of prostate cancer: results of radiology diagnostic oncology group project comparison of three MR imaging techniques. *Radiology* 192:47–54.

40. Husband E, Padhani AR, Macvicar AD, et al. (1998) Magnetic resonance imaging of prostate cancer: Comparison of image quality using endorectal and pelvic phased array coils. *Clin Radiol* 53:673–681.

41. Kaji Y, Kurhanewicz J, Hricak H, et al. (1998) Localizing Prostate Cancer in the Presence of Postbiopsy Changes on MR images: Role of proton MR spectroscopic imaging. *Radiology* 206:785–790.

42. D'Amico AV, Schnall M, Whittington R, et al. (1998) Endorectal coil magnetic resonance imaging identifies locally advanced prostate cancer in select patients with clinically localized disease. *Urology* 51:449–454.

43. Yu KK, Hricak H, Alagappan R, et al. (1997) Detection of extracapsular extension of prostate carcinoma with endorectal and phased-array coil MR imaging: Multivariate feature analysis. *Radiology* 202:697–702.

44. Ikonen S, Karkkainen P, Kivisaari L, et al. (1998) Magnetic resonance imaging of clinically localized prostatic cancer. *J Urol* 159:915–919.

45. Chelsky MJ, Schnall MD, Seidmon EJ, et al. (1993) Use of endorectal surface coil magnetic resonance imaging for local staging of prostate cancer. *J Urol* 150:391–395.

46. Schnall MD, Imai Y, Tomaszewski J, et al. (1991) Prostate cancer: local staging with endorectal surface coil MR imaging. *Radiology* 178:797–802.

47. D'Amico AV, Whittington R, Malkowicz SB, et al. (1997) Combined modality staging of prostate carcinoma and its utility in predicting pathologic stage and postoperative prostate specific antigen failure. *Urology* 49(Suppl 3A):23–30.

48. D'Amico AV, Whittington R, Schnall M, et al. (1995) The impact of the inclusion of endorectal coil magnetic resonance imaging in a multivariate analysis to predict clinically unsuspected extraprostatic cancer. *Cancer* 75:2368–2372.

49. D'Amico AV. (1997) Letters to the editor re: endo-rectal coil magnetic resonance imaging in clinically localized prostate cancer: is it accurate? *J Urol* 157:1371.

50. Carter HB, Brem RF, Tempany CM, et al. (1991) Nonpalpable prostate cancer: detection with MR imaging. *Radiology* 178: 523–525.

51. Vihko P, Heikkila J, Kontturi M, et al. (1984) Radioimaging of the prostate and metastases of prostatic carcinoma with 99mTc-labelled prostatic acid phosphatase-specific antibodies and their fab fragments. *Ann Clin Res* 16(1):51–52.

52. Ahonen A, Kairemo K, Karnani P, et al. (1993) Radioimmunodetection of prostate cancer by 111In-labeled monoclonal antibody against prostatic acid prosphatase. *Acta Oncologica* 32(7–8):723–727.

53. Leroy M, Teillac P, Rain JD, et al. (1989) Radioimmunodetection of lymph node invasion in prostatic cancer. The use of iodine 123 (^{123}I)-labeled monoclonal anti-prostatic acid phosphatase (PAP) 227 A F(ab')2 antibody fragments in vivo. *Cancer* 64(1):1–5.

54. Fair WR, Israeli RS, Heston, WDW (1997) Prostate-specific membrane antigen. *Prostate* 32:140–148.

55. Barren RJ III, Holmes EH, Boynton AL, et al. (1997) Monoclonal antibody 7E11.C5 staining of viable LNCaP cells. *Prostate* 30:65–68.

56. Troyer JK, Beckett ML, Wright GL Jr. (1997) Location of prostate-specific membrane antigen in the LNCaP prostate carcinoma cell line. *Prostate* 30:232–242.

57. Sodee DB, Ellis RJ, Samuels MA, et al. (1998) Prostate cancer and prostate bed SPECT imaging with ProstaScint: semiquantitative correlation with prostatic biopsy results. *Prostate* 37:140–148.

58. Israeli RS, Grob M, Fair WR. (1997) Prostate-specific membrane antigen and other prostatic tumor markers of the horizon. *Urol Clin North Am* 24(2):439–448.

59. Babaian RJ, Sayer J, Podoloff DA, et al. (1994) Radioimmunoscintigraphy of Pelvic Lymph Nodes with 111-Indium-Labeled Monoclonal Antibody CYT-356. *J Urol* 1952–1955.

60. Hinkle GH, Burgers JK, Neal CE, et al. (1998) Multicenter radioimmunoscintigraphic evaluation of patients with prostate carcinoma using indium-111 capromab pendetide. *Cancer* 83(4):739–747.

61. Miller PD, Eardley I, Kirby RS. (1992) Prostate specific antigen and bone scan correlation in the staging and monitoring of patients with prostatic cancer. *Br J Urol* 70:295–298.

62. Lee CT, Oesterling JE. (1997) Using prostate-specific antigen to eliminate the staging radionuclide bone scan. *Urol Clin North Am* 24(2):389–394.

63. Hoh CK, Seltzer MA, Franklin J, et al. (1998) Positron emission tomography in urological oncology. *J Urol* 159:347–356.

64. Hara T, Kosaka N, Kishi H. (1998) PET imaging of prostate cancer using carbon-11-choline. *J Nucl Med* 39:990–995.

65. Carlin BI, Resnick MI, Faulhaber, et al. (1998) Alteration in PET scanning technique increases accuracy in detecting the lymphatic spread of prostate cancer. *J Urol* 159(5):289.

66. Niemczyk P, Cummings KB, Sarvazyan AP, et al. (1998) Correlation of mechanical imaging and histopathology of radical prostatectomy specimens: a pilot study for detecting prostate cancer. *J Urol* 160:797–801.

67. Sarvazyan A. (1998) Mechanical imaging: a new technology for medical diagnostics. *Int J Med Inform* 49(2):195–216.

9 Risk Factors for Prostate Cancer

David L. Shepherd, M.D.

INTRODUCTION

Prostate cancer is the most frequently diagnosed noncutaneous male cancer in the United States and the second most common cause for cancer-related deaths in this population. In 1999, new diagnoses of prostate cancer included 179,000 cases, representing 29% of all male cancer diagnoses *(1)*. The cause of prostate cancer, however, remains largely unknown. The identification of risk factors for this cancer is therefore based on the evaluation of populations recognized through epidemiological studies as being at a unique risk level. Such studies have produced certain demographic, dietary, genetic, histological, and biochemical features that identify patients at an elevated risk for prostate cancer. In addition, these observations have produced current theories on promoters of prostate cancer progression and prevention that are currently being evaluated in large-scale national studies.

From: *Current Clinical Urology: Prostate Cancer Screening*
Edited by: I. M. Thompson, M. I. Resnick, and E. A. Klein
© Humana Press Inc., Totowa, NJ

AGE AS A RISK FACTOR

Many prostate cancers are small (<0.5 cm^3), well-differentiated and clinically undetected during the life of patients. The incidence of these autopsy-detected cancers is directly proportional to the patient's age. Sakr et al. discovered that microfocal prostate cancer actually begins in the fourth decade of life and increases with each successive decade. In his autopsy survey of 152 men, histologic prostate cancer was found incidentally in 0%, 27%, and 34% of specimens of patients in the third, fourth, and fifth decades, respectively (2). By the eighth decade, histologic evidence of prostate cancer is present in greater than 80% of men (3).

Clinically significant prostate cancer is felt to be potentially invasive and to carry the threat for local progression and metastasis. These tumors are defined by a volume of greater than 0.5 cm^3 and greater than a Gleason grade 2 (4). The incidence of these tumors is also strongly associated with and directly proportional to age. Prostate-specific antigen (PSA) screening now permits the early detection of these tumors before the development of invasive disease.

Criticism of PSA screening claims that tumors detected in this manner are similar to clinically insignificant "autopsy cancers" of the aging male. Histologic evaluations of screening-detected tumors, however, demonstrate that the majority of these tumors have features of clinically significant cancers. In a review of 100 whole-mount prostatectomy specimens from men with a mean age of 62.8 yr, 68% of the cancers were larger than 0.5 cm^3 and the mean Gleason score was 5.7. Only 6% of the cancers were well-differentiated (5). Other researchers reported similar findings in the initial PSA-driven prostate screening efforts (6,7). More recent evaluations demonstrate that the majority of prostatectomy specimens from men with preoperative indicators suggesting insignificant tumors such as a PSA less than 4 ng/mL or a "minimal" amount of cancer on needle-biopsy cores actually have clinically significant disease as well (8,9).

Age is, therefore, a major risk for the development of prostate cancer. With increasing age, well-differentiated small cancers represent a "normal" histological finding. These tumors are, however, only detected on autopsy and remain undiagnosed by prostate screening efforts during the life of most patients. Since the advent of PSA-driven prostate cancer screening in 1988, the cancers detected in the majority of aging men are histologically distinct from "autopsy cancers" and represent the early stages of potentially invasive disease (10).

FAMILY HISTORY AS A RISK FACTOR

Evidence that individuals with a family member with prostate cancer are at an elevated risk for the development of prostate cancer was first established in epidemiologic studies of the Utah Mormon population. Subsequent studies consistently observe similar findings in populations of different regions and various races. The risk of prostate cancer diagnosis is elevated twofold to threefold by a family history of prostate cancer *(11,12)*. As a general risk factor, a family history of prostate cancer may indicate the transference of certain genetic factors or an exposure to similar environmental factors such as diet.

The likelihood of inheriting a genetic predisposition for prostate cancer seems most likely in relatives of men who were diagnosed at an early age *(13,14,12)*. In a review of 302 Finnish families with 2 or more affected relatives, 209 asymptomatic men 45–75 yr of age were identified for screening. Ten percent of these men had an elevated PSA and 3% were diagnosed with prostate cancer. Compared to men with a family member diagnosed with prostate cancer after the age of 60 yr, the men with relatives diagnosed at a younger age were nearly three times more likely to have a PSA elevation and five times more likely to be diagnosed with cancer *(15)*. PSA screening is therefore particularly important in men with this history.

Because hereditary prostate carcinoma is characterized by an early age at onset, patients with first-degree relatives with prostate cancer should begin screening before 50 yr of age. This is most important for men with an affected brother. Men who have a brother with prostate cancer have a risk ratio of 3.0–4.5 compared to a risk ratio of 1.9–2.3 if they have a father with prostate cancer *(12,16)*. The combined history of several affected relatives with a relative diagnosed at an early age identifies an exceptionally high-risk population *(17)*.

RACE AS A RISK FACTOR

The definitions of specific racial groups are unclear. Racial groups include individuals of tremendous genetic and social diversity. Despite this intragroup diversity, certain general observations concerning the risk for prostate cancer can be appreciated. Each race has a different level of risk for the clinical diagnosis of prostate cancer. This has led to the evaluation of molecular, genetic, and dietary differences of these groups to determine potential causes of the unique prostate cancer risk levels of certain racial groups *(18)*.

African-American men are at the highest risk for clinically significant prostate cancer. The 1990–1995 Surveillance, Epidemiology, and

End-Results Program (SEER) data demonstrate that the incidence of prostate cancer in African-American men is 50% greater than that of the next highest risk group, Caucasian-American men. The difference is most striking for African-American men younger than 65 yr of age when the incidence of prostate cancer is twice that of Caucasian men in the same age group *(19)*. Hispanic, Asian, and Native American men are at the lowest risk for prostate cancer. Compared to African-American men, Hispanics have only half of the incidence of prostate cancer and Asians and Native Americans have only one-third the incidence. When these four race groups are ranked by the incidences of cancers of other body sites, a similar order is seen. However, the relative difference between the incidence of cancers other than prostate cancer for each ethnic group is less dramatic. For example, the incidence of prostate cancer in African-American men is 234% that of men of all other American races considered collectively *(20)*. By comparison, the incidence of colon cancer in African-American men is only 59% greater than that of American men of all other races. The overall risk for clinically detected prostate cancer is, therefore, dependent on race, and the differences seen in these incidence rates is dramatically greater than that seen for cancers of other sites in American males.

Interestingly, this dramatic difference in prostate cancer incidence for each race group is seen in clinically detected prostate cancer only. The incidence of autopsy-detected prostate cancer appears to be similar for all races. Sakr et al. *(3)*, however, demonstrate that African-American men more commonly have multiple foci of cancer within a single specimen. Men with multifocal tumors would theoretically have a higher probability of experiencing subsequent cellular events leading to tumor progression and clinically detectable disease. In addition, the reason is most likely a combination of genetic differences and cultural differences linked to diet and environmental exposures that affect the cellular environment and events to promote prostate cancer progression.

Immigrants of a single race provide an interesting study population to investigate the impact of environment on the promotion of "autopsy tumors" to clinically evident prostate cancer. Shimizu et al. compared the age-adjusted incidence rates of prostate cancer in immigrants with Japanese and Spanish surnames to Los Angeles County to the incidence seen in representative "homeland" populations and native county residents. The incidence of prostate cancer in Los Angeles immigrants was much higher than that of "homeland" individuals and approximated that of American-born residents of the county with surnames of the same origin *(21)*. Similar studies are rare and difficult to control because of the differences in access to health care, prostate cancer screening practices, and tumor registries in the regions compared.

DIETARY RISK FACTORS

Dietary Fat

The examination of the typical diet of racial groups epidemiologically identified as having a unique risk level for prostate have identified several dietary factors that are potentially important to prostate cancer risk and prevention. For example, Asians are at the lowest risk for prostate cancer, and the typical Asian diet is low in animal fat and rich in soy-based products and vegetables. This observation led to the study of dietary fat content of Chinese men with prostate cancer compared to that of age-matched controls without prostate cancer. Chinese prostate cancer patients were statistically more likely to consume foods with fat from animal sources than age-matched controls without prostate cancer *(22)*. Conversely, African-Americans are at the highest risk for prostate cancer development. The consumption of a diet high (grams of fat/day) in animal fat was linked to prostate cancer in African-Americans but not Caucasian-Americans. Other studies of predominately Caucasian populations of North America and Europe demonstrate a modest, if any, relationship between dietary fat consumption and the incidence of prostate cancer *(23–25)*. By comparison, African-Americans in the upper two quartiles for animal fat consumption had an odds ratio for prostate cancer of 2.0 compared to odds ratios of 1.0 and 1.5 for the lowest two quartiles, respectively *(26)*.

Interestingly, the strongest association between a high-fat diet and prostate cancer is seen in men with aggressive cancers *(26,27)*. In addition, saturated-fat consumption appears to negatively impact the disease-specific survival of prostate cancer patients. In comparing patients of similar tumor grade, stage, age, and initial treatment, men in the upper tercile of saturated-fat consumption are three times as likely to die of prostate cancer than men in the lower tercile *(28)*. Wang and associates reproduced these observations by feeding groups of athymic nude mice with LNCAP xenografts 2.3, 11.6, 21.2, or 40.5 kcal% fat diets *(29)*. Serum PSA, tumor growth rates, final tumor weights, and ratios of final tumor weights to animal weights were significantly greater in the mice fed a 40.5 kcal% fat diet than the other three groups. These tumor parameters were statistically similar in the later three groups. Therefore, significantly different tumor growth rates are seen between mice eating a 40.5 kcal% fat diet and a 21.2 kcal% diet. Reduction of dietary fat below 21.2 kcal%, however, did not provide additional retardation of tumor growth.

All available studies of high-fat diets and prostate cancer indicate that it is a modest risk factor for African-American and Asian males. A high-fat diet is most strongly associated with aggressive prostate cancers in all races. Therefore, the reduction of dietary fat may have some value in prostate cancer prevention or modify the course of established prostate tumors.

Micronutrients

Emerging evidence suggests that a diet rich in selenium, vitamin E, and phytoestrogens is associated with a lower risk for prostate cancer. These observations are the basis for several ongoing national prostate cancer chemoprevention trials.

BODY HABITUS AS A RISK FACTOR

Measures of somatic features such as mass index, lean body mass, and male-pattern baldness may be connected to factors such as diet or reflect androgenic and estrogenic balance and are, therefore, linked to prostate cancer development. Studies investigating these hypotheses fail to support them. Men with vertex balding have a higher free-testosterone level than men with little hair loss, but this did not correlate with an increased incidence of prostate cancer (30). A 12-yr prospective study of 22,248 Norwegian men failed to demonstrate any association between these anthropomorphic features and the development of prostate cancer (31).

MOLECULAR MARKERS OF PROSTATE CANCER RISK
PSA

The first definitive clinical study to investigate the associations between PSA and prostate cancer was conducted by Stamey and associates at Stanford University (32). Brawer and Lange (33) and Catalona et al. (34) initially used serum PSA to screen men and establish values to identify patients at an elevated risk for prostate cancer. These two studies demonstrated that men 50 yr of age or older with a PSA greater that 4.0 ng/mL have a 33% chance of prostate cancer detection on their initial transrectal needle biopsy (33,34). Men with benign pathology on this biopsy but a persistent PSA elevation above 4.0 ng/mL on follow-up are still at significant risk for prostate cancer and therefore undergo at least one rebiopsy. A cancer yield of 19% can be anticipated in these patients. If this second biopsy is benign, the anticipated cancer yield for men with a persistent abnormality is 7–8% on subsequent serial biopsies (35).

Total serum PSA remains one of the most sensitive factors to assess one's risk of prostate cancer. However, a greater than 50% false-positive rate for a PSA elevation greater than 4.0 ng/dL and the management dilemma for the patient with a persistent abnormality and at least two negative biopsies demonstrated the need for more specificity. PSA derivatives are useful to assess the prostate cancer risk in these patients. Numerous studies demonstrate that a PSA velocity >0.75 ng/mL/yr as determined by three serial tests at 3–6 mo intervals or a PSA density >0.10 ng/mL/cm^3 of prostate indicates a significant risk of undetected prostate cancer and therefore warrants the consideration of a third biopsy. PSA derivatives as a primary screening tool to determine the necessity of an initial prostate biopsy by definition, will result in a lower cancer-detection rate and leave potentially curable cancers undetected. Therefore, PSA derivatives are most commonly reserved to assess the risk of cancer in the patient with PSA elevations or prostate nodules that persist after two negative biopsies *(36)*. If the application of new, more aggressive biopsy protocols on the initial biopsy produce a cancer yield similar to two sessions of the sextant protocol, PSA derivatives could be safely employed after the initial biopsy increase while increasing the specificity. Currently, the PSA free-to-total ratio is used to more specifically assess a patient's risk of prostate cancer.

The determination of free-to-total PSA ratio provides the greatest ability to more specifically assess the risk of prostate cancer in exchange for a minimal decrease of the cancer detection rate established by the total PSA alone. Catalona et al. showed in a national, multi-institutional study that using a cutoff of 25% free PSA would prompt 95% of positive biopsies and avoid 20% of negative biopsies indicated by total PSA alone in the range of 4.0–10.0 ng/mL *(37)*. In a multivariate analysis, the percentage of free PSA was a stronger independent predictor of prostate cancer risk than age or total PSA. Lower free PSA percentages directly correlated with a higher risk for prostate cancer in that study. Subsequent studies indicate that less conservative cutoff points may result in even greater specificity while preserving acceptable sensitivity *(38)*. However, larger studies continue to support the finding that if the percentage of free PSA is greater than 25%, the total PSA is between 4.0 and 10.0, and the rectal examination is benign, then the cancer-detection rate that would be established by using total PSA alone will decrease by only 4–5% *(37,39)*. Therefore, assessing prostate cancer risk with this cutoff value to determine the need for an initial prostate biopsy in such patients seems reasonable.

Insulin Growth Factor-1

Insulin-like growth factor (IGF)-1 is a mitogen for prostate epithelial cells and other cell types by allowing progression from the G1 to S cell-cycle phase. The resultant increase in cell division could theoretically increase chances for cell transformation. Insulin-like growth factor binding protein (IGFBP) directly inhibits this effect by decreasing the bioactivity of IGF-1. Several epidemiologic evaluations of IGF-1 and its binding protein in men clearly demonstrate that a low serum IGFBP, high IGF-1, and high IGF-1/IGFBP ratio is associated with a greater risk of prostate cancer (40,41).

Increased IGF-1 levels are associated with an increased risk for prostate cancer. Prostate cancer patients have a 7–8% higher serum insulin-like growth factor (IGF)-1 level than men without prostate cancer (40). Men with IGF-1 levels in the upper quartile of the population distribution have an approximately twofold higher risk of prostate cancer than men of the three lower quartiles and a fourfold higher risk than men in the lower quartile (42,43). This assessment of risk was independent of men's serum PSA value (43). However, when used with PSA to calculate a IGF-1/PSA ratio, the specificity of prostate cancer screening is significantly enhanced over either value considered alone (41). In a prospective screening study measuring serum IGF-1 and PSA values, 245 men were biopsied to diagnosis 71 cancers. An IGF-1/PSA ratio cutoff of 25 significantly enhanced the specificity of either PSA or IGF-1 alone. Employment of this cutoff would detect 95% of the identified cancers and avoid 24.1% of the negative biopsies (41).

Several theories are currently under investigation to explain the association between IGF-1 bioactivity and prostate cancer. In addition to promoting transformation, increased IGF-1 bioactivity may also be the result of IGF-1 production by prostate cancer or derived by the proteolysis of IGFBP by PSA (44). Demonstration of a causal relationship between IGF-1 bioactivity and prostate cancer could provide a unique avenue for prostate cancer prevention such as a 60% reduction in caloric intake, which reduces IGF-1 levels (45).

Androgenic Stimulation

The development of prostate cancer is androgen dependent. Androgen stimulation of the prostate epithelium results in an increased risk for prostate cancer. Eunuchs provided the most dramatic example of this theory. They never achieve pubertal testosterone levels after birth and never developed prostate cancer. One's risk for prostate cancer is most likely directly proportional to the androgenic drive of the prostate epithelium. The androgenic drive may be increased through exogenous exposure or physiological differences such as baseline androgen levels, testosterone conversion to dihydrotestosterone, and androgen receptor transcription. Unique molecular features in each of these areas now identify individuals at a higher risk for prostate cancer.

Elevated baseline serum androgen levels and the exogenous administration of androgens are not conclusively linked to an elevated risk for prostate cancer *(46–48)*. However, differences in androgenic drive could exist for men with the same serum androgen levels but with differences in androgen metabolism. For example, a missense substitution in the human prostatic type II 5 α-reductase gene produces a variant enzyme with an increased capacity to convert testosterone to dihydrotestosterone. Makridakis et al. screened 388 African-American and Hispanic men with prostate cancer and 461 matched controls for this specific mis-sense substitution. The substitution was associated with a significant 7.2 times and 3.6 times increased risk for prostate cancer in African-American and Hispanic men, respectively.

Heritable differences in the androgen receptor transcription rate correlate with prostate cancer risk and may provide a partial explanation for the racial differences in clinical evident prostate cancer. The human androgen receptor (*hAR*) gene is on the X chromosome and encodes for a protein with three structural regions: the protein-binding region, the DNA-binding region, and the transactivation domain. The first exon of the *hAR* for the receptor transactivation region has variable numbers of trinucleotide repeats—$(CAG)_n$ coding for glutamine residues and $(GGC)_n$ coding for glycine residues. The number of these repeats can be determined by the polymerase chain reaction (PCR) of peripheral lymphocyte DNA and is indirectly proportional to the transcriptional activity of the gene *(50)*. The mean number of CAG repeats in exon 1 of the *hAR* is 11–31. A higher number of CAG repeats result in a lower transcription activity of the gene and is clinically manifested as androgen insensitivity *(51,52)*. A lower number or absence of CAG repeats in exon 1 results in increased transcriptional activity of the *hAR (53)*. Conversely, one would expect an increased sensitivity to androgen and perhaps a greater risk for the development of prostate cancer *(54)*.

Giovannucci et al. and Hardy et al. demonstrated that the number of CAG repeats correlates with the incidence of prostate cancer. Men with <20 CAG repeats in exon 1 have a 1.5–2 times relative risk of prostate cancer compared to men with a greater number of repeats *(55,56)*. Men with <17 repeats have a 1.6 times relative risk of prostate cancer as compared to men with 17 or more repeats. Shorter CAG or GGC repeat segments also identify patients at risk for more aggressive prostate cancer. Kakimi examined the number of CAG repeats in patients undergoing radical prostatectomy and pelvic lymph node dissection for clinical stage T2 prostate cancer to demonstrate that men with lymph node positive disease were eight times as likely to have < 18 CAG repeats as compared to men with lymph-node-negative disease *(56)*. Similarly, the number of GGC repeats is directly proportional to the disease-free survival (DFS) and overall survival (OS). Prostate cancer patients with T1–2 tumors and <16 GGC repeats had a relative risk of relapse (DFS) of 3.56 *(57)*. Therefore, the trinucleotide repeats in exon 1 of the androgen receptor is a modest molecular risk factor of prostate cancer.

HISTOLOGY MARKERS OF PROSTATE CANCER RISK

Prostatic Intraepithelial Neoplasia

Prostatic intraepithelial neoplasia (PIN) is identified in up to 16% of men undergoing needle biopsy of the prostate *(58)*. PIN is characterized by a distinctive architectural arrangement of cellular proliferations within preexisting ducts and glands, as in prostatic carcinoma, but lacks the complete disruption of the basal cell layer and stromal invasion seen in carcinoma. With increasing grades of PIN, there is increasing cytologic aberration and basal cell layer disruption.

High-grade PIN is a putative premalignant epithelial change. It is identified in 2–3% of men that undergo a needle biopsy of the prostate for an elevated PSA or suspicious prostate examination. The association with high-grade PIN with concurrent prostate cancer is well-established. Rebiopsy of the prostate will identify cancer in 33–100% of men found to have isolated high-grade PIN on their initial biopsy *(59)*. Immediate, multi-core, systematic biopsy of the entire prostate is therefore recommended for patients in this high-risk group.

Isolated low-grade PIN and adenomatous hyperplasia on needle biopsy of the prostate do not indicate the concurrent presence of cancer *(60,61)*. Rebiopsy in such patients should therefore be based on follow-up serum PSA values and prostate examinations *(62)*.

Prostatic Atypia

Prostatic atypia is diagnosed when the cytological or architectural criteria for prostate cancer or high-grade PIN are suggested but not clearly met. The risk for prostate cancer on subsequent biopsy is not as clearly defined as high-grade PIN. The decision for rebiopsy is therefore left to the urologist. In two retrospective reviews of subsequent biopsies in patients identified with isolated prostatic atypia, cancer was diagnosed in 29–49% of cases *(63,64)*. This represents a substantially greater cancer yield than one would expect from a patient with a persistent PSA abnormality and/or suspicious digital rectal examination and a benign initial biopsy *(65)*. Interestingly, men with a PSA less than 4 ng/mL and isolated prostatic atypia had a 33% chance of cancer on rebiopsy *(63)*. These two studies raise ample concern for the man with isolated prostatic atypia, and rebiopsy is encouraged irrespective of his follow-up serum PSA and prostate examination.

SUMMARY

Future calculations of patient's risk for prostate cancer will likely be calculated from a compilation of defined risk factors, including demographic, dietary, and molecular data. Presently, the independent consideration of major risk factors such as patients' age, race, and family history should guide prostate cancer screening. The most reliable criteria for identifying the patient at a risk level to justify a prostate biopsy are the serum PSA, prostate examination findings, and the pathology of previous prostate biopsies. In the near future, emerging molecular risk factors such as serum IGF-1, IGFBP-3, and androgen receptor CAG repeats will be added to demographic and dietary data to calculate individuals' prostate cancer risk and potentially guide the intensity of their screening. In addition, further identification of dietary risk factors will provide an intriguing opportunity to prevent prostate cancer development. The likely prevention diet to arise from our initial epidemiologic observations would be rich in vegetables, low in animal fat, and supplemented with selenium and vitamin E. This diet is also consistent with our current understanding of a diet that promotes overall good health and, therefore, a reasonable goal while ongoing prostate cancer prevention trials determine its actual effect on prostate cancer development.

REFERENCES

1. Landis SH, Murray T, Bolden S, and Wingo PA. (1999) Cancer Statistics, *CA Cancer J Clin* 49:8–31.
2. Sakr WA, Hass GP, Cassin BF, et al. (1993) The frequency of carcinoma and intraepithelial neoplasia of the prostate in young male patients. *J Urol* 150:379.
3. Sakr WA, Grignon DJ, Haas GP. (1998) Pathology of pre-malignant lesions and carcinoma of the prostate in African-American men. *Semin Uol Oncol* 16:214.
4. Stamey TA, Freiha FS, McNeal JE, et al. (1993) Localized prostate cancer. Relationship of tumor volume to clinical significance for treatment of prostate cancer. *Cancer* 71:933.
5. Humphrey PA, Keetch DW, Smith DS, Shepherd DL, Catalona WJ. (1996) Prospective characterization of pathological features of prostatic carcinomas detected via serum prostate specific antigen based screening. *J Urol* 155(3):816.
6. Brawer MD, Beatie J, Wener MH, et al. (1993) Screening for prostatic carcinoma with prostate specific antigen: results of the second year. *J Urol* 150:106.

7. Mettlin C, Murphy GP Lee F, et al. (1993) Characteristics of prostate cancers detected in a multimodality early detection program. *Cancer* 72:1701.

8. Thorson P, Vollner RT, Arcangeli C, et al. (1998) Minimal carcinoma in prostate needle biopsy specimens: diagnostic features and radical prostatectomy follow-up. *Mod Pathol* 11(6):543.

9. Ladding P, Aus G, Bergdahl S, et al. (1998) Characteristics of screening detected prostate cancer in men 50 to 66 years old with 3 to 4 ng./ml. Prostate specific antigen. *J Urol* 159(3):899.

10. Stamey TA, Donaldson AN, Yemoto EC, et al. (1998) Histological and clinical findings in 896 consecutive prostates treated only with radical retropubic prostatectomy: epidemiologic significance of annual changes. *J Urol* 160(6 Pt 2):2412.

11. Ghadirian P, Howe GR, HIslop TG, Maisonneuve P. (1997) Family history of prostate cancer: a multi-center case-control study in Canada. *Int J Cancer* 70(6):679.

12. Lesko SM, Rosenberg L, Shapiro S. (1996) Family history and prostate cancer risk. *Am J Epidemiol* 144(11):1041.

13. Bratt O, Kristoffersson U, Lundgren R, Olsson H. (1999) Familial and hereditary prostate cancer in southern Sweden. A population-based case-control study. *Eur J Cancer* 35(2):272.

14. Schuurman AG, Zeegers MP, Goldhohn RA, vander Brandt PA. (1999) A case-cohort study on prostate cancer risk in relation to family history of prostate cancer. *Epidemiology* 10(2):192.

15. Matikainen MP, Schleutker J, Morsky P, Kallioniemi OP, Tammela TL. (1999) Detection of subclinical cancers by prostate-specific antigen screening in asymptomatic men from high-risk prostate cancer families. *Clin Cancer Res* 5(6):1275.

16. Cerhan JR, Parker AS, Putnam SD, et al. (1999) Family history and prostate cancer risk in a population-based cohort of Iowa men. *Cancer Epid. Biomarkers Prev* 8(1):53.

17. Gronberg H, Wiklund F, Damber JE. (1999) Age specific risks of familial prostate carcinoma: a basis for screening recommendations in high risk populations. *Cancer* 86(3):477.

18. McDonald C. (1999) Cancer statistics 1999: Challenges in minority populations. *CA: Cancer J Clin* 49(1).

19. Brawley OW, Knopf K, Merrill R. (1998) The epidemiology of prostate cancer part I: descriptive epidemiology. *Semin Urol Oncol* 16:187.

20. Merrill RM, Weed DL, Feuer EJ. (1997) The lifetime risk of developing prostate cancer in white and black men. *Cancer Epidemiol Biomarkers Prev* 6(10):763.

21. Shimzu H, Ross RK, Bernstein, L, Yatani R, Henderson BE, Mack TM. (1991) Cancers of the prostate and breast among Japanese and white immigrants in Los Angeles County. *Br J Cancer* 63(6):963.

22. Lee M. (1998) Case-control study of diet and prostate cancer in China. *Cancer Causes Control* 9(6):545.

23. Shuurman AG, van der Brandt PA, Dorant E, Brants HA, Goldbohm RA. (1999) Association of energy and fat intake with prostate carcinoma risk: results from The Netherlands Cohort Study. *Cancer* 86(6):1019.

24. Andersson SO, Wolk A, Bergstrom R, et al. (1996) Energy, nutrient intake and prostate cancer risk: a population-based case-control study in Sweden. *Int J Cancer* 68(6):716.

25. Rohan TE, Howe GR, Burch JP, Jain M. (1995) Dietary factors and risk of prostate cancer: a case-control study in Ontario, Canada. *Cancer Causes Control* 6(2):145.
26. Hayes RB, Ziegler RG, Gridley G, et al. (1999) Dietary factors and risks for prostate cancer among blacks and whites in the United States. *Cancer Epidemiol Biomarkers Prev* 8(1):25.
27. West DW, Slattery ML, Robison LM, French TK, Mahoney AW. (1991) Adult dietary intake and prostate cancer risk in Utah: a case-control study with special emphasis on aggressive tumors. *Cancer Causes Control* 2(2):85.
28. Meyer F, Bairati I, Shadmani R, Fradet Y, Moore L. (1999) Dietary fat and prostate cancer survival. *Cancer Causes Control* 10(4):245.
29. Wang Y, Corr JG, Thaler HT, Tao Y, Fair WR, Heston WK. (1995) Decreased growth of established human prostate LNCaP tumors in nude mice fed a low-fat diet. *J Natl Cancer Inst* 87(19):1456.
30. Demark-Wahnefried W, Halabi S, Paulson DF. (1997) Serum androgens: associations with prostate cancer risk and hair patterning. *J Androl* 18(5):495.
31. Nilsen TI, Vatten LJ. (1999) Anthropometry and prostate cancer riesk: a prospective study of 22,248 Norwegian men. *Cancer Causes Control* 10(4):269.
32. Stamey TA, Yang N, HayAR, et al. (1987) Prostate-specific antigen as a serum marker for adenocarcinoma of the prostate. *N Engl J Med* 137:909.
33. Brawer MK, Lange PA. (1989) PSA in the screening, staging and follow up of early-stage prostate cancer: A review of recent developments. *World J Urol* 7:7.
34. Catalona WJ, Smith DS, Ratliff TL, et al. (1991) Measurement of prostate specific antigen in serum as a screening test for prostate cancer. *N Engl J Med* 324:1156.
35. Keetch DW, Catalona WJ, Smith DS. (1994) Serial prostatic biopsies in men with persistently elevated serum prostate specific antigen values. *J Urol* 151(6):1571.
36. Keetch DW, Hum 0phry PA. (1997) Patient age and prostate cancer. *Am J Clin Path* 107 (3):265.
37. Catalona WJ, Partin AW, Slawin KM, et al. (1998) Use of the percentage of free prostate-specific antigen to enhance differentiation of prostate cancer from benign prostatic disease: a prospective multicenter clinical trial. *JAMA* 279(19):1542.
38. Trinkler FB, Schmid DM, Hauri D, Pei P, Maly FE, Sulser T. (1998) Free/total prostate-specific antigen ratio can prevent unnecessary prostate biopsies. *Urology* 52(3):479.
39. Thiel RP, Oesterling JE, Wajno KJ, et al. (1996) Multicenter comparison of the diagnostic performance of free prostate-specific antigen. *Urology* 48(6A Suppl):45.
40. Shaneyfelt T, Husein R, Bubley G, Mantzoros CS. (2000) Hormonal predictors of prostate cancer: a meta-analysis. *J Clin Oncol* 18(4):847.
41. Djavan B, Bursa B, Seitz C, et al. (1999) Insulin-like growth factor 1 (IGF-1), IGF-1 density, and IGF-1/PSA ratio for prostate cancer detection. *Urology* 54(4):603.
42. Wolk A, Mantzoros CS, Andersson SO, Bergstrom R, et al. (1998) Insulin-like growth factor 1 and prostate cancer risk: a population-based, case-control study. *J Natl Cancer Inst* 90(12):911.
43. Chan JM. (1998) Plasma insulin-like growth factor-1 and prostate cancer risk: a prospective study. *Science* 279(5350):563.
44. Giovannuci E. (1999) Insulin-like growth factor-1 and binding protein-3 and risk of cancer. *Horm Res* 51(suppl S3):34.

45. Sonntag WE, Lynch CD, Cefalu WT, et al. (1999) Pleiotropic effects of growth hormone and insulin-like growth factor (IGF-1) on biological aging: inferences from moderate caloric restricted animals. *J Gerontol A Biol Sci Med Sci* 54(12):B521-38.

46. Heikkila R, Aho K, Heliovaara M, et al. (1999) Serum testosterone and sex hormone-binding globulin concentrations and the risk of prostate carcinoma: a longitudinal study. *Cancer* 86(2):312.

47. Vatten L. (1997) Androgens in serum and the risk of prostate cancer: a nested case-control study from the Janus serum bank in Norway. *Cancer Epidemiol Biomarkers Prev* 6(11):967.

48. Gann PH. (1996) Prospective study of sex hormone levels and risk of prostate cancer. *J Natl Cancer Inst* 88(16):1118.

49. Makridakis NM, Ross RK, Pike MC, et al. (1999) Association of mis-sense substitution in SRD5A2 gene with prostate cancer in African-American and Hispanic men in Los Angeles, USA. *Lancet* 354(9183):975.

50. Chang C, Kokentris J, Liao St. (1988) Molecular cloning of human and rat complementary DNA encoding androgen receptors. *Science* 240:324-326.

51. Choong CS, Kemppaines JA, Zhou ZX, Wilson LM. (1996) Reduced androgen receptor gene expression with first exon CAG repeat expansion. *Mol Endocrinol* 10:1527.

52. Sobue G, Dayu M, Morishima T, et al. (1994) Aberrant androgen action and increased size of tandem CAG repeat in androgen receptor gene in X-linked recessive bulbospinal neuropathy. *J Neurol Sci* 121:167.

53. Chamberlain NL, Driver ED, Miesfeld RL. (1994) The length and location of CAG trinucleotide repeats in the androgen receptor N-terminal domain affect transactivation function. *Nucleic Acids Res* 22:3181.

54. Ingles SA, Ross RK, Yu MC, et al. (1997) Association of prostate cancer risk with genetic polymorphisms in vitamin D receptor and androgen receptor. *J Natl Cancer Inst* 89:166.

55. Giovannucci E, Stampfer MJ, Krithivas K, et al. (1997) The CAG repeat within the androgen receptor gene and its relationship to prostate cancer. *Proc Natl Acad Sci* 94:3323.

56. HardyDO, Scher HI, Bagenreider T, et al. (1996) Androgen receptor CAG repeat lengths in prostate cancer: correlation with age of onset. *J Clini Endrocrinol Metab* 81:4400.

57. Edwards SM, Badzioch MD, Minter R, et al. (1999) Androgen receptor polymorphisms: association with prostate cancer risk, relapse and overall survival. *Int J Cancer* 84(5):458–65.

58. Bostwick DG, Quain J, Frankel K. (1995)The incidence of high-grade prostatic intraepithelial neoplasia in needle biopsies. *J Urol* 154:1791.

59. Weinstein MH, Greenspan DL, Epstein JJ. (1995) Diagnoses rendered in prostate needle biopsy in community hospitals. *Mod Path* 8:85A.

60. Shepherd D, Keetch DW, Humphrey PA, Smith DS, Stahl D. (1996) Repeat biopsy strategy in men with isolated prostatic intraepithelial neoplasia on prostate needle biopsy. *J Urol* 156(2 Pt 1):460.

61. Sakr WA, Grignon DJ. (1998) Prostatic intraepithelial neoplasia and atypical adenomatous hyperplasia: relationship of pathologic parameters, volume and spatial distribution of carcinoma of the prostate. *Anal Quant Cytol Histol* 20(5):417.

62. Epstein JI, Grignon DJ, Humphrey PA, et al. (1995) Interobserver reproducibility in the diagnosis of prostatic intraepithelial neoplasia. *Amer J Surg Path* 19:873.
63. Chan TY, Epstein JJ. (1999) Follow-up of atypical prostate needle biopsies suspicious for cancer. *Urol* 53(2):351.
64. Ellis WJ, Brawer MK. (1995) Repeat prostate needle biopsy: who needs it? *J Urol* 153(5):1496.
65. Keetch DW, Catalona WJ, Smith DS. (1994) Serial prostatic biopsies in men with persistently elevated serum prostatic specific antigen values. *J Urol* 151(6):1571.

10 Transrectal Ultrasound and Artificial Neural Networks in the Diagnosis of Prostate Cancer

Tillmann Loch, MD

Contents

INTRODUCTION

Prostate cancer is currently the most commonly diagnosed malignancy in the United States. Approximately 39,000 men will have died of this potentially curable disease in 1998. Digital rectal examination (DRE) yields only a low detection rate, and more than half of the palpable tumors have already extended outside the capsule. With the isolation and purification of a glycoprotein, later called prostate-specific antigen (PSA), by Wang et al. in 1979, the world of early detection of prostate cancer changed dramatically.

However, as a result of the enhanced clinical application of PSA, an increasing number of men are becoming candidates for prostate cancer workup. A high PSA value over 20 ng/mL is a good indicator of the presence of prostate cancer, but within the range of 4–10 ng/mL, it is rather unreliable *(1–4)*. Although PSA is capable of indicating a statistical risk of prostate cancer in a defined patient population, it is not able

From: *Current Clinical Urology: Prostate Cancer Screening*
Edited by: I. M. Thompson, M. I. Resnick, and E. A. Klein
© Humana Press Inc., Totowa, NJ

to localize cancer within the prostate gland or guide a biopsy needle to a suspicious area. This necessitates an additional effective diagnostic technique that is able to localize or rule out a malignant growth within the prostate.

It has therefore become a routine procedure to perform 4–18 systematic random biopsies of the prostate under transrectal ultrasound (TRUS) guidance in patients with a PSA value above 4 ng/mL (5–7). The results of six random biopsies performed in men with a value of 4–10 ng/ml were positive in only one out of four men, (8) an accuracy rate of 25%. A study of 101 men subjected to at least six systematic random biopsies revealed benign histology in 86% of the 611 biopsies, a total of 519 biopsies that neither confirmed nor excluded the presence of prostate cancer (8).

Even more alarming is the fact that prostate cancer has been found in 12–37% of patients with a "normal" PSA value of under 4 ng/mL (Hybritech) (9). The methods available for the detection of these prostate cancers are DRE and TRUS. DRE is not suitable for *early* detection, because, as already mentioned, about 70% of the palpable malignancies have already spread beyond the prostate (10).

The classic problem of visual interpretation of TRUS images is that hypoechoic areas suspected of cancer may be either normal or cancerous histologically. They are not differentiable when examined visually or when further analyzed by the objective gray scale. Although about 75% of the cancerous regions appear hypoechoic, many other hypoechoic regions, such as benign prostatic hyperplasia (BPH) nodules, vessels, focal prostatitis, shadows, artifacts, and so forth, are not cancerous. Moreover, about 25% of all cancers have been found to be isoechoic and therefore not distinguishable from normal-appearing areas (11,12). None of the current biopsy or imaging techniques are able to cope with this dilemma.

Artificial neural networks (ANN) are complex nonlinear computational models, designed much like the neuronal organization of a brain. These networks are able to model complicated biologic relationships without making assumptions based on conventional statistical distributions. Applications in medicine and urology have been promising. One example of such an application will be discussed in detail: A new method of artificial neural network analysis (ANNA) was employed in an attempt to obtain existing subvisual information, (13–15) other than the gray scale, from conventional TRUS and improve the accuracy of prostate cancer identification (16).

PATIENTS AND METHODS

This prospective blinded study evaluated 61 patients with clinically localized cancer of the prostate diagnosed by positive needle biopsy. All men were referred to the Kiel University Urology Department and underwent radical prostatectomy between January 1995 and March 1996. The patients ranged between 46 and 89 yr of age, with a median of 67 yr.

Each patient underwent DRE by two urologists. Ambulatory serum PSA was determined prior to DRE, TRUS, or biopsy. PSA levels were ascertained by monoclonal–monoclonal assay (Hybritech Inc., Tandem-E). Each patient was examined by TRUS 1 or 2 days prior to surgery, digitally storing the transverse images on the computer at 4-mm intervals. Computerized image analysis (CIA) then extracted and evaluated subvisual texture information other than the visual gray level.

Transrectal Ultrasound and Computer Analysis

All transrectal ultrasound examinations were performed with a Bruel & Kjear 1846 console (Naerum, Denmark). Each patient was initially scanned transversely with the 7.0-MHz axial transducer (Bruel & Kjear Model 1850). A water balloon stand-off filled with degassed water was always used for optimized focal zone resolution. System settings were a near gain of 5.7 dB, a far gain of 50.1 dB, and a slope of 9.0 dB/cm. Contour and contrast were set at 3, image size was 1, and a frame rate of 14/s was used. The focal point was set at 2.3 cm with a focal range of 1.5–6 cm. The entire procedure was recorded on video tape.

The digitally stored transverse TRUS images (8-bit gray scale: TIFF) were labeled from the apex of the prostate (00) in 4-mm increments (04, 08, 12, etc.) to the base *(15)*. A total of 312 preoperative TRUS transverse images were obtained from the 61 patients, an average of five per patient. The computer evaluated subvisual texture information of all 312 digitally stored TRUS images, establishing six different statistical "descriptors" of image granularity. These descriptors are defined as follows: E- Number of edges, g- dispersion of edge intensity, L- average size of edges, l- dispersion of edge size, D- contrast intensity of edges, and d-dispersion of edge contrast. They all are expressed in absolute numbers, each number representing a square of 2 mm on the TRUS image.

Radical Prostatectomy Specimen

Bilateral staging lymphadenectomy followed by radical retropubic prostatectomy was performed in all patients. The prostate specimens were fixed in 37% formalin and serially cut at 4 mm intervals perpendicular to the rectal surface in correlation with the corresponding TRUS plane.

The paraffin blocks were sectioned at 5 µm, whole-mounted, and stained with hematoxylin and eosin. A total of 289 sections from 61 radical prostatectomy specimens cut at 4 mm intervals were mounted whole and otherwise processed according to the McNeal procedure *(17)*. During microscopic study by one pathologist, individual foci of the cancer were outlined in ink, as were prostatic capsule, transition-zone boundary, ejaculatory ducts, and urethra. Positive margins, capsular penetration and seminal vesicle invasion were assessed quantitatively. Each individual cancerous area was outlined. Carcinoma grade was determined by the Gleason Grading System *(18)*. Areas of well to moderate differentiation (Gleason grade 1–3) were marked with black ink dots and undifferentiated areas (Gleason grade 4/5) were marked with red ink dots.

"Transparent Projection": Computer Correlation of Prostate Whole Mounts and Ultrasound

The 289 pathologically reviewed whole-mount slices were scanned (Hewlett-Packard HP IV) and individually saved as digital files on the computer. Using a new computerized technique of "transparent projection," the pathology whole mounts were virtually overlaid on the TRUS images and aligned so that formalin shrinkage of the pathology specimen was compensated. Additionally, lesion location was confirmed by distinguishing marks obtained from pathology and TRUS, such as calcification, cysts, and zonal anatomy, using a "landmark technique" allowing for approximately 2 mm accuracy in correlation.

As strict quality control was performed, all questionable whole-mount pathology/TRUS matches were discarded, resulting in 188 unquestionably correlated matches used for generating the study results. The 188 completely pathology-confirmed whole-mount sections were classified into benign regions of low- or high-grade cancers. Classification was performed solely by means of the histopathologic marks superimposed upon the TRUS images, disregarding echogenicity. In addition, the anatomical zone of origin (peripheral or transition) of each cancer was identified.

Using a digital light pen, benign regions of low- and high-grade cancers with a minimum size of 4 mm were sectioned by following the transparent ink dots of the pathologist. A total of 553 of these small TRUS samples with the representative descriptor information were then crypted and saved individually as digital files.

Artificial Neural Network Analysis

An artificial neural network analysis (ANNA) was used that allows evaluation of numeric data problems that would otherwise be processed by regression analysis. The independent variables used in the regression became the input and the dependent variables the output. Descriptive statistics were determined for all preoperative and postoperative parameters. Benign, Gleason grades 1–3 and grades 4/5 descriptor samples (input variables) of five randomly selected patients (53/553 samples) were chosen. The computer-generated, pathologically confirmed numeric descriptor data of these 53 known samples were then used to train ANNA.

RESULTS AND COMMENTS

To generate the results of the *blinded* study, a total of 500 pathology-confirmed samples from 61 prostectomized patients was used. Of these, 381 were benign and 119 of malignant histology. Of the 119 malignant samples, 84 (71%) were hypoechoic, 35 (29%) isoechoic, and none were hyperechoic. Of the 68 (57%) Gleason grades 1–3 samples, 44 (65%) were hypoechoic and 24 (35%) isoechoic. Of the 51 (43%) Gleason grades 4/5 samples, 40 (78%) were hypoechoic and 11 (22%) isoechoic (*see* Table 1).

Of the 381 benign pathology-confirmed samples, ANNA classified 378 (99%) correctly as benign and 4 (1%) as malignant. Of the 119 malignant samples, 94 (79%) were correctly classified as cancers and 25 (21%) were falsely classified as benign. Of the 68 Gleason grades 1–3 samples, 61 (90%) were correctly and 7 (10%) were falsely classified. Of the 51 Gleason grades 4/5 samples, 33 (65%) were identified as such and 18 (35%) were not (*see* Table 2).

Subdividing the malignant samples further by the computer-generated average gray level, there were 84 hypoechoic and 35 isoechoic samples. ANNA classified 60 (71%) of the hypoechoic cancers as malignant and 24 (29%) as false negatives. In the isoechoic group, ANNA unexpectedly classified 34 (97%) correctly as cancers, missing only one sample.

Of the 44 hypoechoic pathology-confirmed Gleason grades 1–3 samples, 38 were classified as true positives and 6 as false negatives. Of the 40 hypoechoic pathology-confirmed Gleason grades 4/5 samples, 22 were classified as true positives and 18 as false negatives. ANNA classified 23 out of 24 isoechoic pathology-confirmed Gleason grades, 13 samples, and all 11 isoechoic Gleason grades 4/5 samples correctly (Table 2). Cancerous areas in individual whole-mount sections were missed, but at least one malignant area was identified in each of the cancer patients.

The vast majority of biopsy samples taken from asymptomatic men will not contain cancer. Moreover, in the clinically significant PSA

Table 1
Hypoechoic and Isoechoic Distribution of ANNA Classification
of the 119 Pathology-confirmed Malignant Samples

Gray level intensity	Hypoechoic (84)		Isoechoic (35)	
	True positive	False negative	True positive	False negative
All cancers (119)	60 (71%)	24 (29%)	34 (97%)	1 (3%)
Gleason grade 1–3 (68)	38	6	23	1
Gleason grade 4/5 (51)	22	18	11	0

Table 2
ANNA Classification Results of All Pathology-confirmed TRUS
Samples Regardless of Gray Level.

	True positive	False positive	True negative	False negative
Benign (381)	N/A	4 (1%)	378 (99%)	N/A
Cancers (119)	94 (79%)	N/A	N/A	25 (21%)
Gleason grade 1–3 (68)	61 (90%)	N/A	N/A	7 (10%)
Gleason grade 4/5 (51)	33 (65%)	N/A	N/A	18 (35%)

range of 4.0–10 ng/mL, an estimated 75% of all men will have 4 to 18 histologically benign biopsy samples *(2,8)*, that do not necessarily rule out the presence of prostate cancer.

With the use of CIA and ANNA of TRUS images, a significant reduction of false positives (1%) and false negatives (21%) could be achieved in this prospective study. Although not all cancer samples were detected, all patients with cancer had at least one positive ANNA sample so that none of the 61 patients would have been missed. In addition, clinically significant cancerous regions were detected that otherwise would have been missed.

Most important, 97% of the not visible *isoechoic* pathology-confirmed cancers could be identified. The distribution of hypoechoic (71%) and isoechoic (29%) cancerous regions in this study group are in agreement with prior reports *(11)*. Gleason grades 4/5 were measured as hypoechoic in 80% of the cases, whereas Gleason grades 1–3 only presented hypoechoic in 65% of the cases. Interestingly, ANNA had better predictive values in the isoechoic (97%) than in the hypoechoic (71%) group. Samples consisting of grades 4/5 had significant texture differences vs Gleason grade 3 samples.

These findings support the proposed hypothesis of the presence of additional information in the subvisual aspects of the ultrasound image *(15)*. Only "transparent projection" of the whole mounts and TRUS images with the help of the "landmark technique" enabled the close correlation between pathological and ultrasound findings. All samples analyzed underwent a strict quality control eliminating all questionable findings. Generating one pathology-confirmed sample (n = 553) took approximately 15 min. This meticulous process of correlating pathology and TRUS findings irrespective of the echoic appearance within 2 mm accuracy led to the high specificity of the ANNA classification. Moreover, it enabled detection of the isoechoic lesions, potentially leading to new biopsy strategies. The result of the computation can be projected upon the conventional TRUS image by red boxes, allowing guidance of one needle into the marked area even if it is isoechoic.

CONCLUSIONS AND OUTLOOK

Regardless of peripheral or transition-zone tumor location ANNA findings significantly increased the diagnostic accuracy of visual TRUS interpretation. Although not all cancers were detected, cancerous regions were detected in all of the patients. The objective of the first phase of this ongoing study was to design a highly specific ANNA classification system. Additional research is being carried out to improve the detection of Gleason grades 1–3 and hypoechoic cancers. The distinct ability of ANNA to detect isoechoic tumors appears to be the essential improvement as compared to conventional TRUS. It remains to be seen in clinical prospective studies whether ANNA can replace random by targeted biopsies. In an ongoing study, the subvisual information has been transferred into a three-dimensional prostate model in order to demonstrate improved needle guidance and staging information.

The application of ANNs has not been limited to prostate cancer. Models have been used successfully in many fields of medicine: Diagnosis of Alzheimer's disease *(19)*, bladder cancer *(20)*, breast cancer *(21)*, hepatitis *(22)*, myocardial infarction *(23,24)*, prostate *(25–30)* and ovarian cancer *(31)*, psychiatric emergencies *(32)*, and vasculitis *(33)*; imaging of bone lesions *(34)*, breast *(35)*, chest *(36)*, cerebral perfu-

sion *(37)*, kidney *(38)*, stones *(40)*, prostate cancer *(16,39)*, outcome
prediction of breast, colorectal *(41)*, prostate *(42)* and testis cancer *(43)*,
length of hospital stay *(44)*, cytology *(45)*, histology *(46)*, and quality
of life *(47)*.

ANNs have just begun to enter the world of medicine. This powerful
tool will enable new perspectives in predicting a patient's response to
various treatments and predicting an individual's outcome based on his
specific medical history.

REFERENCES

1. Potosky AL, Miller BA, Albertson PC, Kramer BS (1995) The role of increasing detection in the rising incidence of prostate cancer. *JAMA*, 273, 7:548.
2. Cooner WH, Mosley BR, Rutherford C, Beard JH, Pond HS, Terry WJ, et al. (1990) Prostate cancer detection in a clinical urological practice by ultrasonography, digital rectal examination and prostate specific antigen. *J Urol* 143:1146.
3. Oesterling JE. (1991) Prostate specific antigen: a critical assessment of the most useful tumor marker for adenocarcinoma of the prostate. *J Urol* 145:907.
4. Stamey TA, Yang N, HayAR, McNeal JE, Freiha FS, Redwine E. (1987) Prostate-specific antigen as a serum marker for adenocarcinoma of the prostate. *New Engl J Med* 317:909.
5. Hodge KK, McNeal JE, Terris MK, Stamey TA. (1989) Random systematic versus directed ultrasound-guided transrectal core biopsies of the prostate. *J Urol* 142:71.
6. Nava L, Montorsi F, Consonni P, Scattoni V, Guazzoni G, Rigatti PJ. (1997) Results of a prospective randomized study comparing 6, 12 and 18 transrectal, ultrasound guided, sextant biopsies in patients with elevated PSA, normal DRE, and normal prostatic ultrasound. *J Urol* 157(4):59 (abstract).
7. Vashi AR, Wojno KJ, Gillespie B, Oesterling JE. (1997) Patient age and prostate gland size determine the appropriate number of cores per prostate biopsy. *J Urol* 157(4):365 (abstract).
8. Loch T, Bertermann H, Wirth B, Wand H. (1993) Klinische Bedeutung von RT und PSA für die Erkennung des Prostatakarzinoms. *Urologe A* 32:69.
9. Noldus J, Stamey TA. (1996) Histological characteristics of radical prostatectomy specimens in men with a serum prostate specific antigen of 4 ng./ml or less. *J Urol* 155:441.
10. Catalona WJ, Smith DS, Ratliff TL, Basler JW. (1993) Detection of organ-confined prostate cancer is increased through prostate-specific antigen-based screening. JAMA 270(8):948.
11. Shinohara K, Scardino PT, Carter SC, Wheeler TM. (1989) Pathologic basis of the sonographic appearance of the normal and malignant prostate. *Urol Clin Amer* 16:675.
12. Lee F, Gray JM, McLeary RD,Meadows TK, Kumasaka GH, Borlasa GS, et al. (1985) Transrectal ultrasound in the diagnosis of prostate cancer: Location, echogenicity, histopathology, and staging. *Prostate* 7:117.
13. Loch T, Gouge J, Bertermann H. (1987) Rechnergestützte Realtime-Farbsonographie zur objektiven Bildanalyse. *Ultraschall Klin Prax* 2:242.

14. Loch T, Cochran JS, Fulgham PF, Gettys T, Bertermann H. (1989) Computer assisted image analysis of prostate ultrasound in the diagnosis of carcinoma of the prostate. *J Urol* 141(Suppl.):256A.
15. Loch T, Gettys T, Cochran JS, Fulgham PF, Bertermann H. (1990) Computer-aided image-analysis in transrectal ultrasound of the prostate. *World J Urol* 8:150.
16. Loch T, Leuschner I, Brüske T, Küpper F, Stöckle M, Genberg C. (1997) Neural network analysis of subvisual transrectal ultrasound data: Improved prostate cancer detection. *J Urol* 157(4):364 (abstract).
17. McNeal JE, Redwine E, Freiha FS, Stamey TA. (1989) Zonal distribution of prostatic adenocarcinoma. Correlation with histopathologic pattern and direction of spread. *Am J Surg Pathol* 12:897.
18. Gleason DF. (1977) Histologic grading and staging of prostate carcinoma. In: *Urologic Pathology: The Prostate.* Tannenbaum M, ed. Philadelphia: Lea & Febiger, pp.171–187.
19. Kippenhan JS, Barker WW, Pascal S, et al. (1992) Evaluation of neural-network classifier for PET scans of normal and Alzheimer's disease subjects. *J Nucl Med* 33:1459–1467.
20. Schweiger CR, Maenner GA, Soeregi G, et al. (1994) Neural network evaluation of multiple tumor markers for diagnosis of urinary bladder cancer using three different sets of patients (abstract). Third International Conference of the Mediterranean Society of Tumor.
21. Astion ML, Wilding P. (1992) Application of neural networks to the interpretation of laboratory data in cancer diagnosis. *Clin Chem* 38:34–38.
22. Reibnegger G, Weiss G, Werner-Felmayer G, et al. (1991) Neural networks as a tool for utilizing laboratory information: comparison with linear discriminant analysis and with classification and regression trees. *Proc Natl Acad Sci USA* 88:1426–1430.
23. Baxt WG. (1991) Use of an artificial neural network for the diagnosis of myocardial infarction. *Ann Intern Med* 115:843–848.
24. Baxt WG, Skora J. (1996) Prospective validation of artificial neural network trained to identify acute myocardial infarction. *Lancet* 347:12–15.
25. Snow PB, Smith DS, Catalona WJ. (1994) Artificial neural networks in the diagnosis and prognosis of prostate cancer: a pilot study. *J Urol* 152:1923–1926.
26. Barnhill S, Stamey T, Zhang Z, et al. (1997) The ability of the ProstAsureTM Index to identify prostate cancer patients with low cancer volumes and a high potential for cure. *J Urol* 157:63–67.
27. Babaian RJ, Fritsche HA, Zhang Z, et al. (1998) Evalution of prostAsure index in the detection of prostate cancer: a preliminary report. *Urology* 51:132–136.
28. Tisman G, Strum S, Scholz M, et al. (1997) Pre-therapy prediction of the duration of post-therapy non-detectable PSA for prostate cancer patients considering intermittend combined hormonal blockade by use of computerized neural net modeling. (abstract). Proceedings of the American Society of Clinical Oncology Meeting.
29. Stamey TA, Barnhill SD, Zhang Z, et al. (1996) Effectiveness of ProstAsureTM in detecting prostate cancer (PCa) and benign prostatic hyperplasia (BPH) in men age 50 and older. *J Urol* 155:436A.
30. Snow P, Crawford D, De Antoni E, et al. (1997) Prostate cancer diagnosis from artificial neural networks using the prostate cancer awareness week database. *J Urol* 157:365.

31. Wilding P, Morgan MA, Grygotis AE, et al. (1994) Application of back propagation neural networks to diagnosis of breast and ovarian cancer. *Cancer Lett* 77:145–153.

32. Somoza E, Somoza JR. (1993) A neural-network approach predicting admission decisions in a psychiatric emergency room. *Med Decis Making* 13:273–280.

33. Astion ML, Wener MH, Thomas RG, et al. (1994) Application of neural networks to the classification of giant cell arteritis. *Arthritis Rheum* 37:760–770.

34. Reinus WR, Wilson AJ, Kalman B, et al. (1994) Diagnosis of focal bone lesions using neural networks. *Invest Radiol* 29:606–611.

35. Kalman BL, Reinus WR, Kwasny SC, et al. (1997) Prescreening entire mammograms for masses with artificial neural networks: preliminary results. *Acad Radiol* 4:405–414.

36. Lin JS Ligomenides PA, Freedman MT, et al. (1993) Application of artificial neural networks for reduction of false positive detections in digital chest radiographs. *Proc Annu Symp Appl Med Care* 434–438.

37. Chan KH, Johnson KA, Becker JA, et al. (1994) A neural network classifier for cerebral perfusion imiging. *J Nucl Med* 35:771–774.

38. Maclin PS, Dempsey J, Brooks J, et al. (1991) Using neural networks to diagnose cancer. *J Med Syst* 15:11–19.

39. Prater JS, Richard WD. (1992) Segmenting ultrasound images of the prostate using neural networks. *Ultrason Imaging* 142:159–185.

40. Niederberger CS, Michaels DK, Cho L, et al. (1996) A neural computational model of stone recurrence after ESWL. Proceedings of the International Conference on Engineering Applications of Neural Networks, pp. 423–426.

41. Burke HB, Goodman PH, Rosen DB, et al. (1997) Artificial neural networks improve the accuracy of cancer survival prediction. *Cancer* 79:857–862.

42. Douglas T, Connelly R, McLeod D, et al. (1996) Neural network analysis of preoperative and post-operative variables to predict pathological stage and recurrence. *J Urol* 155:487A.

43. Moul JW, Snow PB, Fernandez EB, et al. (1995) Neural network analysis of quantitative histological factors to predict pathological stage in clinical stage I nonseminomatous testicular cancer. *J Urol* 153:1674–1677.

44. Davis GE, Lowell WE, Davis GL. (1993) A neural network that predicts psychiatric length of stay. *MD Comput* 10:87–92.

45. Mango LJ. (1997) Reducing false negatives in clinical practice: the role of neural network technology. *Am J Gynecol* 175:1114–1119.

46. Stotzka R, Manner R, Bartels PH, et al. (1995) A hybrid neural and statistical classifier system for histopathologic grading of prostatic lesions. *Analytic Quant Cytol Histol* 17:204–218.

47. Krongrad A, Granville LJ, Burke MA, et al. (1997) Predictors of general quality of life in patients with benign prostate hyperplasia or prostate cancer. *J Urol* 157:5534–5538.

11 Evidence of the Effectiveness of Prostate Cancer Screening

*Chris Magee, MD
and Ian M. Thompson, MD*

CONTENTS

INTRODUCTION

Technological advances in medicine often precede parallel advances in knowledge. Such is the fundamental problem with the early detection and screening for prostate cancer. Until the mid-to late 1980s, rarely was prostate cancer screening an issue. Prior to this time, the only method to diagnose prostate cancer was to use digital rectal examination (DRE)—a test of some specificity but very poor sensitivity. Indeed, we previously found that many a patient who ultimately died of prostate cancer *never was found to have an abnormal rectal examination (1).* With DRE used as the only method of early diagnosis, as many as 30–35% of men diagnosed were found to have frank bony metastases, as many as 45–50% were found to have nodal disease, and only about one-third of men with clinically organ-confined disease were proved to have pathologically organ-confined disease at the time of radical prostatectomy *(2,3).* With tumors detected at such a late stage (many of the

From: *Current Clinical Urology: Prostate Cancer Screening*
Edited by: I. M. Thompson, M. I. Resnick, and E. A. Klein
© Humana Press Inc., Totowa, NJ

patients being incurable), little hubbub was raised over efforts to detect the disease at an earlier stage.

Enter prostate-specific antigen (PSA). The time was the mid- to late 1980s. Little was known initially regarding normal ranges and the performance of this test in an early detection setting. Simultaneously, engineers had designed the first automated, smaller-gauge needle-biopsy "guns." The result was an extraordinary surge in the number of prostate tumors detected. Indeed, never in the experience of the monitoring system set up by the National Cancer Institute (the Surveillance, Epidemiology, and End Results program or SEER) had such an increase in disease incidence been witnessed. Little was understood regarding the yield, performance characteristics, and type of tumors that would be detected using the combination of PSA and spring-loaded biopsy guns.

A number of innovative and pioneering urologists recognized the potential of this combination for the early detection of prostate cancer. The experiences at the University of Washington and at Washington University in St. Louis gave both an impetus for early diagnosis efforts around the nation and provided a guide for how PSA should be interpreted. As a result of this phenomenon, the United States was a participant in the largest *natural experiment of PSA testing* for the early diagnosis of prostate cancer, beginning in 1987–1988. Recognizing the potential confounds with PSA screening, the National Cancer Institute developed the most ambitious screening study ever mounted in the world—the PLCO (Prostate, Lung, Colorectal Cancer, and Ovarian Cancer screening) Study. This study was designed to enroll 148,000 men and women, half of whom would be screened and half who would receive only "standard community care." The study continues to enroll patients and to steadily move towards its accrual goal with publication of final results sometime about the year 2010 *(4)*.

In the meantime, technology marched on. Over the course of the 12 yr since the onset of screening, major changes have been witnessed. Effectively, what has occurred has been a nonrandomized study of screening. It is the impression of many experts in the field that this natural study provides us with a glimpse into the potential effectiveness of PSA screening. It is the focus of this chapter to outline the growing body of evidence that suggests that screening for prostate cancer using both PSA and DRE will result in a fall in prostate cancer mortality and that it should be offered to the general public as a routine health promotion test.

WHAT SHOULD WE EXPECT TO WITNESS IF AN EFFECTIVE SCREENING TEST IS INCREASINGLY USED FOR THE GENERAL POPULATION?

To understand the epidemiologic and clinical observations that provide the background of this chapter, two issues must be clarified. The first is the natural history of adenocarcinoma of the prostate. The second is the anticipated consequences of early detection. With a clear understanding of these two issues, a series of expected observations can be anticipated.

The Natural History of Prostate Cancer

Before the 1980s, many an article was written on the rather innocuous natural history of prostate cancer. Many early series that included patients first diagnosed in the 1940s were notable for rapid development of metastases and death. One such example was that of Hanash and colleagues, the last patient of which was diagnosed in 1942 *(5)*. In this series, the authors reported 10-yr survivals for 50 and 129 patients with stage A and B disease, respectively. These 10-yr survivals of 52% and 4% (considerably different from today's experience) are almost certainly the result of the poor staging methods available at the time. Effectively, the only tools available for staging these patients were plain radiographs and physical examination. With only a DRE to identify "localized" prostate cancer and such poor staging modalities, it is little wonder that most of these patients probably had occult metastases and would be classified as D2 (or M+) today.

More recently, Chodak and colleagues conducted a meta-analysis of six series of patients with localized disease, constituting 828 patients who were followed with surveillance alone *(6)*. Unlike the earliest series, Chodak et al. found 10-yr disease-specific survival for well-differentiated and moderately-differentiated tumors to be 87%, whereas survival for poorly differentiated tumors was only 34% at the 10-yr mark. Of interest, anticipating subsequent studies, the authors found that 10-yr metastasis-free survivals for well-differentiated and moderately-differentiated and poorly differentiated tumors were 81%, 58%, and 26% respectively. As the median survival of patients with metastatic disease is approx. 2–3 yr, this final conclusion is a sobering observation suggesting that younger men with localized disease are at a very high risk of death from the disease.

Chodak et al's observation was recently supported by an independent study by Albertsen and colleagues who analyzed the results of observation for 767 men followed in the Connecticut Tumor Registry *(7)*. The authors published a series of very informative graphics that displayed a patient's risk of dying of prostate cancer or another cause at 5, 10, and 15 yr, based on the age of the patient at diagnosis and the grade of the tumor. (See Fig 3, Chapter 2.) Demonstrating that older men are at a lesser risk of dying from the disease, the authors found 5-, 10-, and 15-yr survivals of a 70 to 74 yr-old male with Gleason score 7 tumor were 60%, 24%, and 9%, respectively. The corresponding 5-, 10-, and 15-yr *disease-specific* survivals were 84%, 48%, and 60%, respectively. On the other hand, results for younger men were much less favorable, if treatment was not provided. A 55-59 year old man with a Gleason 2-4 score tumor was found to have 5, 10, and 15-year disease specific survivals of 98%, 96%, and 95%. The corresponding survivals of moderately differentiated tumors (Gleason 7) were 75%, 48%, and 30% while the survivals for poorly-differentiated tumors were 58%, 23%, and 14%, respectively.

With better staging, improved grading, and better follow-up of patients with localized prostate cancer, we now have tremendous insight into the natural history of the disease. Although patients with well-differentiated disease seem to be destined to "do well" almost regardless of treatment, these patients now constitute a very small fraction of newly diagnosed prostate cancers *(8,9)*. For the remainder of patients with moderately or poorly differentiated disease, their risk of disease progression, metastases, and death from the disease within a 10-year time frame is substantial.

Anticipated Results of a Program of Early Detection

Given the natural history of prostate cancer described, what then should be the results of the implementation of a program of early detection—especially a program based on prostate-specific antigen for detection? Fig. 1 helps us to understand the impact of such a program. The figure is a theoretical display of the natural history of prostate cancer, given a wide range of biologic tumor activities, and compares these with methods of detection. On the y-axis of the figure, it can be seen that the tumor would develop at a size that detection is not possible (microscopic, normal PSA). The tumor subsequently grows to such a size that the PSA is above the "normal level." Thereafter, with further growth, the tumor may ultimately become palpable. Increased growth then leads to extraprostatic disease, nodal metastases, bone metastases, and, ultimately, death from the disease. We have somewhat arbitrarily shaded an area of a range of tumor volumes at which the tumor is detectable and has not spread so far as to be incurable. (Ideally, tumor detection should occur within this range.) An abnormal DRE has been placed

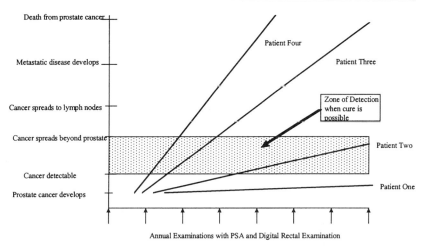

Fig. 1. Theoretical display of the natural history of prostate cancer.

outside the "window of cure" as we have previously demonstrated that over two-thirds of tumors detected with DRE alone are pathologically beyond the confines of the prostate *(3)*.

Given this paradigm, there are several growth rates of prostate tumors. Some may grow at such a slow rate as to never become detectable during the individual's life-span (Patient One). Indeed, autopsy series suggest that the majority of prostate tumors are of this variety, and reviews of tumors detected through screening suggest that early detection does not detect these indolent, well-differentiated, and microscopic tumors except under very rare circumstances *(10,11)*. A second form of tumor is one that is detected by virtue of an abnormal PSA or DRE (Patient Two). Although this tumor is generally of a larger volume, this hypothetical patient will ultimately die of another disease process without succumbing to prostate cancer. Such a patient does not benefit from screening or treatment. A third patient (Patient Three) is destined to die from prostate cancer if not diagnosed early. With serial screening examinations, he can be diagnosed while the disease is confined to the prostate and can be cured. Such a patient meets the criteria of Whitmore: Having a disease for which a cure is both *necessary and possible (12)*. A final, unusual, patient (Patient Four) has a rapidly growing tumor that is destined to cause his demise. Unfortunately, during annual examinations, the tumor is first undetectable, but in the interval between examinations, it grows to such an extent so as to be incurable at the next visit when it is detected. We have demonstrated that such a problem may occur when DRE alone is used for prostate cancer detection *(13,14)*.

This description of the methods of detection of prostate cancer and how early detection practices may affect different types of tumors helps us to predict what should happen over the course of time after proliferation of an *effective* screening test for prostate cancer—a test that ultimately affects mortality from the disease. Let us now examine what we would expect to occur with the proliferation of PSA testing.

Prior to the advent of PSA screening, two patterns of clinical activity were prevalent: (1) The only method of prostate cancer screening used employed DRE, a very insensitive screening test, and (2) very few men participated in prostate cancer screening. Since the advent of PSA screening, many men, indeed a majority of some socioeconomic groups, depending on patterns of screening, have had not just a PSA but *annual* PSA testing, a practice that has led to a dramatic change in the type of tumors detected in the United States. Before we observe what happened in the United States, let us consider what would be *expected* to occur, should an *effective* screening test be implemented before its efficacy was known. We shall hypothesize a series of observations that would be seen upon the proliferation of this test.

Phase One: Dramatic Increase in Incidence Rate. With the first proliferation of PSA testing, it would be expected that a large group of men with previously undiagnosed prostate cancer would be identified. From studies of serum banks, comparing men who ultimately developed prostate cancer to those who did not develop this disease, we know that an increase in the rate of increase in PSA occurs some 5 yr prior to the clinical diagnosis of the disease if symptoms intervene *(15)*. Before PSA screening, the only test available was DRE, a test that detected prostate cancer in only about 2% of men and, in these patients, detected them late. Thus, a tremendous number of men with early and locally advanced prostate cancers existed in the US population, all undiagnosed owing to a lack of symptoms. Thus, the first effect that should be seen with the proliferation of an *effective* screening test would be an increase in prostate cancer detection.

Phase Two: Initial Detection of Men with All Stages of the Disease. For a prostate cancer screening test to be ultimately effective, it must detect the disease long before extraprostatic spread developed. Unfortunately, many undiagnosed prostate cancers at the inception of PSA testing would be expected to be locally advanced or, as a minimum, of high volume, as these tumors would be diagnosed in men who previously had not undergone screening with a sensitive test. Few should exhibit metastatic disease, but a wide range of pathologic disease stages should be seen—all asymptomatic—but would include node-positive disease, extracapsular spread, and pathologically localized disease.

Phase Three: Stage Shift—Fall in Percentage and Number of Men with Advanced Disease. As men with pathologically advanced prostate cancer that had been present for many years were identified during the first few cycles of prostate cancer screening, it would be expected that men tested during subsequent years should be more likely to have disease confined to the prostate. Thus, after the first few years of prostate cancer screening, a significant stage shift should be recognized with not only a fall in the *percentage* of men with pathologically advanced disease but also a fall in the *absolute number* of men with such incurable disease.

Phase Four: Significant Fall in Prostate Cancer Incidence. As the fraction of men in the United States who underwent PSA screening increased and as the large numbers of those who had preexisting disease were identified, it would be expected that a fall in the number of men diagnosed with the disease would be seen. This fall in the number of men diagnosed should follow a dramatic increase in disease detection and, if PSA screening were widely practiced, should ultimately approach disease prevalence rates seen prior to the development of PSA or slightly greater because of a greater fraction of the disease detected with PSA than with DRE.

Phase Five: Decrease in Number of Men with Metastatic Disease. Assuming that the tumors detected by prostate cancer screening were clinically important and would have progressed to metastatic disease if not recognized and thereby left untreated, it would be expected that a fall in the number of men with metastatic disease would be the next observation in this natural experiment.

Phase Six: Initial Fall in Population Prostate Cancer Mortality. Following on the heels of a fall in the number of cases of metastatic disease, it would be expected that a fall in prostate cancer mortality would follow this event by 2–4 yr. Initially, a small reduction in prostate cancer mortality should be witnessed within 5–7 yr of the inception of screening. The men whose lives would be expected to be saved during this time frame would be the 10–20% of men with high-grade tumors in whom death resulting from the disease is frequently witnessed within 5–10 yr of diagnosis, if left untreated *(16)*. Additionally, the men who would benefit from this effect would only be those who actually underwent disease screening; those who did not would continue to present with high-stage disease and would not be expected to have any improvement in mortality.

Phase Seven: Continued fall in Mortality. Again, assuming that PSA screening effectively identified those men with prostate tumors destined to cause their demise and identified them soon enough for cure, after another 10–15 yr, a major reduction in prostate cancer mortality would thereafter be witnessed. As moderately and well-differentiated tumors detected during screening examinations, if otherwise not detected and treated, would cause death of the patient some 8–15 yr later, this continued fall in mortality should be expected for perhaps two decades after the initial proliferation of screening. As in Phase Six, we would never expect screening and treatment to prevent all deaths resulting from the disease as (1) no screening test can detect *all* tumors sufficiently early for cure and (2) not all men will participate in screening or would delay PSA testing until the disease is no longer curable.

The Alternative Scenario

Phases One through Seven speculate on what might occur with an *effective* prostate screening test if gradually disseminated across the United States. Two alternate hypotheses could be advanced. One is that the test is insensitive to prostate tumors, similar to the deficiencies of DRE, and that the test only detected tumors when the disease was too advanced to be treated effectively. In such a scenario, one would expect a different series of events, such as (1) an increased number of cases detected, (2) a similar stage distribution initially, (3) with time, no decrease in pathologically advanced disease, and (4) no change in mortality. Another possible result might be that the screening effort would detect only those tumors that were indolent and did not pose a threat to patient survival. If this hypothesis proved correct, the "natural experiment" would witness the following phases: (1) detection of an increased number of cases, (2) a lower-stage distribution (as a result of the detection of indolent disease), (3) no change in the absolute number of pathologically advanced tumors, (4) no fall in the number of cases of metastatic disease, and (5) ultimately, no change in mortality. Indeed, under these circumstances, mortality rates could actually increase because of the application of treatments (that have a small yet measurable mortality rate) to a disease of no consequence.

It is the contention of this chapter that the "natural experiment" of the dissemination of PSA screening has witnessed Phases One through Six outlined earlier. Phase Seven is anticipated in the next 5–10 yr. Specific, irrefutable documentation is available that provides evidence of these effects.

PHASE ONE: DRAMATIC INCREASE IN INCIDENCE RATE

The rise in prostate cancer incidence seen in the United States after the introduction of PSA was the greatest increase ever seen for any tumor at any organ site. In the SEER tumor registry system, disease incidence increased from 84.4/100,000 population to 163/100,000 population between the years 1984 and 1991. In some regions, such as Utah, the rate increased even higher—in Utah, reaching 236.2/100,000 in 1992 *(17)*.

An increase in prostate cancer incidence after the proliferation of PSA screening was not seen only in the United States and Canada but also has been seen in other countries that have adopted some degree of PSA screening. In Switzerland, where prostate cancer mortality rate was one of the highest in the world (20.3 deaths per 100,000 population annually), the introduction of early detection practices led to an increase in prostate cancer incidence from 33.1 per 100,000 in 1974 to 48.6 per 100,000 in 1994 *(18)*.

Somewhat of concern was that the types of tumors detected by PSA screening would be those of no consequence—the so-called "autopsy tumors." Evidence is growing that such is not the case and comes from several areas. The first was the observation that clinical T1c tumors (detected by PSA screening and with a normal DRE) were of similar volume and grade as clinical T2 tumors (those tumors with abnormal DRE). Additionally, growing evidence suggests that these tumors are of *lower* pathologic stage. [In the series of Ghavamian and colleagues, the rate of pT3 disease was 76% among T1c tumors compared to 54% among T2 tumors *(19)*.] Finally, an interesting observation has been made by our group and that of Schwartz. It appears that through PSA screening *in combination with the development of α-blockers and finasteride*, the majority of prostate cancers now diagnosed are those of the peripheral zone (PZ), and tumors of the transition zone (TZ) have all but disappeared as the number of transurethral resection of the prostate (TURPs) have fallen to all-time lows. Our group has demonstrated that these PZ tumors are almost two full Gleason score values greater than TZ tumors (6.2 vs 4.5) and both Sakr's group and our group have demonstrated that well-differentiated disease—a disease primarily of the TZ—has all but disappeared *(20,21)*.

Further evidence to support the concept that with the advent of PSA screening more biologically significant tumors were being detected comes from an analysis of the SEER database between 1973 and 1994. Perrotti and colleagues found that not only did high-grade (grade 3) tumors remain relatively constant, despite the dramatic increase in number of tumors detected after 1988 (grade 3 tumors comprised 24.4% of all tumors between 1980 and 1994 and 21.4% of all tumors between 1990 and 1994), but they were noted to be much more likely to be organ confined (and therefore *curable*) in the latter period (82.6% vs 66.9%, respectively) *(22)*.

PHASE TWO: INITIAL DETECTION OF MEN
WITH ALL STAGES OF THE DISEASE

Initial use of PSA for the detection of prostate cancer led to the "harvest" of a large number of men who had never undergone early detection in any fashion. As a result, some men were detected with levels in excess of 100 ng/mL in the first vist. Petros and Catalona's report in 1992 of the frequency of node-positive disease between 1983 and 1991 spans the time of introduction of PSA but gives insight into this effect (23). Although some 20–30% of patients prior to the advent of PSA were found to have nodal disease, Catalona's group found that nodal disease was found in 3.3%, 5.3%, and 9.7% of patients with stage A2, B1, and B2 disease, respectively (23). We subsequently found that rates were under 5% overall and that for patients who were found with PSA values in the low-elevated range, rates could be predicted to be lower than 2-3% (24).

PHASE THREE: STAGE SHIFT—FALL IN PERCENTAGE
AND NUMBER OF MEN WITH ADVANCED DISEASE

Results of the dramatic stage migration in prostate cancer after the inception of PSA screening can be found in many series from individual institutions and from population-based studies. Of the more important effects that should be sought is a desired decrease in the rate of pathologically advanced disease—disease that has a much greater likelihood of association with recurrence, progression, and death (25). The results from one of the largest prostate cancer screening programs is illustrative of the effect on the rate of locally advanced disease. Smith et al. reported on the results from Washington University in 10,248 volunteers who participated in annual PSA screening (26). Over a period of 4 yr, the rate of elevated PSA and the rate of cancer diagnosis fell precipitously. Pathologically advanced disease fell from 33% to 27% among this population.

The series of patients treated with radical prostatectomy at Stanford is also instructive of the results of PSA screening and the fall in pathologic stage (27). Between 1988 and 1996, a total of 896 patients underwent radical prostatectomy at Stanford. Most importantly, all prostate specimens were examined in the same manner by the same pathologist during this period. Notably, there were no changes over this period of time in the percentage of high-grade disease, preoperative PSA, and tumor volume. Germane to this discussion, the proportion of organ-confined tumors increased from 40% at the outset of the study period to 75% at the end of the period, seminal vesicle invasion decreased from 18% to 5%, and positive margins fell from 30% to 14%. All of these changes suggest that the PSA screening period continued to identify aggressive tumors but, through earlier diagnosis, identified these tumors sufficiently early so as to allow a greater likelihood of cure with treatment.

Whereas the general experience in the United States has been the largest series to demonstrate a fall in tumor stage, smaller but proportional to the population, a potentially larger experience in Austria has been reported from Tyrol *(28)*. In this region, PSA screening was provided to 21,079 volunteers, of whom 1618 (8%) were found to have an elevated PSA. One hundred ninety seven of these men were found to have prostate cancer and 135 underwent radical prostatectomy. Of these 135 men, 95 were found to have organ-confined disease. However, when analyzing the rates of pathologically advanced tumors diagnosed over the 5-yr period of screening, the authors found that the rate of pathologically advanced disease fell from 71.3% in 1993 to 34.3% in 1997.

It is important to recognize that the fall in pathologically advanced prostate tumors occurred as pathologic evaluation of radical prostatectomy specimens became much more sophisticated. Previously, prostatectomy specimens were sampled in a relatively haphazard fashion, allowing pathologically involved margins to go without being recognized. As pathologists became more sophisticated, the use of whole mounts with thin sectioning allowed a greater fraction of pathologically involved margins to be recognized *(29)*. Thus, despite this closer attention to margin and seminal vesicle status, it is truly impressive that pathologic T3 rates continue to fall.

PHASE FOUR: SIGNIFICANT FALL IN PROSTATE CANCER INCIDENCE

One of the first regions of the country to recognize the fall in prostate cancer incidence was the SEER registry in Connecticut. As one might expect, after men who were at the highest risk and who had never been subjected to as sensitive a screening test as PSA presented for evaluation and were diagnosed, these men were no longer at risk for incident disease. Thus, after an initial rise in incidence rates between 1988 and 1992, incidence rates fell significantly for men over age 64 *(30)*. Of interest is that, as of 1997, no decline had yet been witnessed for men under 65 yr of age, perhaps as a result of the slower rate of participation in PSA screening and the "annual entry" into the "screening age" of men in these group. In Utah, a state that witnessed one of the greatest increases in tumor incidence, the incidence rate peaked in 1992 at 236.2/ 100,000 population, and in the subsequent 2 years, it fell to 195/100,000 and 164/100,000 population *(31)*.

PHASE FIVE: FALL IN NUMBER OF MEN WITH METASTATIC DISEASE

A few registries in the United States have summarized their results with the diagnosis of metastatic prostate cancer before and after the inception of PSA screening, and the SEER surveillance system has provided an insight into the impact of PSA screening on the diagnosis of metastatic disease. The importance of this observation cannot be overstressed, as it is generally those men who are found to have metastatic disease at the time of initial prostate cancer diagnosis who are most likely to die of their disease. Smart summarized SEER data from 1973 and 1993 and found a significant fall in the number of men diagnosed with metastatic disease while also noting that the increase in prostate cancer incidence was primarily the result of an increased diagnosis of moderately differentiated and poorly differentiated disease while the frequency of diagnosis of well-differentiated disease was essentially unchanged *(32)*.

A similar observation was made in the Seattle–Puget Sound region. Newcomer and colleagues followed population diagnosis patterns and noted that prostate cancer incidence rose from 230/100,000 in 1984 to 486/100,000 in 1991 and thereafter declined back to 293/100,000 in 1994 *(33)*. The authors found that all stages of the disease followed the incidence trends except for metastatic disease which peaked in 1986 and thereafter *declined* by greater than 60%. An earlier fall in metastatic disease rates was identified in Detroit, where the fall was first appreciated in 1989*(34)*. Within the context of a randomized, prospective trial of prostate cancer screening, Labrie and colleagues compared the rate of metastatic disease detected in a group of men undergoing their first screening with the rate of metastases among men undergoing *subsequent* screening examinations *(35)*. The rate among initially examined men was 8% compared to 0.9% among follow-up examinations.

PHASE SIX: INITIAL FALL IN POPULATION PROSTATE CANCER MORTALITY

Probably the most accepted source of data testifying to a fall in prostate cancer mortality, beginning several years after the inception of prostate cancer screening, is from SEER of the National Cancer Institute. Through monitoring a 10–12% sample of the United States, this program can obtain relatively rapid insight into the changes in prostate cancer mortality. Through this program, it has been identified that a 6% fall in prostate cancer mortality has been witnessed over the first half of the 1990s with as much as a 12% fall among men under the age of 75 *(36)*.

An additional source, supporting the conclusions of the SEER program *vis à vis* the national fall in prostate cancer mortality, has been the National Cancer Database program of the American College of Surgeons and the American Cancer Society. Surveying data from 1114 hospitals and 103,979 patients diagnosed with prostate cancer in 1992 and from 1144 hospitals and 72,337 patients diagnosed in 1995, the NCDB program found that (1) the average age at diagnosis fell by almost 2 yr, (2) the proportion of patients diagnosed with prostate cancer who were African-Americans increased from 8.8% to 11.8%, and (3) the annual rate of fall in prostate cancer mortality has been approximately 1% per year since 1990 *(37)*.

One location where a population has been followed on a very careful basis is Olmsted County, MN–the home of the Mayo Clinic. There, Roberts and colleagues have tracked the changes in prostate cancer mortality before and after the onset of PSA screening. They recently described trends in prostate cancer mortality between 1980 and 1997 *(38)*. The authors found that age-adjusted mortality rates within this community increased initially from 25.8/100,000 men in 1980–1984 to 34/100,000 in 1989–1992. Subsequently, the authors found that these rates fell to 19.4/100,000 in the period 1993–1997. These changes reflected a 22% fall in mortality (with 95% confidence intervals of a 17% increase to a 49% fall).

Canada has witnessed a revolution in the diagnosis and treatment of prostate cancer in much the same manner as the United States PSA screening has grown in interest among both health care professionals and patients, perhaps due to the public education efforts in the U.S. that "spill over" the border. In Quebec, Meyer and colleagues analyzed the changes in mortality rates from prostate cancer between 1979 and 1996 *(39)*. They found that mortality rates increased until 1989, were stable between 1989 and 1995, and dropped thereafter by 15%. Incidence rates, as in the United States, rose steadily until 1993. Meyer's group continued this analysis for Canada as a whole and found that mortality fell by 9.6% between 1991 and 1996 *(40)*. As was witnessed in the United States, the mortality decline was seen for all age groups but was most pronounced among men under age 75.

Etzioni and colleagues have conducted a computer simulation model based on population-based PSA testing patterns, cancer detection rates, average lead time (the time by which diagnosis is advanced by screening), and projected decreased risk of death associated with early diagnosis of prostate cancer through PSA testing *(41)*. Using a relatively conservative estimate of the efficacy of prostate cancer screening from the PLCO screening study of the NIH, she and her colleagues anticipated that prostate cancer mortality *would have increased* after 1991 (during a period when mortality actually *decreased*) if a lead time (the time by which diagnosis is moved forward by screening) of 3 yr or less would be expected.

Using the PLCO estimates, the investigators found that other causes (other than the proliferation of PSA) may have been operational in the fall in prostate cancer mortality. Some have suggested that the reason for this effect may have been the stage shift toward higher-grade tumors using screening and the detection of tumors of clinical importance that, indeed, have rapid biologic growth rates.

Although a significant fall in mortality from prostate cancer has been seen from various areas of North America, this has not been witnessed in the US neighbor to the south–Mexico. In this country, where PSA screening is used for only a fraction of the population, the crude mortality rate rose from 3.16 per 100,000 to 6.75 per 100,000 between the years 1980 and 1995 *(42)*.

Obviously, if the early diagnosis of prostate cancer is to be effective in the reduction of mortality from prostate cancer, we must be assured that the treatment itself will cure the disease in those men who are diagnosed. There is a growing body of evidence that contemporary treatment, most notably radical prostatectomy, is an effective method to prevent a man with prostate cancer from dying of his disease. Catalona and colleagues reviewed a series of 1778 men who underwent radical prostatectomy, generally for PSA-detected prostate cancer, and found that cancer-specific survival at 7 yr was 96% *(43)*.

It is appropriate to mention the randomized, prospective study of screening among 46,193 men from Quebec City and the metropolitan area of Quebec conducted by Labrie and colleagues between 1988 and 1996 *(44)*. The authors prospectively offered screening to one group of individuals and, through telephone directories, identified another group for follow-up who were not offered screening. The authors subsequently analyzed these two groups, *not* on the basis of which of the two arms of the study to which they were randomized but based on whether they received screening. (It should be noted that the *proper* method of analysis is based on the *intent-to-treat* and, in this study, an intent-to-treat analysis revealed no benefit to screening.) An intriguing observation, however was that among the 38,056 men who ultimately were not screened, 137 deaths were recorded, whereas among the 8137 men who did undergo screening, only 5 deaths were noted. Because of the poor compliance of the two groups to the study "treatment" (screening or no screening), this study will not answer the screening question for most experts but will serve to "stir the fire" in the screening debate.

PHASE SEVEN: CONTINUED FALL IN MORTALITY

The seventh phase of the effect of PSA screening has not yet been witnessed as of the publication of this text. We have witnessed a 6%

overall reduction in prostate cancer mortality and a 12–15% fall in mortality among men under age 65. If, indeed, we witness the continued, durable effects of PSA screening and if this screening test is truly effective, we should expect that mortality should fall considerably over the next decade.

CONCLUSIONS

The data we have presented provide clear and compelling witness to the effectiveness of PSA screening in the "natural experiment" of its widespread adoption during the 1990s. Advances arising from ongoing clinical trials may alter our method of screening over the years to come. One such advance has been the suggestion that replacing DRE with a lower PSA cutpoint (3.0 ng/ml) will result in a decrease of detected cancers by 7.6% but will decrease the number of biopsies by 12% and result in a much simpler screening procedure *(45)*. Although clinical trials will be essential in the determination of which men benefit most from these efforts and in better estimating the degree of improvement in survival, it can be expected that these studies will confirm these results. Assuming that they do and that there will be a continued fall in mortality, the primary challenge facing the medical community and those public institutions and bodies entrusted with maintaining the health of the nation will be to ensure wide distribution of this knowledge and availability of screening and treatment to all men of the United States.

REFERENCES

1. Thompson IM, Zeidman EJ. (1991) Presentation and clinical course of patients ultimately succumbing to carcinoma of the prostate. *Scand J Urol Nephrol* 25:111.
2. Droller MJ. (1980) Adenocarcinoma of the prostate: an overview. *Urol Clin North Am* 7:579–581.
3. Thompson IM, Ernst JJ, Gangai MP, Spence CR. (1984) Adenocarcinoma of the prostate: Results of routine urological screening. *J Urol* 132:690.
4. Gohagan JK. Prorok PC. Kramer BS. Cornett JE. (1994) Prostate cancer screening in the prostate, lung, colorectal and ovarian cancer screening trial of the National Cancer Institute. *J Urol* 152(5 Pt 2):1905–1909.
5. Hanash KA, Utz DC, Cook EN, et al. (1972) Carcinoma of the prostate: a 15-year followup. *J Urol* 107:450–453.
6. Chodak GW, Thisted RA, Gerber GS, et al. (1994) Results of conservative management of clinically localized prostate cancer. *New Eng J Med* 330:242-248.
7. Albertsen PC, Hanley JA, Gleason DF, Barry MJ. (1998) Competing risk analysis of men aged 55 to 74 years at diagnosis managed conservatively for clinically localized prostate cancer. *JAMA* 280:975–980.
8. Schwartz KL, Grignon DJ, Sakr WA, Wood DP Jr. (1999) Prostate cancer histologic trends in the metropolitan Detroit area, 1982 to 1996. *Urology* 53(4):769–774.

9. Endrizzi J, Optenberg SA, Byers R, Thompson IM. The disappearance of the well-differentiated prostate cancer. Presented at the 1999 meeting of the American Association of Genitourinary Surgeons.

10. Sakr WA, Haas GP, Cassin BF, Pontes JE, Crissman JD. (1996) The frequency of carcinoma and intraepithelial neoplasia of the prostate in young male patients. *J of Urol* 150(2 Pt 1):379–385.

11. Dugan JA, Bostwick DG, Myers RP, Qian J, Bergstralh EJ, Oesterling JE. (1996) The definition and preoperative prediction of clinically insignificant prostate cancer. *JAMA.* 275(4):288–294.

12. Whitmore WF Jr. (1994) Localised prostatic cancer: management and detection issues. *Lancet.* 343(8908):1263–1267.

13. Gerber GS, Thompson IM, Thisted R, Chodak GW. (1993) Disease specific survival following routine prostate cancer screening by digital rectal examination. *JAMA* 269:61–64.

14. Thompson IM, Zeidman EJ. (1991) Presentation and clinical course of patients ultimately succumbing to carcinoma of the prostate. *Scand J Urol and Nephrol* 25:111.

15. Carter HB, Pearson JD, Metter JE, et al. (1992) Longitudinal evaluation of prostate-specific antigen levels in men with and without prostate disease. *JAMA.* 267:2215–2220.

16. Albertsen PC, Hanley JA, Gleason DF, Barry MJ. (1998) Competing risk analysis of men aged 55 to 74 years at diagnosis managed conservatively for clinically localized prostate cancer. *JAMA* 280:975–980.

17. Stephenson RA, Smart CR, Mineau GP, James BC, Janerich DT, Dibble RL. (1996) The fall in incidence of prostate carcinoma. On the down side of a prostate specific antigen induced peak in incidence—data from the Utah Cancer Registry. *Cancer* 77(7):1342–1348.

18. Levi F, La Vecchia C, Randimbison L, Erler G, Te VC, Franceschi S. (1998) Incidence, mortality and survival from prostate cancer in Vaud and Neuchatel, Switzerland, 1974-1994. *Ann Oncol*(1):31–35.

19. Ghavamian R, Blute ML, Bergstralh EJ, Slezak J, Zincke H. (1999) Comparison of clinically nonpalpable prostate-specific antigen-detected (cT1c) versus palpable (cT2) prostate cancers in patients undergoing radical retropubic prostatectomy. *Urology* (1):105–110.

20. Endrizzi J, Thompson IM, Optenberg SA. (1998) Disappearance of well-differentiated disease with the advent of PSA screening. 1998 Kimbrough Urological Seminar.

21. Schwartz KL, Grignon DJ, Sakr WA, Wood DP Jr. (1999) Prostate cancer histologic trends in the metropolitan Detroit area, 1982 to 1996. *Urology* (4):769–774.

22. Perrotti M, Rabbani F, Farkas A, Ward WS, Cummings KB. (1998) Trends in poorly differentiated prostate cancer 1973 to 1994: observations from the Surveillance, Epidemiology and End Results database. *J Urol* 160(3 Pt 1): 811–815.

23. Petros JA, Catalona WJ. (1992) Lower incidence of unsuspected lymph node metastases in 521 consecutive patients with clinically localized prostate cancer. *J Urol* 147(6):1574–1575.

24. Bishoff JT, Reyes A, Thompson IM, Harris MJ, St Clair SR, Gomella L, Butzin CA. (1995) Pelvic lymphadenectomy can be omitted in selected patients with carcinoma of the prostate: development of a system of patient selection. *Urology* 45(2):270–274.

25. Paulson DF, Moul JW, Walther PJ. (1990) Radical prostatectomy for clinical stage T1-2N0M0 prostatic adenocarcinoma: long-term results. *J Urol* 144(5): 1180–1184.
26. Smith DS, Catalona WJ, Herschman JD. (1996) Longitudinal screening for prostate cancer with prostate-specific antigen. *JAMA* 276(16):1309–1315.
27. Stamey TA, Donaldson AN, Yemoto CE, McNeal JE, Sozen S, Gill H. (1998) Histological and clinical findings in 896 consecutive prostates treated only with radical retropubic prostatectomy: epidemiologic significance of annual changes. *J Urol* 160(6 Pt 2):2412–2417.
28. Horninger W, Reissigl A, Rogatsch H, Volgger H, Studen M, Klocker H, Bartsch G. (1999) Prostate cancer screening in Tyrol, Austria: experience and results. *Eur Urol* 35(5-6):523–538.
29. Sakr WA, Grignon DJ. (1999) Prostate. Practice parameters, pathologic staging, and handling radical prostatectomy specimens. *Urol Clin North Am* 26(3):453–463.
30. Polednak AP. (1997) Trends in prostate carcinoma incidence in Connecticut (1988-1994) by age and race. *Cancer* ;79(1):99–103.
31. Stephenson RA, Smart CR, Mineau GP, James BC, Janerich DT, Dibble RL. (1996) The fall in incidence of prostate carcinoma. On the down side of a prostate specific antigen induced peak in incidence—data from the Utah Cancer Registry. *Cancer* 77(7):1342–1348
32. Smart CR. (1997) The results of prostate carcinoma screening in the U.S. as reflected in the surveillance, epidemiology, and end results program. *Cancer* 80(9):1835–1844.
33. Newcomer LM, Stanford JL, Blumenstein BA, Brawer MK. (1997) Temporal trends in rates of prostate cancer: declining incidence of advanced stage disease, 1974 to 1994. *J Urol* 158(4):1427–1430.
34. Schwartz KL, Severson RK, Gurney JG, Montie JE. (1996) Trends in the stage specific incidence of prostate carcinoma in the Detroit metropolitan area, 1973-1994. *Cancer* 78(6):1260–1266.
35. Labrie F, Candas B, Cusan L, Gomez JL, Diamond P, Suburu R, et al. (1996) Diagnosis of advanced or noncurable prostate cancer can be practically eliminated by prostate-specific antigen. *Urology* 47(2):212–217.
36. Mettlin CJ, Murphy GP. (1998) Why is the prostate cancer death rate declining in the United States? *Cancer* 82(2):249–251.
37. Mettlin CJ, Murphy GP, Rosenthal DS, Menck HR. (1998) The National Cancer Data Base report on prostate carcinoma after the peak in incidence rates in the U.S. The American College of Surgeons Commission on Cancer and the American Cancer Society. *Cancer* ;83(8):1679–1684.
38. Roberts RO, Bergstralh EJ, Katusic SK, Lieber MM, Jacobsen SJ. (1999) Decline in prostate cancer mortality from 1980 to 1997, and an update on incidence trends in Olmsted County, Minnesota. *J Urol* 161(2):529–533.
39. Meyer F, Moore L, Bairati I, Fradet Y. (1998) Quebec prostate cancer mortality dropped in 1996. *Cancer Prev Control* 2(4):163–166.
40. Meyer F, Moore L, Bairati I, Fradet Y (1999) Downward trend in prostate cancer mortality in Quebec and Canada. *J Urol* 161(4):1189–1191.
41. Etzioni R, Legler JM, Feuer EJ, Merrill RM, Cronin KA, Hankey BF. (1999) Cancer surveillance series: interpreting trends in prostate cancer—part III: Quantifying the link between population prostate-specific antigen testing and recent declines in prostate cancer mortality. *J Natl Cancer Inst* ;91(12):1033–1039.

42. Tovar-Guzman V, Hernandez-Giron C, Lopez-Rios O, Lazcano-Ponce EC (1999) Prostate cancer mortality trends in Mexico, 1980-1995. *Prostate* 39(1):23–27.
43. Catalona WJ, Smith DS. (1998) Cancer recurrence and survival rates after anatomic radical retropubic prostatectomy for prostate cancer: intermediate-term results. *J Urol* 160(6 Pt 2):2428–2434.
44. Labrie F, Candas B, Dupont A, Cusan L, Gomez JL, Suburu RE, Diamond P, Levesque J, Belanger A.(1999) Screening decreases prostate cancer death: first analysis of the 1988 Quebec prospective randomized controlled trial. *Prostate* 38(2):83–91.
45. Beemsterboer PM, Kranse R, de Koning HJ, Habbema JD, Schroder FH. (1999) Changing role of 3 screening modalities in the European randomized study of screening for prostate cancer (Rotterdam). *Int J Cancer* 84(4):437–441.

12 Prostate Cancer Screening
A Note of Caution

Otis W. Brawley, MD

CONTENTS

INTRODUCTION

The argument against prostate cancer screening is not really an argument against, but an argument for extreme caution in its advocacy. It is a fact that screening *may* save lives, but it is also a fact that screening has not been proven to save lives and that there are some definite harms associated with screening. Although it is often emphasized that many medical experts believe screening and treatment of early-stage disease saves lives, rarely is it emphasized that the definitive studies of prostate cancer screening have not been done. Indeed, it is important that phy-

Statements made are those of the author and should not be implied as the official policies of the National Cancer Institute or the Department of Health and Human Services.

From: *Current Clinical Urology: Prostate Cancer Screening*
Edited by: I. M. Thompson, M. I. Resnick, and E. A. Klein
© Humana Press Inc., Totowa, NJ

sicians and advocates for screening realize that most expert organizations (American and foreign) that publish cancer screening recommendations have taken a position against recommending prostate cancer screening until the definitive studies are completed *(1–3)*. A few organizations have advocated that men be informed of the potential risks and potential benefits and be allowed to make a choice *(4,5)*. Over-enthusiasm for screening actually raises serious ethical and moral questions *(6–8)*.

It is important to recognize that there is scientific evidence to suggest that prostate cancer screening is beneficial. American prostate cancer rates have changed dramatically over the past 15 yr, in which screening has been widely available. Most notably, there is a 16% decline in mortality from 1991 to 1997 for men age 50 yr and older *(9)*. There has also been an increase in the proportion of localized cancers at diagnosis; a decrease in the incidence of distant cancers at diagnosis and prostate-cancer-specific survival after diagnosis has increased *(10,11)*.

These findings are not definitive evidence that screening saves lives. The most definitive evidence that screening saves lives is through a well-designed and well-analyzed randomized clinical trial *(12)*.

In the annals of medicine, there have been cancers for which the evidence supporting screening was as strong as it currently is for prostate cancer, but, ultimately, randomized clinical trials demonstrated that these screening techniques did not decrease the cancer-specific mortality rate *(13,14)*. Even if screening decreases mortality, it is possible that the morbidities associated with screening and treatment might be so great that screening is simply not reasonable.

Through the study of prostate cancer epidemiologic trends and the application of the principles of cancer screening, it is possible to see that the positive data supporting screening is by no means definitive and the efficacy of screening is a legitimate question *(15)*.

The decline in prostate-cancer-specific mortality among Americans is often cited as reason for screening to continue. The decline actually began within 2 yr of screening becoming popular *(16)*. This is likely too soon for the decline to be the result of screening and treatment of localized disease *(17)*. The decline in mortality might be attributable to artifact or it might be attributable to the changing use of hormonal therapy. The cause of the decline is an open question and it is premature to attribute it to screening and treatment of localized prostate cancer.

THE PRINCIPLES OF SCREENING

Screening can produce a shift in stage and an increase in survival without reducing mortality. An increase in cancer survival can be the result of *lead-time bias (12)*. *Lead-time bias* occurs when the patient is diagnosed earlier and treatment does not impact on the natural history of the disease, meaning the patient does not live longer. When lead-time bias occurs, the screening test only prolongs the time the subject is aware of the disease.

Length bias occurs when slower growing, less aggressive cancers are detected during screening. It has been noted in a number of cancers that those diagnosed as a result of the onset of symptoms between scheduled screenings are generally more aggressive and treatment outcomes are less favorable *(18)*. Overdiagnosis which is also referred to as "detection of pseudodisease," is an extreme form of length bias. Overdiagnosis occurs when disease is detected, diagnosed and treated that would not have caused death if never detected, diagnosed, or treated.

When length bias and overdiagnosis are significant factors in a screened population, a large number of cured individuals exist who did not need to be cured *(19)*. This will artifactually increase cancer specific survival. The affect of lead-time bias and length bias can be minimized in a randomized clinical trial assessed by intention to screen.

In the United States, lung cancer screening was widely advocated from the early 1950s into the mid-1970s *(13,14)*. Arguments for lung cancer screening and against a clinical trial to assess it included findings that there was an increase in the proportion of localized disease at diagnosis, a decrease in the amount of distant disease at diagnosis, and an increase in survival. Four clinical trials were eventually completed *(20,21)*. These trials all confirmed that screening found more localized disease that could be surgically treated and that those screened and diagnosed had an increase in lung cancer survival. Importantly, there was no improvement in mortality. Indeed, in two of four randomized trials of screening vs no screening, there was a small but statistically insignificant increase in mortality in the screened populations when compared to the control populations.

Similar data have been observed in screening for neuroblastoma in children with a urine test for vanillylmandilic acid *(22,23)*. Both lung and neuroblastoma screening led to increased numbers of cancers diagnosed at a stage more amiable to surgical intervention. The number of surgical procedures increased in both diseases, but the mortality rates were not positively affected.

THE SCREENING PRINCIPLES AND CLINICAL DATA

There is evidence that lead-time bias exists in prostate cancer screening. Among prostate cancer patients, a number of men detected early and treated with radical prostatectomy for presumed localized disease ultimately relapsed by prostate specific antigen (PSA) meaning they had extraprostatic disease *(24,25)*. These men may be victims of lead-time bias. These studies also demonstrate that the reported decline in distant disease at diagnosis may not be as significant as it appears at first glance.

Studies also provide evidence of length bias and overdiagnosis among men with prostate cancer. Many T1C prostate cancers found at autopsy in men dying of noncancer related causes actually fulfill histologic and size criteria for clinically significant disease, but are obviously not clinically significant *(26)*. Cystoprostatectomy specimens from men with bladder cancer also demonstrate that the reservoir of undetected slow-growing tumors is large. Half of all American men diagnosed with prostate cancer are 71 yr of age or older and over 80% are 65 or older *(17)*. This is a population for which competing causes of death, especially cardiovascular disease are significant. Many prostate tumors that would be clinically relevant to younger or healthy men are not clinically significant to older men.

In a case series of men treated for diagnosed prostate cancer, pathologists estimated that 15% of men with T1C stage cancers had tumors that did not fulfill histologic criteria for clinically significant prostate cancer *(27)*. In other words, pathologists looking at a group of men diagnosed through screening and treated with radical prostatectomy believe that at least one in seven received unnecessary treatment based on histologic criteria for malignancy and aggressiveness. Given the additional considerations of competing causes of death in an elderly population, this is likely to be a minimum proportion rather than maximum proportion *(27,28)*.

Case series of men diagnosed with clinically localized prostate cancer and treated with observation demonstrate that a number of diagnosed tumors do not need definitive therapy *(19)*. In a Swedish study of men diagnosed with clinically stage A and B prostate cancer and observed, only 8.5% of patients were dead after 10 yr of follow-up and only 15% of the deaths in the series were the result of prostate cancer. In a series of 50 patients diagnosed and treated with observation, Adolfsson *(29)* reported that 12% of men with stage C disease at diagnosis had died at 5 yr and 30% at 9 yr.

Epidemiologic data also demonstrate that cancer makes screening very prone to lead-time bias and length bias (including overdiagnosis). Prostate cancer survival rates in Sweden increased dramatically from 1960 to the early 1980s as methods of diagnosis changed. Through analysis of incidence and mortality, the investigators estimate that at least one-third of cancers diagnosed in 1980–1984 were of the nonlethal type if all cancers diagnosed from 1960–1964 were of the lethal type.

Prostate cancer screening is relatively uncommon in Europe. Despite consistently higher incidence rates in the United States with a more recent dramatic rise and fall in incidence compared to the United Kingdom, mortality rates are extremely similar from the 1960s to the 1990s *(30)*. This again suggests that screening in the U.S. is diagnosing a group of men whose tumors are not clinically significant to the individual man. Even within United States cancer registries, there are highly variable age-adjusted incidence rates among white males and the registries have strikingly similar age-adjusted mortality rates *(15)*. The varying incidence rates have been attributed to varying rates of screening. The fact that these registries have similar mortality rates again suggests that there is length bias.

THE UNCERTAIN EFFECTIVENESS OF THERAPY FOR LOCALIZED PROSTATE CANCER

Screening cannot decrease mortality unless treatment of localized disease prolongs lives or prevents death. Two separate reviews of the medical-outcomes literature have found that the literature is inadequate to make valid comparisons of treatment of localized prostate cancer *(31,32)*. Unfortunately, the status of the prostate cancer-treatment literature is such that a large number have weak study designs, allowing biases affecting choice of treatment and patient selection. Only one small randomized prospective trial—assessing radical prostatectomy—has been completed. This trial involved 111 men with early-stage prostate cancer randomized to radical prostatectomy and placebo vs placebo alone. This trial, of small size and low power, showed a statistically indistinguishable life expectancy in both arms *(33)*.

The uncertainty about the efficacy of treatment of localized prostate cancer has led to varied patterns of cancer care in the United States. There is a 20-fold difference in prostatectomy rates per 100,000 among states in the United States. Rhode Island and Alaska have very differing prostatectomy rates and even with such a varied rate of treatment, the age-adjusted mortality rates for white males are very similar *(34,35)*.

The effectiveness of radical prostatectomy in localized disease is being addressed in a major national trial *(36)*. The Prostate Intervention Versus Observation Trial began in 1993. It compares radical prostatectomy to palliative expectant management for clinically localized prostate cancer. The study will enroll approx 1200 men and is expected to have a 90% power to detect a 15% reduction in all-cause mortality. Similar trials are underway in Europe.

THE ADVERSE CONSEQUENCES OF TREATMENT

The enthusiasm for screening stems from the hope that it will decrease the suffering from advanced prostate cancer. Screening and subsequent treatment, however, definitely cause considerable morbidity. Those who are treated are at risk for the morbidities of therapy, including those who are cured unnecessarily and those who need to be cured but cannot be with current therapy. These men experience all the morbidities of local therapy but none of the benefits. Many actually experience them sooner, and for a longer time, because screening advances the date of diagnosis without extending the life span. A study of Medicare beneficiaries treated with radical prostatectomy from 1985 to 1991 found that less than 60% had pathologically organ-confined disease *(25)*. More than one-third were administered additional therapy within 5 yr after surgery. Even in men with pathologically confined cancer, the cumulative incidence of additional prostate cancer treatment 5 yr after radical prostatectomy was 25%.

Ironically, the morbidities of prostate cancer treatment are better defined than the efficacy of the treatment *(37,38)*. Both radical prostatectomy and external beam radiation have been linked to sexual dysfunction (primarily impotence), rectal injury, urinary incontinence and urethral stricture. A review of the medical literature concerning outcomes in men treated for localized prostate cancer found that up to 60% have complete impotence and an additional 30% may have some sexual dysfunction. There were rectal injury rates of 1–3%, urinary incontinence rates of up to 30% and urethral stricture rates of 8–18%. Morbidity from radiation therapy was at the lower range compared to surgery *(39,38)*. Morbidity is a very subjective factor, and patient-reported morbidities from surveys are substantially higher than physician-reported morbidity rates. It is not at all clear that the nerve-sparing prostatectomy procedure has improved the overall self-reported rates of sexual dysfunction and urinary dysfunction (37,40).

In a study of Medicare beneficiaries treated with radical prostatectomy, the surgical mortality rate was 2%, and 8% suffered major cardiopulmonary complications after surgery *(25)*. Some series published by individual surgeons have reported death rates of less than 0.5%. These results are likely the result of patient selection and the surgeon's skill. Medicare studies include only men aged 65 and over; however, this age group does include more than 80% of all men with prostate cancer. In all fairness, it should be noted that prostatectomy-related morbidity may be declining *(41)*.

THE ECONOMIC COSTS OF SCREENING

It has been estimated that prostate cancer screening could add up to $26 billion per year in health-care costs. This is a substantial portion of America's healthcare expenditure *(42–44)*. If screening saves lives, it is the author's belief that the cost is well worth it, but it would be a shame if known effective medical procedures such as smoking cessation or screening mammography were sacrificed to pay for a procedure that does not work.

DETERMINING THE EFFECTIVENESS OF SCREENING

Screening is a public health intervention intended to cause a decline in mortality *(44)*. The ability to detect disease does not mean that a screening test is effective in decreasing mortality. Ultimately, the effectiveness of screening can only be determined through well-designed properly analyzed clinical screening studies. Such a trial must be randomized and analyzed by intention (i.e., as randomized) with a mortality end point. Such a trial as was done in lung cancer screening with chest X-ray and sputum cytology would minimize many of the biases of screening.

No such randomized clinical trial in prostate cancer screening has been completed. A randomized trial of prostate cancer screening began in the United States in 1993 *(45)*. The Prostate, Lung, Colon, and Ovarian Cancer Screening Trial is enrolling 74,000 men and women. The men are randomized to annual screening with serum PSA and digital rectal examination (DRE) or usual care. Several other screening trials are underway in Europe *(20,46)*.

Recently, LaBrie and colleagues *(46)* published results of a trial that some believed answered the screening question. However, this study has significant weaknesses in design and analysis. It was prone to bias by not being truly randomized and was not analyzed on the basis of intention-to-screen. Indeed, when the data were analyzed by intention-to-screen, the relative risk of death from prostate cancer in the screened group was 1.16 times greater than the control group (Dr. Peter Boyle, unpublished data). This trial and the findings of its subsequent analysis demonstrate the complexity of the prostate-cancer-screening question.

Comparison of long-term prostate cancer mortality rates of screened populations to similar populations that have not been screened may provide some clues as to the effectiveness of screening. Such ecologic studies are not nearly as definitive as a randomized trial and can be very difficult to interpret, as the two populations may have multiple differences.

CONCLUSION

The current state of knowledge does not permit a truly informed decision with regard to routine prostate cancer screening and subsequent treatment. Whether screening saves lives is a real question that desperately needs to be answered. This disease is very prone to lead-time bias, length bias, and overdiagnosis, and there is substantial debate among experts as to whether prostate cancer screening saves lives. Some experts are concerned that prostate cancer screening, more than screening for other cancers, may cause net harm. Professional organizations taking a skeptical view of prostate cancer screening include the US Preventive Services Task Force, the American College of Physicians, and the Canadian Task Force on the Periodic Health Examination *(1,3,46,48,49)*.

Whereas there is reason to believe and hope that screening saves lives, overenthusiasm and lack of understanding of the complexities of screening can lead to misinformation and mislead the patients we serve. Prostate cancer screening clearly detects many asymptomatic cancers, but the ability to reliably distinguish tumors that are lethal, but still curable, from those that are of little or no threat to health is limited. No well-designed trial has been completed to test the true benefit of prostate cancer screening and treatment, but trials are in progress. While results of these trials are pending, health professionals should inform each man about the current state of knowledge, detail the known risks and theoretical benefits, encourage participation in clinical trials whenever possible, and reassure him that, for now, there is no-clear cut right or wrong choice regarding the individual decision to be screened or not.

REFERENCES

1. Rose VL. (1997) ACP issues guidelines on the early detection of prostate cancer and screening for prostate cancer. *Am Fam Physician* 56:1674–1675.
2. Woolf SH. (1997) Should we screen for prostate cancer? *Br Med J* 314:989-990.
3. Denis LJ, Murphy GP, Schroder FH. (1995) Report of the consensus workshop on screening and global strategy for prostate cancer. *Cancer* 75:1187–1207.
4. Brown V. (1996) Informed consent for PSA testing. *J Fam Pract* 43:234–235.
5. Review of current data impacting early detection guidelines for prostate cancer. Proceedings of an American Cancer Society workshop. Phoenix, Arizona, March 10–11, 1997. *Cancer* 80:1808–1881.
6. Taube A. (1996) Screening with PSA (prostate specific antigen) raises ethical questions. *Lakartidningen* 93:3341.
7. Glode LM. (1994) Prostate cancer screening: a place for informed consent? *Hosp Pract* (Off. Ed.) 29:8, 11–8, 12.

8. Mandelson MT, Wagner EH, Thompson RS. (1995) PSA screening: a public health dilemma. *Annu Rev Public Health* 16:283–306:283–306.
9. Tarone R, Chu K, Brawley OW. (2000) Implications of Stage-Specific Survival Rates in Asssessing Recent Declines in Prostate Cancer Mortality Rates. *Epidemiology* 11:1–5.
10. Feuer EJ, Merrill RM, Hankey BF. (1999) Cancer surveillance series: interpreting trends in prostate cancer—part II: Cause of death misclassification and the recent rise and fall in prostate cancer mortality. *J Natl Cancer Inst* 91:1025–1032.
11. Hankey BF, Feuer EJ, Clegg LX, Hayes RB, Legler JM, Prorok PC, et al. (1999) Cancer surveillance series: interpreting trends in prostate cancer—part I: Evidence of the effects of screening in recent prostate cancer incidence, mortality, and survival rates. *J Natl Cancer Inst* 91:1017–1024.
12. Kramer BS, Brown ML, Prorok PC, Potosky AL, Gohagan JK. (1993) Prostate cancer screening: what we know and what we need to know. *Ann Intern Med* 119:914–923.
13. Eddy DM. (1989) Screening for lung cancer. *Ann Intern Med* 111:232–237.
14. Collins MM, Barry MJ (1996) Controversies in prostate cancer screening. Analogies to the early lung cancer screening debate. *JAMA* 276:1976–1979.
15. Brawley OW. (1997) Prostate carcinoma incidence and patient mortality: the effects of screening and early detection. *Cancer* 80:1857–1863.
16. Legler JM, Feuer EJ, Potosky AL, Merrill RM, Kramer BS. (1998) The role of prostate-specific antigen (PSA) testing in the recent prostate cancer incidence decline in the U.S.A. *Cancer Causes Control* 9:519–527.
17. Feuer EJ, Merrill RM, Hankey BF. (1999) Cancer surveillance series: interpreting trends in prostate cancer—part II: Cause of death misclassification and the recent rise and fall in prostate cancer mortality. *J Natl Cancer Inst* 91:1025–1032.
18. Gerber GS, Thisted R, Chodak GW, Thompson IM. (1993) Disease-specific survival following routine prostate cancer screening by digital rectal examination: corrected patient classification. *JAMA* 270:2437.
19. Chodak GW, Thisted RA, Gerber GS, Johansson JE, Adolfsson J, Jones GW, et al. (1994) Results of conservative management of clinically localized prostate cancer. *N Engl J Med* 330:242–248.
20. Fontana RS, Sanderson DR, Woolner LB, Taylor WF, Miller WE, Muhm JR. (1986) Lung cancer screening: the Mayo program. *J Occup Med* 28:746–750.
21. Petty TL (1997) Is prostate cancer screening analogous to lung cancer screening?. *JAMA* 277:1120–1121.
22. Philip T. (1999) Early detection of neuroblastoma in infants: Research? Yes. Routine Screening? *No Med Pediatr Oncol* 33:355–356.
23. Ajiki W, Tsukuma H, Oshima A, Kawa K. (1998) Effects of mass screening for neuroblastoma on incidence, mortality, and survival rates in Osaka, Japan. *Cancer Causes Control* 9:631–636.
24. Lu-Yao GL, Potosky AL, Albertsen PC, Wasson JH, Barry MJ, Wennberg JE. (1996) Follow-up prostate cancer treatments after radical prostatectomy: a population-based study. *J Natl Cancer Inst* 88:166–173.
25. Fowler FJJ, Barry MJ, Lu-Yao G, Roman A, Wasson J, Wennberg JE. (1993) Patient-reported complications and follow-up treatment after radical prostatectomy. The National Medicare Experience: 1988-1990 (updated June 1993). *Urology* 42:622–629.

26. Albertsen PC. (1996) Defining clinically significant prostate cancer: pathologic criteria versus outcomes data . *J Natl Cancer Inst* 88:1177–1178.

27. Hoedemaeker RF, Rietbergen JB, Kranse R, van der Kwast TH, Schroder FH. (1997) Comparison of pathologic characteristics of T1c and non-T1c cancers detected in a population-based screening study, the European Randomized Study of Screening for Prostate Cancer. *World J Urol* 15:339–345.

28. Albertsen PC. (1996) Defining clinically significant prostate cancer: pathologic criteria versus outcomes data. *J Natl Cancer Inst* 88:1177–1178.

29. Adolfsson J. (1993) Deferred treatment of low grade stage T3 prostate cancer without distant metastases. *J Urol* 149:326–328.

30. Shibata A, Ma J, Whittemore AS. (1998) Prostate cancer incidence and mortality in the United States and the United Kingdom. *J Natl Cancer Inst* 90:1230–1231.

31. Wasson JH, Cushman CC, Bruskewitz RC, Littenberg B, Mulley AGJ, Wennberg JE. (1993) A structured literature review of treatment for localized prostate cancer. Prostate Disease Patient Outcome Research Team. *Arch Fam Med* 2:487–493; erratum: *Arch Fam Med* 2(10):1030 (1993).

32. Middleton RG, Thompson IM, Austenfeld MS, Cooner WH, Correa RJ, Gibbons RP, et al. (1995) Prostate Cancer Clinical Guidelines Panel Summary report on the management of clinically localized prostate cancer. The American Urological Association. *J Urol* 154:2144–2148.

33. Graversen PH, Nielsen KT, Gasser TC, Corle DK, Madsen PO. (1990) Radical prostatectomy versus expectant primary treatment in stages I and II prostatic cancer. A fifteen-year follow-up. *Urology* 36:493–498.

34. Lu-Yao GL, McLerran D, Wasson J, Wennberg JE. (1993) An assessment of radical prostatectomy. Time trends, geographic variation, and outcomes. The Prostate Patient Outcomes Research Team . *JAMA* 269:2633–2636.

35. Lu-Yao GL, Greenberg ER. (1994) Changes in prostate cancer incidence and treatment in USA. *Lancet* 343:251–254.

36. Moon TD, Brawer MK, Wilt TJ. (1995) Prostate Intervention Versus Observation Trial (PIVOT): a randomized trial comparing radical prostatectomy with palliative expectant management for treatment of clinically localized prostate cancer. PIVOT Planning Committee. *J Natl Cancer Inst Monogr* 69–71.

37. Litwin MS, Hays RD, Fink A, Ganz PA, Leake B, Leach GE, et al. (1995) Quality-of-life outcomes in men treated for localized prostate cancer. *JAMA* 273:129–135.

38. Stanford JL, Feng Z, Hamilton AS, Gilliland FD, Stephenson RA, Eley JW, et al. (2000) Urinary and sexual function after radical prostatectomy for clinically localized prostate cancer: the Prostate Cancer Outcomes Study. *JAMA* 283:354–360.

39. Jonler M, Ritter MA, Brinkmann R, Messing EM, Rhodes PR, Bruskewitz RC. (1994) Sequelae of definitive radiation therapy for prostate cancer localized to the pelvis. *Urology* 44:876–882.

40. Demers RY, Swanson GM, Weiss LK, Kau TY. (1994) Increasing incidence of cancer of the prostate. The experience of black and white men in the Detroit metropolitan area. *Arch Intern Med* 154:1211–1216.

41. Thompson IM, Middleton RG, Optenberg SA, Austenfeld MS, Smalley SR, Cooner WH, et al. (1999) Have complication rates decreased after treatment for localized prostate cancer? *J Urol* 162:107–112.

42. Lubke WL, Optenberg SA, Thompson IM. (1994) Analysis of the first-year cost of a prostate cancer screening and treatment program in the United States. *J Natl Cancer Inst* 86:1790–1792.

43. Optenberg SA, Thompson IM. (1990) Economics of screening for carcinoma of the prostate. *Urol Clin North Am* 17:719–737.

44. Woolf SH. (1994) Public health perspective: the health policy implications of screening for prostate cancer. *J Urol* 152:1685–1688.

45. Gohagan JK, Prorok PC, Kramer BS, Cornett JE. (1994) Prostate cancer screening in the prostate, lung, colorectal and ovarian cancer screening trial of the National Cancer Institute. *J Urol* 152:1905–1909.

46. Shroder FH, Damhuis RA, Kirkels WJ, De Koning HJ, Kranse R, Nus HG, et al. (1996) European randomized study of screening for prostate cancer—the Rotterdam pilot studies. *Int J Cancer* 65:145–151.

47. Labrie F, Candas B, Dupont A, Cusan L, Gomez JL, Suburu RE, et al. (1999) Screening decreases prostate cancer death: first analysis of the 1988 Quebec prospective randomized controlled trial. *Prostate* 38:83–91.

48. Woolf SH. (1997) Should we screen for prostate cancer? *Br Med J* 314:989–990.

49. Ramsey EW. (1994) Early detection of prostate cancer. Recommendations from the Canadian Urological Association. *Can J Oncol* 4 (Suppl1):82–5;82–85.

13 Quality of Life and Health Behavior in Prostate Cancer Screening Populations

Mark S. Litwin, MD, MPH
and Kristen A. Reid, BA

CONTENTS

INTRODUCTION

The controversy surrounding prostate cancer screening divides experts and practicing clinicians into believers and nonbelievers. Those in favor of screening argue that it leads to early diagnosis, which saves lives through early intervention. The validity of this argument is grounded in the observation that advanced disease is incurable and kills many patients each year. Indeed, it is the second leading cause of cancer death in American men. Those opposed to screening ardently contend that it is plagued by too many deficiencies, such as lead-time bias and length bias, to be recommended routinely. This argument is bolstered by the idea that any potential gains in survival are canceled out by quality-of-life impairments that may result from aggressive treatment *(1)*.

From: *Current Clinical Urology: Prostate Cancer Screening*
Edited by: I. M. Thompson, M. I. Resnick, and E. A. Klein
© Humana Press Inc., Totowa, NJ

Patients who have spoken out on the issue tend to be those who have individually benefited from screening, early diagnosis, and curative therapy that has proceeded without complications. They are generally satisfied with their care *(2)* and appreciative of the screening effort *(3)*. Occasionally, individual patients have also reported on unhappy outcomes of early intervention for screen-detected tumors *(4)*. In general, the debate centers on the ultimate impact of diagnosis and treatment on quantity and quality of life. Despite the controversy and the recommendations of many preventive medicine organizations, prostate cancer screening is occurring with great frequency and significant cost to health care systems throughout the world *(5)*. It remains unknown whether or not prostate cancer screening is worthwhile *(6)*.

Typically absent from this rhetoric is the impact of screening itself on men at risk for prostate cancer. In fact, screening decisions may themselves have a substantial effect on various aspects of quality of life, irrespective of whether prostate cancer is diagnosed. Prostate cancer screening typically includes measurement of the serum prostate specific antigen (PSA) level and palpation of the prostate by digital rectal examination (DRE). It may also include performance of transrectal ultrasound and obtaining tissue samples through prostate needle biopsies. Prostate cancer screening has the potential to cause anxiety, discomfort, and medical complications. It may also provide reassurance with negative findings or early diagnosis of malignancies that would otherwise have remained undetected. Screening is an example of secondary prevention, a public health approach designed to diagnose disease at an earlier and potentially more curable stage *(7)*. The impact of prostate cancer screening on patient-centered medical outcomes may be considered in two components: quality of life and health behaviors.

Health-related quality of life (HRQOL) comprises a set of measurable variables, now commonly studied under the umbrella of medical outcomes research. It is assessed with questionnaires, often called instruments, that contain items, which are combined into scales to measure various domains of quality of life. HRQOL instruments provide scores that are usually converted into ranges of 0–100, with higher values representing better outcomes. HRQOL instruments must be demonstrated to have important psychometric properties such as reliability, validity, responsiveness, and ease of use. In prostate cancer patients, HRQOL assessment should include general domains, such as physical, emotional, and role function, as well as disease-specific domains, such as urinary, sexual, and bowel impairment *(8,9)*. HRQOL data are best when gathered with written, self-administered instruments and analyzed by objective third parties rather than by the treating physician

(10). Data should be collected at baseline before treatment, then longitudinally over time to detect changes *(11,12).* HRQOL results should be interpreted in the context of what is normal for older men without prostate cancer *(13).* Contemporary interpretations of HRQOL are based on the World Health Organization's 1948 definition of health as not merely the absence of disease but a state of physical, emotional, and spiritual well-being *(14).*

The Health Belief Model, popularized in the 1970s *(15),* maintains that health care decisions may be viewed in terms of knowledge, attitudes, and behaviors. Each of these components may be separately affected by a variety of inputs, such as education, literacy, social or demographic factors, personality, personal/family and community experience, and intervention programs. Although related, health knowledge and health attitudes are independent of each other and may or may not lead to particular health behaviors. Health knowledge and attitudes are also measured with survey instruments. Although they, too, should ideally adhere to the principles of psychometric validation, knowledge and attitude questionnaires are often developed and fielded with somewhat less rigorous techniques.

HEALTH-RELATED QUALITY OF LIFE

Few published studies have attempted to collect and analyze HRQOL data in men undergoing prostate cancer screening. In the Rotterdam Screening Trial for Prostate Cancer, investigators have undertaken a comprehensive quality-of-life evaluation of participants in a large, population-based screening program in Europe. Their goal is to measure the effect of screening on quality of life, using rigorous methodology and established instruments, such as the RAND Medical Outcomes Study 36-Item Health Survey (SF-36) *(16)* and the State-Trait Anxiety Inventory (STAI) *(17).* They recently reported on a longitudinal study of 626 men in the screening program and compared them to 500 unselected non-participants *(18).* Over time, they demonstrated significant but very small decrements in several quality-of-life domains, most notably a 4.2 point worsening (scale range, 0–100) on the bodily pain scale of the SF-36 and a 3.7 point worsening (scale range, 20–80) on the state anxiety scale of the STAI. At the group level, they did not find evidence that screening caused clinically meaningful short-term changes in health status, despite pain associated with the prostate biopsy and anxiety associated with awaiting the results. No substantial quality-of-life differences were seen when comparing screened and unscreened men. They concluded that any significant quality-of-life impairments that result from prostate cancer screening must occur in the posttreatment phase.

In a similar but more biochemically oriented study, Gustafsson and colleagues *(19)* measured anxiety in men screened for prostate cancer. In an innovative approach, they used questionnaires, such as the Sleep Disturbance Index (SDI) *(20)*, to measure psychological reactions and serum cortisol levels to measure physiological stress responses *(21)*. In randomly selected Swedish subjects, they found that screening itself caused mean serum cortisol elevations of more than 30 nmol/L compared with population-based controls (479 vs 447 nmol/L). The authors added context by noting that in prison guards, a particularly stressful occupation, mean serum cortisol levels have been reported at 504 nmol/L *(22)*. In their study population, the highest cortisol levels were seen in postbiopsy subjects 2 wk after screening and immediately prior to learning the biopsy results (496 nmol/L). Measured changes in anxiety and sleep disturbance were minimal, except in men whose biopsies were positive for prostate cancer.

In a project known as the Prostate Cancer Risk Assessment Program (PRAP), investigators at Fox Chase Cancer Center have begun to collect longitudinal data on quality of life, risk perception, and screening behavior among men at high risk for prostate cancer. Using a biopsychosocial model, this study capitalizes on a unique opportunity to evaluate high-risk patients before they are diagnosed with prostate cancer and follow them over time with validated instruments *(23)*. Along with the Rotterdam Screening Trial, the Fox Chase Program should shed valuable new light on the psychosocial implications of prostate cancer screening during the next several years.

PATIENT PREFERENCES

One technique for determining whether or not to screen patients for prostate cancer is to assess their utilities, or preferences, for various outcomes of screening. Patient utilities are individuals' valuations of various health states. A state of perfect health is assigned a utility of 1, whereas death or an extremely poor health state is assigned a utility of 0. Suboptimal states of health resulting from impairment of bodily functions correspond to intermediate values between 0 and 1. By incorporating patient utilities into comparisons of different medical interventions, survival rates and quality of life can be considered simultaneously. Utilities are used to construct estimates of quality-adjusted life-years (QALYs); that is, a year during which a patient is impotent is worth fewer QALYs than a year during which he is potent. If a particular treatment prolongs survival at the expense of quality of life, then QALY measurement can be used to incorporate both components into the same equation. QALYs can be used to evaluate outcomes of treatment modalities, which incur different treatment morbidities. They can also be incorporated into decision-analysis models that are used to develop public health policy.

One possible outcome is a diagnosis of prostate cancer, which would require the patient to make a treatment decision. This could lead to the benefit of cure, but it might also be associated with quality-of-life impairments. Hence, utilities assessment uses established methodologies to help the patient determine how he would feel about the possible outcomes of cancer cure with or without difficulties in the sexual, urinary, or bowel domains. If the patient decides that impotence, incontinence, or radiation proctitis would be so undesirable that he would prefer an early death from prostate cancer than aggressive treatment, then he clearly should not be screened. Conversely, the patient may value length of life relatively more highly than he does the minor inconvenience of occasional mild stress incontinence, or he may already be experiencing age-related erectile dysfunction and thus would not be affected by the possibility of impotence from prostate cancer treatment. In either case, he may conclude that screening is worthwhile for him because it has the potential to lengthen his life without compromising his assessment of its quality.

The virtual absence of literature showing a survival advantage from one form of treatment or another makes utilities assessment particularly sensitive to quality-of-life changes. Hence, men must be fairly insensitive to quality-of-life changes in order for utilities analyses to show a QALY benefit from prostate cancer screening. In one small but particularly well-done study, 10 couples were interviewed in depth to assess their utilities for various possible health state outcomes after screening (24). Interestingly, the husbands reported substantially lower utilities for potential impotence, incontinence, and bowel dysfunction than did their wives. In fact, when the patient preferences were incorporated into a decision model, 7 of 10 men preferred the no-screening strategy, whereas 9 of the 10 wives preferred to have their husbands screened for prostate cancer. When quality-adjusted life expectancies were calculated, screening added 2.5 QALYs when the wives' utilities were used but did not add any QALYs when the husbands' utilities were used. This study illustrates that prostate cancer screening decisions are extremely utility-sensitive.

In another small pilot study of utilities in men screened for prostate cancer, Cantor and colleagues (25) measured preferences for potentially impaired health states in order to create a mathematical model of the outcomes of screening. From this model, they concluded that when quality-of-life preferences of actual patients are considered, routine screening of asymptomatic men is ill-advised.

In 100 unaffected sons of men with prostate cancer, 60% expressed worry about increased risk because of genetics. Nearly 90% of these men wanted more information about inheritability of prostate cancer, whereas a similar proportion were definitely or probably inclined to undergo screening. Sons with more than 12 yr of formal education were less interested in knowing whether prostate cancer was inheritable. Although the reasons behind this are unclear, this observation may reflect a better understanding of the controversies involved in screening *(26)*. Other work has shown that men with a family history of prostate cancer perceive themselves to be at greater risk for the disease, which, in turn, creates a greater level of psychological distress *(27)*. This moderate amount of fear may be useful in encouraging screening behaviors.

INFORMED CONSENT

Some investigators contend that patients are asked to make screening decisions with inadequate information and that if they understood all the potential ramifications, many would say no to prostate cancer screening. In a widely quoted study, Wolf and colleagues *(28)* conducted a randomized, controlled trial to test this hypothesis. They evaluated over 200 men, randomly assigned to receive either a 3-min scripted overview of the risks and benefits of prostate cancer screening or a single sentence about the clinical value of PSA. The main outcome measure was interest in undergoing PSA screening, as measured with a single survey question. Although some critics argue that the intervention was weighted against screening, the reported findings are revealing. The authors concluded that those who received the more detailed information showed much less interest in screening (mean difference, 0.8 points on the 5-point scale) and were much less likely to indicate high interest in screening (odds ratio, 0.34; 95% confidence interval [CI], 0.19–0.60, $p < 0.001$). Advancing age enhanced the observed effect. Family history of prostate cancer wiped out the effect of the intervention (odds ratio, 3.95; 95% CI, 1.52–10.29, $p = 0.005$). This effect was consistent with another study of attitudes, in which Vranicar-Lapka and colleagues *(29)* reported that a family history of cancer increased the proportion of subjects interested in screening from 73% to 86%. Oddly, this effect was greater than that of a personal history of cancer, which increased the proportion of subjects interested in cancer screening only slightly, from 73% to 78%.

The content of shared decision-making sessions has been the topic of much investigation in prostate cancer. Chan and Sulmasy *(30)* conducted a series of expert panels and patient focus groups to determine what information should be conveyed in order to inform men adequately.

They concluded that, at a minimum, patients should be told (1) of the possibility of both false-positive and false-negative tests; (2) of the fact that it is not currently known whether PSA screening reduces population mortality; (3) that PSA screening may cause anxiety; (4) that PSA can detect tumors sooner than DRE; (5) that advanced prostate cancer is considered incurable; and (6) that PSA testing is controversial. These findings support the authors' pleas for individualized doctor–patient communication in cancer screening decisions for prostate and other tumors *(31)*.

Recently, Lee commented that it may be too much to expect busy clinicians to take the time to guide their patients through the "current maze of conflicting recommendations and statistics" when making screening decisions *(32)*. Marshall *(33)* subsequently opined that primary care physicians may simply be so overwhelmed both by the controversial differences in expert opinion and by the deluge of patients interested in screening that they are unable to respond in a well-considered manner. Both authors recommended that adequate informed consent somehow be incorporated into the primary care setting before prostate cancer screening is undertaken.

Many men incorrectly perceive themselves to be at increased risk for prostate cancer when they experience the bothersome urinary symptoms typically associated with benign prostate enlargement *(34)*. Indeed, the knowledge deficits that lead to this misperception provide a valuable opportunity for educating the public. Those who are better informed about prostate cancer are more likely to show interest in PSA screening if they have a positive family history. Those who are less informed tend to base their screening decisions on how serious they consider prostate cancer to be and how willing they are to accept the potential risks of treatment *(35)*. Conversely, the most common reason given by men who choose not to participate in free community screening programs is the lack of urological complaints. These observations reinforce the finding that the specific, known health promotional aspects of prostate cancer screening programs should be carefully considered when determining whether to promote screening in various communities *(36)*.

A variety of educational interventions—including the Wolf script mentioned earlier—have been devised to facilitate informed consent prior to making screening decisions. One of the most useful, though potentially controversial in its content, is a videotape created by investigators on the Prostate Patient Outcomes Research Team (PORT). The work of Flood and colleagues *(37)* with this video in informed medical decision-making has revealed that although patients are remarkably uninformed about the natural history of prostate cancer, they can be educated about the relevant issues before undertaking screening. Furthermore, when queried about their screening preferences, more informed patients are evenly split on the decision of whether to undergo PSA screening. Using another educational videotape, Volk and colleagues *(38)* showed that thoroughly informing patients on the potential benefits and harms of PSA screening is both effective and well received. Core knowledge about the risks and benefits of PSA testing was increased substantially. In a randomized, controlled trial, men who viewed the tape were less likely to express interest in having the PSA test (62% vs 80%, $p = 0.009$) when queried 2 wk later. Unlike other studies, this effect was not mitigated by a family history of prostate cancer. Although critics may question the content of the video, most would agree that the better informed patients are, the better their health care decisions are. Indeed, the goal of educational interventions should not be to decrease interest in prostate cancer screening, but rather, to enhance the value of truly shared decision-making between the patient and his doctor.

KNOWLEDGE AND SCREENING BEHAVIORS

The Health Belief Model *(15)* holds that the determinants of health behaviors include (1) predisposing factors, such as knowledge, attitudes, beliefs, and values; (2) enabling factors, such as access to health care; and (3) reinforcing factors, such as peers, teachers, and health professionals *(39)*. Each of these components is developed independently and may impact actions such as seeking prostate cancer screening. Some individuals' actions may be based on knowledge alone, whereas others may be based on attitudes alone. Still others may have accurate knowledge and positive attitudes but lack the availability of health care resources and, hence, not be screened. A growing body of research in prostate cancer screening has been built on this theoretical framework. Much of this literature has focused on cultural differences in how knowledge and attitudes impact behaviors.

Brown and colleagues *(40)* analyzed data from the National Health Interview Survey (NHIS) to assess levels of knowledge and utilization of DRE for prostate cancer screening. In the Cancer Control Supplement to the 1987 NHIS, more than 22,000 households across the United States were studied, yielding a sample of over 7,000 men over age 40. Of the eligible male participants, 77% had heard of the DRE and 58% had had one performed. In multivariate logistic regression controlling for a variety of factors, family income over $40,000 and greater years of education were positively associated with increased knowledge and use of DRE, whereas large family size was negatively associated with both measures, and marital status had no effect. Minorities and Southerners were less likely to have heard of or have had a DRE. Men who had accurate knowledge of early warning signs of cancer were more likely to have had a DRE performed (odds ratio, 1.40; 95% CI, 1.27–1.55). A personal history of cancer was also associated with greater likelihood of having had a DRE performed (odds ratio, 1.63; 95% CI, 1.38–1.93).

Weinrich and colleagues *(41)* recently reported on a large community-based project in which they assessed prostate cancer knowledge in a group of volunteers, then observed whether or not those volunteers chose to undergo screening. They used a simple, yet reliable and valid, six-item knowledge assessment (Table 1) to determine core prostate cancer knowledge among a predominantly African-American group of 319 participants, who were then referred for free screening with PSA and DRE. After controlling for covariates, such as ethnicity, education, income, and urinary symptoms, the authors showed that a high score on the knowledge questionnaire significantly predicted screening behavior ($p = 0.05$). They also demonstrated that the presence of urinary symptoms was an even stronger predictor of screening ($p = 0.002$). This finding is of concern because prostate cancer typically does not cause any symptoms when it is in its earliest and most curable stages. However, other authors mentioned earlier have reported similar findings. Both of these study conclusions underscore the valuable opportunity for the development of community-based education programs in populations of older men.

KNOWLEDGE AND ATTITUDES
IN AFRICAN-AMERICAN
AND HISPANIC-AMERICAN MEN

Although prostate cancer is considered to be more prevalent and more lethal in African-Americans, numerous studies have demonstrated knowledge deficits in this group. Demark-Wahnefried and colleagues *(42)* used a validated 20-item instrument (Fig. 1) to assess knowledge, attitudes, and behaviors in African-American men. They were less likely than Caucasian-Americans to report knowing someone with prostate cancer (31% vs 58%, $p < 0.001$), but more likely to report their acquaintances dying (38% vs 27%, $p = 0.08$) or becoming impotent (18% vs 10%, $p < 0.03$) from the disease or its treatment. African-Americans were significantly more likely than Caucasian-Americans to know that race is a risk factor (53% vs 33%, $p < 0.001$), however, they were less likely to agree with the statement that men with prostate cancer can lead normal lives. Over 90% of both groups agreed with the statement that prostate cancer can be cured if found early. A two-thirds majority of

Table 1

Knowledge of Prostate Cancer Screening Questionnaire

1. Older men are more likely to get prostate cancer.
2. A man can have prostate cancer and have no symptoms.
3. The only way a man can know if he has prostate cancer is to have a prostate checkup.
4. A man over 40 should have a rectal checkup every year.
5. Pain often in your lower back or upper legs could be a sign of prostate cancer.
6. Finding prostate cancer when it has first started to grow increases the chance of a cure.

All six statements are considered true. Range of possible scores is 0–6.

Source: Reprinted with permission of Oncology Nursing Press, Inc., from Oncology Nursing Forum, The Impact of Prostate Cancer Knowledge on Cancer Screening, Sally P. Weinrich et al., Vol. 25, No. 3, 1998; permission conveyed through Copyright Clearance Center, Inc.

both groups correctly identified that screening included a DRE. Although encouraging, the results of this study suggest that important knowledge differences exist between racial groups.

One reason that medical knowledge is thought to be an important determinant of health behavior is that it is often associated with a trait called self-efficacy. This psychological construct involves the idea that an individual feels not only knowledgeable but also capable of actually carrying out the screening behavior (43,44). In 1995, Boehm and colleagues (45) reported the results of a powerful church-based intervention designed to increase both knowledge and self-efficacy for prostate cancer screening in African-American men in the midwest. Modeling was provided by members of the community who were trained as lay educators to serve as role models of the screening behaviors. To assess knowledge, the investigators used a validated Prostate Cancer Screening Knowledge Inventory (Table 2). To assess self-efficacy, they used a validated set of four items, each of which was scored on a 5-point Likert scale (Table 3). After the intervention, substantial improvements were seen in both knowledge and self-efficacy for prostate cancer screening. The authors contended that by designing an intervention that included testimonials from actual patients who had survived prostate cancer, they were able to overcome a fatalistic and helpless attitude toward health that was often seen in older, African-American men (46). This study, too, demonstrates that men at high risk for prostate cancer can be educated and motivated to seek screening for early detection.

Other studies have confirmed that educational interventions are successful in encouraging screening for this disease in minorities. Myers

This is a survey to find out what men think about prostate cancer. Please help us gain a better understanding of what we can do to improve screening for this disease by completing this questionnaire. Thank you!

1. Do you have a <u>regular</u> doctor who you see when you are sick?

    Yes ☐
    No ☐

2. Do you have health insurance?

    Yes ☐
    No ☐

3. A Digital Rectal Examination is when the prostate is felt by a health professional by inserting a gloved finger into the rectum and gently pressing on the prostate to feel for lumps. Have you ever had a Digital Rectal Exam?

    No ☐
    Yes ☐   If yes,

    ⇓

How long ago?	
within the last year	☐
1 – 2 years ago	☐
2 – 3 years ago	☐
3 – 4 years ago	☐
4 – 5 years ago	☐
more than 5 years ago	☐
don't remember	☐

4. Have you ever "put-off" a digital rectal exam?

    No ☐
    Yes ☐   If yes,

    ⇓

Why did you put off the exam? (check all that apply)	
Didn't feel it was needed	☐
Cost too much	☐
I don't have a doctor	☐
I don't go to doctors unless I have problems	☐
Doctor didn't tell me to have one	☐
Too embarrassing	☐
Too many other health problems	☐
Had trouble fitting it into my schedule	☐
The exam is painful	☐
Other (please tell us)_____	☐

Fig. 1. *(continued on next four pages)* Knowledge and attitude survey used in prostate cancer awareness study by Demark-Wahnefried et al. from refs. *7* and *42*.

and colleagues *(47)* showed that after an enhanced and personalized intervention, men were more likely to believe that prostate cancer screening should be done in the absence of symptoms if they were older than 50 (odds ratio, 1.7; 95% CI, 1.1–2.8) or married (odds ratio, 2.3; 95% CI, 1.3–4.0). Those who received the personally tailored intervention were also more likely actually to undergo prostate cancer screening (odds ratio, 2.6; 95% CI, 1.7–3.9). For the convenience of other researchers, this chapter reproduces the data collection instruments, as well as

5. A Prostate Specific Antigen Test is where blood is drawn and tested for a protein linked to the prostate gland.
    Have you ever had a PSA test?

    No   ☐
    I don't know   ☐
    Yes   ☐   If yes,

                              ⇓

How long ago?	
within the last year	☐
1 – 2 years ago	☐
2 – 3 years ago	☐
over 3 years ago	☐
don't remember	☐

6. Has your doctor ever talked to you about having a test for prostate cancer?

    No   ☐
    Yes   ☐   If yes,

                   ⇓

What tests did your doctor mention? (check all that apply)	
Digital Rectal Examination	☐
Prostate Specific Antigen Testing	☐
Ultrasound	☐
Biopsy	☐
Don't remember	☐

7. Do you know anyone who has had prostate cancer?

    No   ☐
    Yes   ☐   If yes,

                   ⇓

Please check all that apply to that person (those people):	
they lead full, normal lives	☐
they have sexual problems (i.e. unable to have an erection)	☐
they have trouble with bladder control	☐
they are very ill with prostate cancer	☐
they died of prostate cancer	☐
although they have (had) prostate cancer, they have (had) other health problems that are (were) worse	☐
other (please tell us)_____	☐

Fig. 1. *(continued)*

a one-page list of screening pros and cons popularized by Chodak
(Table 4). These results have been confirmed with other patient populations across the United States *(48,49)*, particularly those that employ
community- and church-based educational interventions *(50)*, as well as
newspaper advertising *(51)*. African-American men are twice as likely as
Caucasian-American men to prefer private appointments over mass

8. Do you have a direct blood relative who has or had prostate cancer (i.e. grandfather, father, brother, uncle or son)?

Yes ☐
No ☐

9. One out of 11 American men will develop prostate cancer during his lifetime. What do you think your chances are of getting prostate cancer someday?

less than the average man ☐
the same as the average man ☐
more than the average man ☐

10. Race is a risk factor for some diseases like high blood pressure and diabetes. Who do you think is more likely to get prostate cancer?

white men ☐
black men ☐
race is not a risk factor for prostate cancer ☐
don't know ☐

11. Who do you think is more likely to get prostate cancer?

a man whose father has had prostate cancer ☐
a man whose father has not had prostate cancer ☐
it doesn't make any difference ☐
don't know ☐

12. How often do you think a man over the age of 40 should have a digital rectal exam?

never ☐
once every 5 years ☐
once every 3 years ☐
once every 2 years ☐
once a year ☐
don't know ☐

13. How would you describe your health compared to other men your age?

excellent ☐
above average ☐
average ☐
below average ☐
poor ☐

Fig. 1. *(continued)*

screening clinics (odds ratio, 2.2, $p < 0.001$) *(51)*. Knowledge interventions are equally effective in African-American and Caucasian-American men *(51,52)*.

One factor shown to be strongly and independently associated with African-Americans' willingness to undergo screening is the understanding that they are at increased risk for prostate cancer *(53)*. Furthermore, the perception that African-American men are more averse than others to having a DRE has been proved false in the vast majority of screening candidates between the ages of 40 and 70 *(54)*.

Studies in Hispanic-American men have revealed similar findings, particularly among urban populations. Hispanic-American men may also

14. Do you agree or disagree with the following statements? Please check the appropriate box.

Statement	Agree	Disagree	Don't Know
Prostate cancer can be cured if caught early enough.	☐	☐	☐
A man with prostate cancer can still live a normal life.	☐	☐	☐
With prostate cancer, the cure is worse than the disease.	☐	☐	☐
A man can have prostate cancer without having pain or other symptoms.	☐	☐	☐
It's better to leave well enough alone. If you have prostate cancer, it's better not to know.	☐	☐	☐
I've been pretty healthy all my life. I don't need to have my prostate checked.	☐	☐	☐

15. Have you ever smoked cigarettes?

No ☐
Yes ☐   If yes,

⇓

How many years have (did) you smoke(d)?

_____ years

On the average, how many cigarettes do (did) you smoke each day?

_____ cigarettes

16. What is the highest level of education you have completed?

8th grade or less ☐
some high school ☐
high school graduate ☐
technical school ☐
some college ☐
college graduate ☐
post graduate work/degree ☐

17. What is your race?

white ☐
black ☐
spanish/hispanic ☐
oriental/asian ☐
other: _____ ☐

Fig. 1. *(continued)*

be at increased risk for late presentation because of poor access to care, as well as misconceptions and fatalistic attitudes about cancer. Indeed, Hispanic-American men are twice as likely as whites to report never having had a DRE (42% vs 20%) *(55)*. Zimmerman *(56)* reported on the results of a large, multisite screening project, in which Hispanic-American men were interviewed to study their knowledge, attitudes, and suggestions.

18. What is your marital status?

married ☐
widowed ☐
divorced ☐
single ☐

19. What were the most important reasons you came in for screening?
(check all that apply to you)

It was free ☐
I was worried about cancer ☐
For peace of mind ☐
Doctor told me to come ☐
Relative/friend told me to come ☐
Friend or relative has had prostate cancer ☐
I felt it was time for a check-up ☐
I have had problems (problems with
    urination, back pain, etc.)
    which I wanted "checked-out." ☐
Second opinion ☐
Prostate cancer has been in the news lately
    and I felt I should check it out. ☐
Other (please tell us)_____ ☐

20. How did you find out about this screening clinic? (check all that apply)

Doctor ☐
Friend/Relative ☐
Television ☐
Radio ☐
Newspaper
Poster (please write where you saw it) ☐
_____
Flyer/Bulletin (please write where you got it) ☐
_____
Other (please tell us) ☐
_____

Fig. 1. *(continued)*

One-third felt that promotion from within the community was the best method of outreach and that modes should include English and Spanish newspapers, radio, and television. Participants reported that the most important factors impacting their screening behavior were learning about their own health and screening clinic convenience. Embarrassment about the DRE was described as not important by more than 80%.

SCREENING BEHAVIORS

Not all patients pursue prostate biopsy after an abnormal PSA or DRE. Krongrad and colleagues (57) have shown that as few as 57% of veterans in south Florida follow up with further diagnostic workup after abnormal screening tests. The reasons for such high diagnostic dropout rates are unclear. Other studies have shown that transrectal ultrasound and prostate biopsy are generally well-accepted by patients and are

Table 2
Prostate Cancer Screening Knowledge Inventory

TRUE or FALSE. Some of the statements below are true; some are false. Please circle **T** for each statement that you think is **TRUE**; circle **F** for each one that you think is **FALSE**.

1. The prostate gland is a small walnut shaped gland that is located below the bladder and connected to the penis.	T	F
2. The prostate gland makes some of the fluid that is part of the semen or come.	T	F
3. Any man over the age of 40 is at risk for prostate cancer.	T	F
4. More African American men are diagnosed with prostate cancer than whites.	T	F
5. Finding prostate cancer early can help with the treatment and cure of prostate cancer.	T	F
6. African American men who have fathers or brothers with prostate cancer are more likely to get prostate cancer than those who do not.	T	F
7. An exam every 5 years to check for prostate cancer is the best way to find prostate cancer early.	T	F
8 Warning signs of prostate cancer are having a hard time passing urine; passing urine often, especially at night; blood or pus in the urine; and pain or burning when passing urine.	T	F
9. The warning signs of prostate cancer are always present with prostate cancer.	T	F
10. A PSA blood test can be done to check for prostate cancer.	T	F
11. A digital rectal exam or DRE can be done to check for prostate cancer.	T	F

Source: Ref. *45*; reprinted with permission.

Table 3
Prostate Cancer Screening Self-Efficacy Scale

1. How sure are you that you can have a PSA blood test to check your prostate for cancer?
2. How sure are you that you can have a DRE to check your prostate for cancer?
3. How sure are you that you can have an examination every year to check your prostate for cancer?
4. How sure are you that you can recognize the warning signs of prostate cancer?

Note: Each item is scored on a 5-point Likert scale.
Source: Ref. *45*; reprinted with permission.

Table 4
Pros and Cons of Prostate Cancer Screening[a]

The case *for* screening

1. Advanced prostate cancer is incurable
2. Without screening, few patients are diagnosed early
3. PSA improves early detection

The case *against* screening

1. No studies have shown that screening decreased mortality
2. Many men with prostate cancer will die of comorbid diseases
3. Current therapies may cause significant morbidity
4. Improved early detection does not guarantee that cancer deaths can be prevented

[a]Adapted from Chodak.

associated with minimal disruption in quality of life, other than transient discomfort and anxiety *(58–62)*. Complications are rare *(63)*.

McKee *(64)* reported that the most important cues to action in prostate cancer screening were specific appointments, reminder cards, having a friend or family member with cancer, and newspaper promotion. No cue to action was more effective in older versus younger men. Barriers to early cancer detection in older men are thought to emanate from deeply ingrained attitudes, such as fear of vulnerability, dependence on female caretakers, and frustration by conflicting media messages. Each of these must be addressed in order to encourage more accurate health knowledge, better attitudes, and stronger self-efficacy for prostate cancer screening *(65)*.

SUMMARY

Clearly, quality of life must be considered when designing screening trials for prostate cancer. Although the few published studies in this area suggest that the quality-of-life effects are fairly mild and temporary, more work is needed. There is a need for a uniformly accepted, validated quality-of-life measure to be used in large and small screening trials throughout the world *(66)*. By the very nature of the demographics of prostate cancer, any impact of screening will affect a large segment of the population. Those who test positive for cancer will likely find the discomfort and anxiety to have been worthwhile, but the two-thirds of men whose biopsies are negative may feel differently *(67)*. The human costs of screening accrue to the rest of the population for whom there has been no direct health benefit. In addition, screening subjects who are found to have asymptomatic but untreatable disease will spend more of their lives as cancer patients, a state known to be associated with increased psychological distress *(68)*. Although these factors may or may not alter individual screening decisions, the development of a sound and rational health policy should entail comprehensive attention to both major and minor outcomes of screening.

The effect of prostate cancer screening on quality of life is a prime example of what has been called the sociology of medical technology. This framework is presented by Willis *(69)* in a fascinating discussion of the psychosocial and sociopolitical context that surrounds prostate cancer screening in postmodern America. How much harm and how much benefit? When approaching the issue of prostate cancer screening, both of these questions must be addressed with great attention to the many intricacies of human behavior. Clearly, screening saves many lives, but it also may lead to a cascade of events that is costly in both human and financial terms *(70)*. In a provocative and thoughtful essay, Meador *(71)* describes his prediction for the last well person in the world, the one who has defied all odds and escaped all diagnoses despite extensive and frequent screening. As more and more conditions become detectable by screening, he spends more and more of his time in screening clinics, undergoing screening for more and more diseases. Finally, his entire life is overtaken by screening. He remains healthy, but his life is devoid of quality.

REFERENCES

1. Saksela E. (1998) A guinea pig's view on prostate cancer screening trials. *Acta Oncol* 37:533–537.
2. Carvalhal GF, Smith DS, Ramos C, et al. (1999) Correlates of dissatisfaction with treatment in patients with prostate cancer diagnosed through screening. *J Urol* 162:113–8.

3. Gray RE, Philbrook A. (1997) Prostate cancer: 13. Whose prostate is it anyway? The view from the other side of the examining table. *CMAJ* 160:833–6.
4. Korda M (1997) *Man to man: surviving prostate cancer.* New York: Vintage Books.
5. Perkins JJ, Sanson-Fisher RW, Clarke SJ, Youman P. (1998) An exploration of screening practices for prostate cancer and the associated community expenditure. *Br J Urol* 82:524–9.
6. Rietbergen JB, Schroder FH. (1998) Screening for prostate cancer —more questions than answers (see comments). *Acta Oncol* 37:515–32.
7. Demark-Wahnefried W, Catoe KE, Paskett E, Robertson CN, Rimer BK. (1993) Characteristics of men reporting for prostate cancer screening. *Urology* 42:269–74; discussion 274–5.
8. Patrick DL, Deyo RA. (1989) Generic and disease-specific measures in assessing health status and quality of life. *Med Care* 27:S217–32.
9. Litwin MS (1994) Measuring health related quality of life in men with prostate cancer. *J Urol* 152:1882–7.
10. Litwin MS, Lubeck DP, Henning JM, Carroll PR. (1998) Differences in urologist and patient assessments of health related quality of life in men with prostate cancer: results of the CaPSURE database. *J Urol* 159:1988–92.
11. Litwin MS, McGuigan KA, Shpall AI, Dhanani N. (1999) Recovery of health related quality of life in the year after radical prostatectomy: early experience. *J Urol* 161:515–9.
12. Litwin MS, Shpall AI, Dorey F, Nguyen TH. (1998) Quality-of-life outcomes in long-term survivors of advanced prostate cancer. *Am J Clin Oncol* 21:327–32.
13. Litwin MS. (1999) Health related quality of life in older men without prostate cancer. *J Urol* 161:1180–4.
14. WHO. (1948) *Constitution of the World Health Organization, Basic Documents.* Geneva: WHO.
15. Rosenstock I. (1974) Historical origins of the Health Belief Model. In: Becker M, ed. *The Health Belief Model and Personal Health Behavior.* Thorafare, NJ: Slack, pp. 1–8.
16. Ware JE Jr, Sherbourne CD. (1992) The MOS 36-item short-form health survey (SF-36). I. Conceptual framework and item selection. *Med Care* 30:473–83.
17. van der Ploeg HM (1980) Validation of the state-trait anxiety inventory. *Ned T Psychol* 35:243–249.
18. Essink-Bot ML, de Koning HJ, Nijs HG, Kirkels WJ, van der Maas PJ, Schroder FH. (1998) Short-term effects of population-based screening for prostate cancer on health-related quality of life. *J Natl Cancer Inst* 90:925–31.
19. Gustafsson O, Theorell T, Norming U, Perski A, Ohstrom M, Nyman CR. (1995) Psychological reactions in men screened for prostate cancer. *Br J Urol* 75:631–636.
20. Akerstedt T, Torsvall L. (1978) Experimental changes in shift schedules—their effects on well-being. *Ergonomics* 21:849–56.
21. Lundberg U, Frankenhaeuser M. (1980) Pituitary–adrenal and sympathetic-adrenal correlates of distress and effort. *J Psychosom Res* 24:125–30.
22. Harenstam A, Theorell T. (1990) Cortisol elevation and serum gamma-glutamyl transpeptidase in response to adverse job conditions: how are they interrelated? *Biol Psychol* 31:157–71.
23. Bruner DW, Baffoe-Bonnie A, Miller S, et al. (1999) Prostate cancer risk assessment program. A model for the early detection of prostate cancer. *Oncology (Huntingt)* 13:325–334; discussion 337–339, 343–344 pas.

24. Volk RJ, Cantor SB, Spann SJ, Cass AR, Cardenas MP, Warren MM. (1997) Preferences of husbands and wives for prostate cancer screening (see comments). *Arch Fam Med* 6:72–76.
25. Cantor SB, Spann SJ, Volk RJ, Cardenas MP, Warren MM. (1995) Prostate cancer screening: a decision analysis (see comments). *J Fam Pract* 41:33–41.
26. Bratt O, Kristoffersson U, Lundgren R, Olsson H. (1997) Sons of men with prostate cancer: their attitudes regarding possible inheritance of prostate cancer, screening, and genetic testing. *Urology* 50:360–365.
27. Taylor KL, DiPlacido J, Redd WH, Faccenda K, Greer L, Perlmutter A. (1999) Demographics, family histories, and psychological characteristics of prostate carcinoma screening participants. *Cancer* 85:1305–1312.
28. Wolf AM, Nasser JF, Schorling JB. (1996) The impact of informed consent on patient interest in prostate-specific antigen screening (see comments). *Arch Intern Med* 156:1333–1336.
29. Vranicar-Lapka D, Barbour-Randall L, Trippon M, et al. (1992) Oncology patients' and their significant others' responses to a proposed cancer prevention/detection program. *Cancer Nurs* 15:47–53.
30. Chan ECY, Sulmasy DP. (1998) What should men know about prostate-specific antigen screening before giving informed consent? *Am J Med* 105:266–274.
31. Wolf AM, Becker DM. (1996) Cancer screening and informed patient discussions. Truth and consequences. *Arch Intern Med* 156:1069–1072.
32. Lee JM (1993) Screening and informed consent (see comments). *N Engl J Med* 328:438–440.
33. Marshall KG. (1993) Screening for prostate cancer. How can patients give informed consent? *Can Fam Physician* 39:2385–2390.
34. Ward JE, Hughes AM, Hirst GH, Winchester L. (1997) Men's estimates of prostate cancer risk and self-reported rates of screening (see comments). *Med J Aust* 167:250–253.
35. Wolf AM, Philbrick JT, Schorling JB. (1997) Predictors of interest in prostate-specific antigen screening and the impact of informed consent: what should we tell our patients? *Am J Med* 103:308–314.
36. Nijs HG, Tordoir DM, Schuurman JH, Kirkels WJ, Schroder FH. (1997) Randomised trial of prostate cancer screening in The Netherlands: assessment of acceptance and motives for attendance. *J Med Screen* 4:102–106.
37. Flood AB, Wennberg JE, Nease RF, Jr., Fowler FJ, Jr., Ding J, Hynes LM. (1996) The importance of patient preference in the decision to screen for prostate cancer. Prostate Patient Outcomes Research Team (see comments). *J Gen Intern Med* 11:342–349.
38. Volk RJ, Cass AR, Spann SJ. (1999) A randomized controlled trial of shared decision making for prostate cancer screening. *Arch Fam Med* 8:333–340.
39. Green LW, Krueter MW, Deeds SG, Partridge KB. (1980) *Health Education Planning: A Diagnostic Approach*. Palo Alto, CA: Mayfield.
40. Brown ML, Potosky AL, Thompson GB, Kessler LG. (1990) The knowledge and use of screening tests for colorectal and prostate cancer: data from the 1987 National Health Interview Survey. *Prev Med* 19:562–574.
41. Weinrich SP, Weinrich MC, Boyd MD, Atkinson C. (1998) The impact of prostate cancer knowledge on cancer screening. *Oncol Nurs Forum* 25:527 534.
42. Demark-Wahnefried W, Strigo T, Catoe K, et al. (1995) Knowledge, beliefs, and prior screening behavior among blacks and whites reporting for prostate cancer screening. *Urology* 46:346–351.
43. Bandura A. (1982) The assessment and predictive generality of self-percepts of efficacy. *J Behav Ther Exp Psychiatry* 13:195–199.

44. O'Leary A. (1985) Self-efficacy and health. *Behav Res Ther* 23:437–451.
45. Boehm S, Coleman-Burns P, Schlenk EA, Funnell MM, Parzuchowski J, Powell IJ. (1995) Prostate cancer in African American men: increasing knowledge and self- efficacy. *J Community Health Nurs* 12:161–169.
46. Scroggins TG, Jr., Bartley TK. (1999) Enhancing cancer control: assessing cancer knowledge, attitudes, and beliefs in disadvantaged communities. *J La State Med Soc* 151:202–208.
47. Myers RE, Chodak GW, Wolf TA, et al. (1999) Adherence by African American men to prostate cancer education and early detection (see comments). *Cancer* 86:88–104.
48. Myers RE, Wolf TA, McKee L, et al. (1996) Factors associated with intention to undergo annual prostate cancer screening among African American men in Philadelphia. *Cancer* 78:471–479.
49. Robinson SB, Ashley M, Haynes MA. (1996) Attitudes of African Americans regarding screening for prostate cancer. *J Natl Med Assoc* 88:241–246.
50. Weinrich SP, Boyd MD, Bradford D, Mossa MS, Weinrich M. (1998) Recruitment of African Americans into prostate cancer screening. *Cancer Pract* 6:23–30.
51. Barber KR, Shaw R, Folts M, et al. (1998) Differences between African American and Caucasian men participating in a community-based prostate cancer screening program. *J Community Health* 23:441–451.
52. Abbott RR, Taylor DK, Barber K. (1998) A comparison of prostate knowledge of African-American and Caucasian men: changes from prescreening baseline to postintervention. *Cancer J Sci Am* 4:175–177.
53. Myers RE, Wolf TA, Balshem AM, Ross EA, Chodak GW. (1994) Receptivity of African-American men to prostate cancer screening. *Urology* 43:480–487.
54. Gelfand DE, Parzuchowski J, Cort M, Powell I. (1995) Digital rectal examinations and prostate cancer screening: attitudes of African American men. *Oncol Nurs Forum* 22:1253–1255.
55. McCoy CB, Anwyl RS, Metsch LR, Inciardi JA, Smith SA, Correa R. (1995) Prostate cancer in Florida: knowledge, attitudes, practices, and beliefs. *Cancer Pract* 3:88–93.
56. Zimmerman SM. (1997) Factors influencing Hispanic participation in prostate cancer screening. *Oncol Nurs Forum* 24:499–504.
57. Krongrad A, Kim CO, Burke MA, Granville LJ. (1996) Not all patients pursue prostate biopsy after abnormal prostate specific antigen results. *Urol Oncol* 2:35–39.
58. Aus G, Hermansson CG, Hugosson J, Pedersen KV. (1993) Transrectal ultrasound examination of the prostate: complications and acceptance by patients. *Br J Urol* 71:457–459.
59. Irani J, Fournier F, Bon D, Gremmo E, Dore B, Aubert J. (1997) Patient tolerance of transrectal ultrasound-guided biopsy of the prostate. *Br J Urol* 79:608–10.
60. Collins GN, Lloyd SN, Hehir M, McKelvie GB. (1993) Multiple transrectal ultrasound-guided prostatic biopsies—true morbidity and patient acceptance. *Br J Urol* 71:460–463.
61. Clements R, Aideyan OU, Griffiths GJ, Peeling WB. (1993) Side effects and patient acceptability of transrectal biopsy of the prostate. *Clin Radiol* 47:125–126.
62. Webb JA, Shanmuganathan K, McLean A. (1993) Complications of ultrasound-guided transperineal prostate biopsy. A prospective study (see comments). *Br J Urol* 72:775–777.
63. Rietbergen JB, Kruger AE, Kranse R, Schroder FH. (1997) Complications of transrectal ultrasound-guided systematic sextant biopsies of the prostate: evalu-

ation of complication rates and risk factors within a population-based screening program. *Urology* 49:875–880.

64. McKee JM. (1994) Cues to action in prostate cancer screening. *Oncol Nurs Forum* 21:1171–1176.

65. Rubenstein L. (1994) Strategies to overcome barriers to early detection of cancer among older adults. *Cancer* 74:2190–3.

66. Iverson D. (1994) The need to measure quality of life in a prostate cancer screening trial. *Can J Oncol* 4 Suppl 1:76–77.

67. Stewart-Brown S, Farmer A. (1997) Screening could seriously damage your health (editorial) (see comments). *Br Med J* 314:533–534.

68. Wardle J, Pope R. (1992) The psychological costs of screening for cancer. *J Psychosom Res* 36:609–624.

69. Willis E. (1997) The prostatic imperative and the social relations of medical technology. *Int J Technol Assess Health Care* 13:602–612.

70. Marshall KG. (1996) Prevention. How much harm? How much benefit? 3. Physical, psychological and social harm. *Cmaj* 155:169–176.

71. Meador CK. (1994) The last well person (see comments). *N Engl J Med* 330:440–441.

14 Prostate Cancer Screening Recommendations from Organized Medicine

Gregory T. Sweat, MD

CONTENTS

INTRODUCTION

Physicians universally believe in disease prevention and the favorability of detecting disease early. Unfortunately, many barriers exist to providing comprehensive clinical preventive care. Insufficient time to provide appropriate counsel with regard to health promotion, inadequate reimbursement for the provision of preventive services, and the paucity of medical training in health promotion and disease prevention have led to uncertainty and confusion regarding the priority of providing these services. The link joining scientific research to clinical application is incomplete in many aspects of modern medicine. Early detection of prostate cancer is one such area that arguably lacks this complete link.

From: *Current Clinical Urology: Prostate Cancer Screening*
Edited by: I. M. Thompson, M. I. Resnick, and E. A. Klein
© Humana Press Inc., Totowa, NJ

This deficiency of proven clinical efficacy also leads to a variety of recommendations from different medical providers. Fortunately, various organizations, government and private, are providing guidelines for screening. As technology advances, the acceptance and, ultimately, the recommendation of newly available tests and procedures will vary. The services provided within routine health maintenance examinations have become increasingly scrutinized. The serum tumor marker, prostate-specific antigen (PSA), has not escaped scrutiny in regard to its ability to detect asymptomatic cancer of the prostate. The evidence trail for prostate cancer early detection is building and should be followed regardless of where it leads.

UNITED STATES
PREVENTIVE SERVICES TASK FORCE

As previously common and debilitating conditions declined after the introduction of certain clinical preventive services, support grew for reliable data surrounding the content of periodic examinations. In 1984, the United States Public Health Service organized the United States Preventive Services Task Force (USPSTF) to provide ongoing evaluation and review of preventive services used by clinicians. The initial review culminated in the first edition of *Guide to Clinical Preventive Services,* which was published in 1989 and contains a discussion regarding prostate cancer detection in asymptomatic men *(1).* Recommendations were then revised and updated in late 1995 in the second edition of the text. The USPSTF was initially guided by the Office of Disease Prevention and Health Promotion and subsequently moved to the Agency for Health Care Quality and Research (AHCQR). The Center for Practice and Technology Assessment assists in coordination within the AHCQR.

In late 1998, the Task Force was reconvened to continue the ongoing critical review of preventive services for clinicians, managed-care professionals, and employers. The Task Force has benefited by partnerships with the Canadian Task Force and the United States Public Health Service, as well as by representation from multiple primary care and subspecialty societies. The utilization of similar framework and analysis and the adoption of parallel guidelines such as the Canadian Task Force creates a synergy that allows for the expeditious delivery of evidence-based clinical guides. Both groups are formulating recommendations based on the quality of published scientific evidence, with attention toward study design and analysis. The independent experts that form the Task Force are appointed by the AHCQR and are federally supported. There are currently 12 evidence-based practice centers, 2 of which bear the responsibility for research (University of North Carolina at Chapel Hill and Oregon Health Sciences in Portland.) In the second edition, more than 6000 citations are used to substantiate their recommendations. The literature cited pertaining to screening for prostate cancer consists of more than 100 citations.

The prostate cancer burden of suffering within the population as well as the accuracy of currently available screening tests and the effectiveness of early detection were issues that directed the group toward consensus.

The recommendation provided by the USPTF for prostate cancer screening is as follows:

> *Routine screening for prostate cancer with digital rectal examination, serum tumor markers (e.g. prostate specific antigen), or transrectal ultrasound is not recommended.*
>
> *Patients who request screening should be given objective information about the potential benefits and harms of early detection and treatment. If screening is to be performed, the best-evaluated approach is to screen with DRE and PSA and to limit screening to men with a life expectancy greater than ten years. There is currently insufficient evidence to determine the need and optimal interval for repeat screening or whether PSA thresholds must be adjusted for density, velocity, or age.*

In 1995, as part of the second edition, available evidence led the USPTF to the classification of efforts to detect prostate cancer as a (D) recommendation. (See Table 1 for the classification system.) Since the release of the second edition, indirect evidence of the strength of PSA screening has been mounting, but it remains doubtful that the Task Force would overlook the current void of rigorously analyzed randomized prospective trials to construct an evidence-based recommendation. Randomized controlled trials of DRE and PSA screening efficacy are currently underway in the United States and in Europe. The data and results of these studies will not be available for some time. The European randomized study of prostate cancer screening based in the Netherlands is currently enrolling more than 190,000 European men with an expected completion by 2008 *(2)*. Initial results from the Finnish cohort after 1 yr and enrolling 20,000 men have shown a 2.1% prostate cancer detection rate. The positive predictive value was 27%, which corresponds to mammography's effectiveness for breast cancer screening *(3)*. In the United States, the National Cancer Institute is conducting the Prostate, Lung, Colorectal, and Ovarian Cancer Screening Trial (PLCO),

Table 1
U.S. Preventive Services Task Force Strength of Recommendations

A:
There is good evidence to support the recommendation that the condition be specifically considered in a periodic health examination.
B:
There is fair evidence to support the recommendation that the condition be specifically considered in a periodic health examination.
C:
There is insufficient evidence to recommend for or against the inclusion of the condition in a periodic health examination, but recommendations may be made on other grounds.
D:
There is fair evidence to support the recommendation that the condition be excluded from consideration in a periodic health examination.
E:
There is good evidence to support the recommendation that the condition be excluded from consideration in a periodic health examination.

which is enrolling approximately 75,000 men, with an expected completion date of 2006 *(4)*.

CANADIAN TASK FORCE

The Canadian Task Force has worked in collaboration with the United States Preventive Task Force since the 1980s to develop comprehensive guidelines *(5)*. The Canadian Task Force was established in 1976 and has served Canada in much the same way that the Preventive Task Force has served American providers, payers, and employers. The Canadian Task Force made its final recommendations with regard to prostate cancer screening in June of 1994 and is looking toward review in the near future. The currently available direction from the task force is as follows:

> *There is insufficient evidence to include prostate specific antigen (PSA) screening in the periodic health examination of men over 50 years of age. Exclusion is recommended on the basis of low predictive value and the known risk of adverse effects associated with therapies of unproven effectiveness. (D) Recommendation*

Although the language regarding screening is identical, the discussion differs slightly and is based on the absence of evidence for effectiveness of therapy and the risk of adverse effects associated with currently available methods of treatment. Little evidence exists to include or exclude

Table 2
Canadian Task Force Grades of Recommendations

A:
Good evidence to support the recommendation that the condition be specifically considered in a PHE.
B:
Fair evidence to support the recommendation that the condition be specifically considered in a PHE.
C:
Poor evidence regarding inclusion or exclusion of a condition in a PHE, but recommendations may be made on other grounds.
D:
Fair evidence to support the recommendation that the condition be specifically excluded from consideration in a PHE.
E:
Good evidence to support the recommendation that the condition be specifically excluded from consideration in a PHE.

Note: PHE = periodic health examination.

DRE as part of any periodic health examination but for the early detection of prostate cancer the evidence receives a grade (C). Furthermore, transrectal ultrasound use in screening for prostate cancer is not recommended. (D) Recommendation. (*See* Table 2 for graded recommendations.) Both the United States and Canadian Task Forces are set to reconvene to review recent findings with regard to prostate cancer screening. New guidelines should be released in the next few years.

AMERICAN CANCER SOCIETY

As a nationwide, community-based voluntary health organization, the American Cancer Society (ACS) has had an impact on the morbidity and mortality of many types of cancer. In 1997, the ACS identified prostate cancer as a priority issue and, as such, has focused substantial attention on its long-term goal of a 50% reduction of age-adjusted mortality by the year 2015. Prostate cancer was one of the first areas in which 20 – 25 million dollars was set aside for requests for proposals to evaluate treatment outcomes and pursue policy and behavioral research *(6)*.

In 1997, the detection and treatment of prostate cancer was reaffirmed as a newly designated core priority issue with updated detection guidelines. A uniform screening program for prostate cancer became increasingly necessary in the late 1980s as the incidence of prostate cancer increased dramatically. This was thought to be attributed to the widespread use and application of PSA testing. During that same time period, the overall 5-yr prostate cancer survival rate had increased. In 1992, the ACS issued the following prostate cancer screening recommendation:

> *Digital rectal examination and prostate specific antigen should be performed on men 50 and older. If either is abnormal, further evaluation should be considered (7).*

In early 1997, a workshop was convened to evaluate the proposal for an updated guideline in light of data from ongoing clinical trials. The updated guideline is as follows:

> *Guideline Statement: Both the Prostate Specific Antigen (PSA) test and Digital Rectal Examination (DRE) should be offered annually, beginning at age 50 years, to men who have at least a ten year life expectancy, and to younger men who are at high risk. Information should be provided to patients regarding potential risks and benefits of intervention (7).*

Although, at first glance, this seems to be similar to the 1992 guideline, the language is remarkably different. Not only has the Society seemingly relaxed its stance by changing the verbiage from *should* be performed annually to *offered* annually, it has also added a critical piece with regard to the provision of information to all men undergoing screening. Furthermore, in the narrative accompanying the guideline, the Society defines those at high risk as men with a strong familial predisposition, e.g., two or more affected first- degree relatives, or African-Americans who should begin screening at a younger age, such as age 45. African-American men seem to have a much higher incidence of prostate cancer. The incidence rate per 100,000 men among African-Americans is 224.3, vs other racial and ethnic groups in the United States, including, white (150.3), Hispanic (104.4), Asians/Pacific Islander (82.2), and American Indian (46.4). The mortality rate for prostate cancer is also dramatically higher: African-American men is 55%, White, 24%, Hispanic, 17%, Asians/Pacific Islander, 11%, American Indian, 14%. African-American men also have a relatively low 5-yr survival rate when contrasted with white men, 81% vs 95% respectively *(8)*.

Also specifically addressed within the main guideline is the issue of informed consent or the provision of information deemed adequate to make an informed decision regarding prostate cancer screening. Many organizations have now addressed the issue of an adequately informed patient. The American College of Physicians has addressed this specifically in their guideline statement, which will be reviewed later in this chapter. The society has provided accompanying information for its guideline that is deemed necessary for men undergoing screening.

1. Some elevations in PSA may be the result of benign conditions of the prostate.
2. Screening for prostate cancer in asymptomatic men can detect tumors at an early stage.
3. DRE of the prostate should be performed by health care workers skilled in recognizing subtle prostate abnormalities.
4. There is a specific need to provide men with greater information about the potential risks of intervention and offer further guidance for men at risk or advanced age.

Although a priority for many organizations, informed consent for prostate cancer screening in its current state does not seem to be effective or widespread. In the July/August 1999 issue of *Effective Clinical Practice*, Federman et al. described data from questionnaires sent to men having had a PSA test ordered for screening purposes. The questionnaire queried the patient's knowledge and attitude toward PSA screening, treatment of prostate cancer, and interactions with their primary care provider. Within several months of having seen their health care provider, only 32% of men were aware of the test having been performed and were able to recall a discussion regarding the risks and benefits of PSA testing. Approximately one-third were completely unaware of the test ever having been ordered. Of those aware of the test and recalling a discussion, fewer than one-third of them knew that treatment of prostate cancer has not been shown to improve survival. Approximately one-half recall the risks of differing therapies for prostate cancer *(9)*. These results are viewed by advocates of informed consent as unsettling. The process of providing information regarding prostate cancer screening certainly seems to be ineffective, if completed at all.

Gabriel Feldman, MD, MPH, National Director of Prostate and Colorectal Cancer Control at the ACS urges that providers, not patients, use the guidelines. He further states that the guidelines are intended to discourage the extremes of prostate cancer screening, such as physicians that universally promote the use of PSA and DRE or those who do not offer the screening test because of the lack of evidence of benefit. The ACS and Feldman are currently attempting to provide consistency in policy statements. There have been discussions among the American College of Preventive Medicine, the American College of Physicians–American Society of Internal Medicine, and the American Academy of Family Physicians to create a uniform statement for primary care physicians *(10)*.

AMERICAN COLLEGE OF PHYSICIANS—
AMERICAN SOCIETY OF INTERNAL MEDICINE

The American College of Physicians released a position paper just before the American Cancer Society did, as a series of three articles in the *Annals of Internal Medicine* in 1997 with recommendations for the early detection of prostate cancer. The first article established the prevalence of clinically relevant prostate cancer and served to evaluate the effectiveness of DRE and PSA to screen for prostate cancer *(11)*. The second identified the benefits, harms, and economic costs of DRE and PSA, then reviewed the utilization of screening programs *(12)*. The third in the series served to review, condense, and clarify the current level of knowledge surrounding early detection of prostate cancer as well as to assist health care providers in adequately informing patients of the risks and benefits of early detection *(13)*. Dr. Chris Coley and colleagues performed a relatively exhaustive search through relevant studies using a MEDLINE search, from 1966 to 1995, specifically concentrating on prospective cohort studies. The document was developed for the Health and Public Policy Committee by the Clinical Efficacy Assessment Subcommittee and approved by the Board of Regents in 1996.

Recommendation 1

> *Rather than screening all men for prostate cancer as a matter of routine, physicians should describe the potential benefits and known harms of screening, diagnosis, and treatment; listen to the patient's concerns; and then individualize the decision to screen.*

Accompanying the recommendation is further narrative describing possible harms and the lack of known benefit from early treatment and that indirect evidence suggests that the most benefit will be served screening men 50–69yr of age. Information pertaining to individually determined risk benefit equations must always be provided.

Recommendation 2

> *The College strongly recommends that physicians help enroll eligible men in ongoing clinical studies.*

The American College of Physicians also chose to focus on the issue of counseling patients and providing informed consent. A strong stance is taken with regard to ensuring that each patient is fully informed. The ACP recommends that the following eight topics be discussed before any testing program.

1. Prostate cancer is an important health problem.
2. Benefits of one time or repeat screening and aggressive treatment of prostate cancer have not yet been proven.
3. DRE and PSA measurement can both have false-positive and false-negative results.
4. Probability that further invasive evaluations will be required as a result of testing is relatively high.
5. Aggressive therapy is necessary to realize any benefit from the discovery of the tumor.
6. A small but finite risk for early death and significant risk for chronic illness, particularly with regard to sexual and urinary function, are associated with these treatments.
7. Early detection may save lives.
8. Early detection and treatment may avert future cancer-related illness.

The entire review was designed for clinicians wishing to have an in-depth background regarding the specific issues and controversies that surround the use of different modalities for prostate cancer screening. This allows the provider to integrate many aspects of the controversy surrounding prostate cancer screening into his or her practice of preventive medicine. Health care organizations and patients will continue to seek increasing amounts of information regarding the quality of health care each receives. The ACP not only provides an informed recommendation but also provides points of contention to be resolved prior to testing.

AMERICAN ACADEMY OF FAMILY PHYSICIANS

The mission of the American Academy of Family Physicians (AAFP) always has been to provide physicians with practical services and information in the clinical setting. Through the recommendations of periodic health examinations, the Academy has provided a uniform body of standards and guidelines that are easily accessible and implemented by any physician. The Academy's Commission on Clinical Policies and Research serves to develop these recommendations for periodic health examinations. They have been updated in June 1995, 1996, and, again, in July 1999. The genesis of the AAFP standards and guidelines is the United States Preventive Task Forces *Guide to Clinical Preventive Services (1)*. There exists in the Academy a working group on periodic health examinations that is currently reviewing and updating its policy regarding prostate cancer screening. The rigorous analysis provided by the USPTF is coupled with consideration of overall cost and patient compliance and preference to provide a substantiated document. With regard to prostate cancer, the group has identified a patient population of men, ages 50–65 yr and advises an intervention of:

Counsel about the known risks and uncertain benefits of screening for prostate cancer. (14)

There is no mention within the guideline of high-risk populations such as men with a strong family history or men with a different ethnicity receiving special consideration.

The act of screening this population is labeled as a "guideline" by the Academy, not a "standard." Interventions receive the label "standard" when sufficient evidence exists, after considering the benefits, risks, and costs, that patients would unanimously prefer the intervention. Recommendations designated as "guidelines" exhibit weaker evidence of benefit and that an appreciable but not unanimous majority of patients would prefer the intervention. The clinical difference is that there should be a stronger effort made to implement "standards." The Academy acknowledges that providing "guidelines" and "standards" is only one element of improving the health care of patients. Implementation must first occur for them to be effective. Together with the Department of Health and Human Services, the Academy has developed the Put Prevention into Family Practice Project to provide a variety of resources to assist implementation of providing satisfactory clinical preventive services. They are taking this one step further by providing a self-assessment as part of a Vital Signs Program *(14)*.

AMERICAN UROLOGIC ASSOCIATION

In 1989, the Board of Directors of the American Urologic Association (AUA) began to develop evidence-based practice guidelines for the care of the urologic patient. The practice parameters, guidelines, and standards committee was developed at that time and has since overseen guidelines developed addressing such issues as benign prostatic hyperplasia, prostate cancer, erectile dysfunction, and female urinary stress incontinence. The AUA guidelines are strictly evidence-based and were created by a panel of 10–15 experts who extensively reviewed the literature pertaining to a specific guideline topic. With regard to the early detection of prostate cancer, there has not been such a guideline developed by the AUA except to note that its Board of Directors endorses the American Cancer Society's policy regarding early detection of prostate cancer. The most recent review and approval occurred in September 1997 *(15)*. Recognizing the need for further urologist and nonurologist guidance with regard to certain urologic topics, the Board of Directors has endorsed the creation of consensus-based guidelines, called Best

Practice Policies. Recently, a multidisciplinary panel was created and convened to develop a resource and guide for the use of PSA testing for specialists and nonspecialists. Although not strictly evidence based, the panel formulated statements and recommendations by consensus after review of the literature and extensive discussion. The document produced was comprehensive in its coverage of issues pertaining to the evaluation of men at risk for prostate cancer, assistance in pretreatment staging, and the posttreatment monitoring and management of men with the disease *(16)*. The document concisely and clearly reviewed topics related to PSA, such as sensitivity and specificity issues relating to its performance, factors affecting it that might impact the interpretation of results, biopsy indications, and its relation to risk and extent of prostate cancer. Although not specifically labeled as recommendations or guidelines, several statements are made regarding the early detection of prostate cancer:

> *The decision to use PSA for the early detection of prostate cancer should be individualized. Patients should be informed of the known risks and the potential benefits.*

> *Early detection of prostate cancer should be offered to asymptomatic men 50 years of age or older with an estimated life expectancy of more than ten years. It is reasonable to offer testing at an earlier age to men with defined risk factors, including men with a first-degree relative who has prostate cancer and African-American men.*

AMERICAN COLLEGE OF RADIOLOGY

The American College of Radiology made formal its approach to policy decisions in the 1950s by creating a council of elected representatives who meet annually to debate and approve resolutions. There are currently more than 250 councillors with representation from each state. In 1991, a resolution was accepted pertaining to the detection of prostate cancer:

> *A combination of digital rectal examination and serum prostate-specific antigen (PSA) level should be used as an initial screening procedure for prostate cancer. The use of prostate ultrasound is best reserved to evaluate those patients who have either an abnormal digital rectal examination or an abnormal PSA level. (Resolution 36) (17)*

This policy statement resides in the Digest of Council Actions 1989–1999 and as part of the bylaws it must be reviewed at 10-yr intervals.

As the ability to detect prostate cancer becomes increasingly exact, so will uniformity among organizations dedicated to providing efficacious modalities for screening to providers and payers. As evidenced by the principles adopted by government-sponsored groups, internists, family physicians, radiologists, urologists, and community-action groups, uniform consensus is on the horizon. Although variance still remains among organizational policy and provider practice, ultimately, patient welfare is the interest to be considered.

REFERENCES

1. U.S. Preventive Services Task Force. (1995) *Guide to Clinical Preventive Services*, 2nd Ed. pp. 119–134.
2. Schroder FH. (1994) The European Screening Study for Prostate Cancer. *Canadian Journal of Oncology* 4(Supp 1):102–109.
3. Maattanen L, Auvinen A, Steman U-H, et al. (1999) European Randomized Study of prostate cancer screening: first year results of the Finnish Trial.
4. Prorkup P: (1994)The National Cancer Institute Multiscreening Trial. *Can J Oncol* 4(Suppl No. 1): 98–101.
5. Canadian Task Force on the Periodic Health Examination. (1994) *Canadian Guide to Clinical Preventive Health Care*. Ottawa: Canada Communication Group, pp. 812–823.
6. Eyre, HJ. (1997) The American Cancer Society's Prostate Cancer Position (editorial). *CA: Cancer J Clin* 47(5):259–260.
7. von Eschenbach A, Ho R, Murphy GP, Cunningham M, Linns N. (1997) American Cancer Society Guidelines for the Early Detection of Prostate Cancer: Update, June 10, 1997. *Cancer* 80(9):1805–1807.
8. Landis SH, Murray T, Bolder S. (1999) Cancer statistics, 1999. *CA Cancer J Clin* 49:8–31.
9. Federman DG, Goyal S, Kamina, A, et al. (1999) Informed Consent for PSA Screening: does it Happen? Am Coll Physicians–Am Soc Intern Med 2(4).
10. Friedrich, MJ. (1999) Issues in prostate cancer screening. *JAMA* 281(17):1573–1575.
11. Anon (1997) Clinical Guideline: Part I. Early Detection of Prostate Cancer. Part I: Prior Probability and Effectiveness of Tests. Annals of Internal Medicine Position Paper, March 1, 1997, *Ann Intern Med* 126:394–406.
12. Anon. (1992) Clinical Guideline: Part II. Early Detection of Prostate Cancer. Part II: Estimating the Risks, Benefits, and Costs. Annals of Internal Medicine Position Paper, March 15, 1997, *Ann Intern Med* 126:468–479.
13. Clinical Guideline: Part III. Screening for Prostate Cancer. Part II: Estimating the Risks, Benefits, and Costs. Annals of Internal Medicine Position Paper, March 15, 1997, 126:480-484.
14. American Academy of Family Physicians, Commission on Clinical Policies and Research. (1996) Summary of Policy Recommendations for Periodic Health Examination, November 1996, Revised July 1999.
15. The American Urological Association, Inc., Policy Statements, Board of Directors, September 1999.
16. AUA Prostate Cancer Panel. (2000) Prostate specific antigen best practice policy. *Oncology* 14;267–280.

17. The American College of Radiology, Digest of Council Actions, Section II: Professional and Public Policy Statements, Letter I: Radiologic Practice and Ethics, Page 9, 1989–1999.

15 Informed Consent and Prostate Specific Antigen Screening

What Patients Ought to Know

Evelyn C. Y. Chan, MD, MS

CONTENTS

INTRODUCTION
JUSTIFICATION FOR INFORMED CONSENT
INFORMED CONSENT
RISK COMMUNICATION
DECISION AIDS
CONCLUSION
REFERENCES

INTRODUCTION

Screening for prostate cancer with prostate-specific antigen (PSA) is controversial. National professional organizations have issued different recommendations. In 1993, the American Cancer Society recommended PSA screening as part of an annual prostate examination in men age 50 yr and older or beginning at age 40 in men at high risk *(1)*. The American Urological Association issued similar recommendations *(2)*. In 1997, both organizations added to their recommendations that men ought to be informed of the risks and benefits of PSA screening *(3,4)*. In contrast, the U.S. Preventive Services Task Force *(5)* and the National Cancer Institute *(6)* have refrained from recommending annual PSA screening.

At the center of the controversy are questions that remain unanswered. Until randomized clinical trials such as the Prostate, Lung, Colorectal,

From: *Current Clinical Urology: Prostate Cancer Screening*
Edited by: I. M. Thompson, M. I. Resnick, and E. A. Klein
© Humana Press Inc., Totowa, NJ

and Ovarian Cancer Trial are complete *(7,8),* whether mass screening
with PSA reduces the morbidity and mortality from prostate cancer will
remain unknown. The overall balance of benefits and harms from widespread screening and its consequences will also remain unclear, along
with the economic implications and the appropriate course of public
health policy that the nation ought to adopt *(9).*

Already, the issue of PSA screening has surfaced in national politics.
In 1999, members of Congress, many of whom included survivors of
prostate cancer, approved legislation for a prostate cancer stamp that
would promote "annual checkups and tests" (10). Soon physicians in
leading medical journals decried the practice of putting a "stamp of
approval" on a screening strategy whose net benefit had not yet been
proven *(11,12).* Their concerns added to the general debate over whether
to endorse PSA screening for all *(9,13–15).*

Because of the growing recognition that there are potential risks and
benefits to PSA screening, several professional organizations and individual physicians support discussing them with patients. In addition to
the American Cancer Society *(3)* and the American Urological Association, *(4)* the American Academy of Family Physicians *(16)* and the
American College of Physicians *(17)* support patient informed decision
making. In effect, informed consent for screening is gaining support
(15,18–20).

JUSTIFICATION FOR INFORMED CONSENT

One of the basic principles of medical ethics is the principle of
nonmaleficence, an obligation not to inflict harm intentionally,
which has been closely associated with the maxim *Primum non nocere*:
"Above all [or first] do no harm" (21). From this, it has been argued that
the practice of recommending PSA screening in the absence of clear
evidence that there is a net benefit has focused primarily on the benefits
for the sick (the "patient") rather than on the healthy and ought not to be
done *(22).*

The assumption that the earlier a disease is detected, the better it is for
the patient is questionable because of several potential risks *(22).* For
diseases for which there is no or only rarely successful treatment, very
early detection may lead to anxiety, because the patient will know for
a longer period of time that he has a disease for which little can be done.
A patient may be subject to the risk of receiving unnecessary treatment
or overtreatment, defined as treatment that he would have never received
had he not been screened and from which he gained no net benefit *(22).*
A patient may also undergo a procedure for the removal of prostate

cancer that was the preferred method at the time of diagnosis, but later was shown to be more aggressive or more damaging than was needed *(22)*. On a societal level, a premature recommendation can reduce the chance that a randomized clinical trial of the test can be completed to determine whether there is a net benefit for everyone. If people come to believe that a test is beneficial, they may be less willing to be assigned to the control group *(22)*. This concern has already been raised with clinical trials for PSA screening *(23)*.

Regardless of whether PSA screening ought to be recommended, the practice of PSA screening is already widespread *(13,24–26)*. This raises the issue of what to do. Without clear evidence of a net benefit for PSA screening from randomized clinical trials and without a clear consensus from experts in the medical community, whether PSA screening ought to be done should be decided with a patient's perspective and choice in mind. Because screening with PSA carries potential benefits and potential harms, a patient in consultation with his personal physician ought to weigh facts and values to arrive at a decision in his best interest *(19,27–30)*.

The process of patient education leading up to patient involvement in shared decision making will be challenging because studies show that many men do not know even the most basic facts about prostate cancer screening or PSA *(31–35)*. For example, in a study conducted from 1993 to 1994 with 369 men at two different Veterans Administration facilities, Diefenbach and colleagues found that only 31% of the men at one site and 16.3% at the other site were aware that they had received a PSA test, even though all eligible subjects in the study had had it. Few men understood what the PSA test measured (<21%) and even fewer (<7%) knew what further workup would be required for an abnormal test result *(31)*. In a statewide telephone survey conducted around the same time, Mainous and Hagen found that men were poorly informed about prostate cancer. Some men even thought that the PSA test is a test for sterility *(33)*.

More recent studies have focused upon whether patients are knowledgeable about the risks and benefits of screening. In 1996, Federman and colleagues found that 69% of 173 men at a university-affiliated Veterans Affairs medical center were aware that their physician had ordered a PSA test. Among the 120 men who were aware of receiving a PSA test, only 47% recalled having a discussion with their primary care provider about the risks and benefits of screening *(32)*. O'Dell and colleagues also found that at a university-based family medicine clinic, aside from college graduates, most patients could not identify the principal advantages and disadvantages of PSA screening *(34)*.

Although African-American men have a higher incidence of prostate cancer, are more likely to be diagnosed at an advanced stage and have higher mortality rates than Caucasian men *(36–39)*, they are less knowledgeable about prostate cancer and screening than Caucasians. In a study of 319 men, 82% of whom were African-American, Weinrich found that on a six-item scale of knowledge, Caucasians had more knowledge about prostate cancer screening than African-Americans (P=0.07) *(40)*. Barbar and colleagues found that African-American men were significantly less likely than Caucasian men to correctly identify facts about risk, symptoms, and screening for prostate cancer *(41)*. Other studies have shown that African-American men remain largely ignorant about prostate cancer and screening *(42,43)*.

Just how much of this situation arises from the extent to which physicians and other health care providers fail to communicate information about it to patients is not clear. Patients may, for example, forget whether a physician discussed PSA screening with them. However, it is clear that physicians and health care providers need to continue improving their educational and research efforts in this area.

INFORMED CONSENT

Implementation: "How Do I Do It?"

There are two models for implementing informed consent: the "event" model and the "process" model. In the event model, a physician, as expert, simply discloses facts to a patient, who then assesses his values to arrive at a decision. This model treats medical decision making as a discrete event that takes place at a single moment in time. In the process model, a physician, as an expert advisor, helps the patient assess facts and values to arrive at a decision through a process of shared decision making. This model treats medical decision making as a process that evolves over time so that a patient can consider the values that he and his physician hold. It also permits patients to reflect upon and discuss issues with spouses, friends, and family *(27–30,44–46)*.

A similar conceptualization of informed consent proposes a graded approach to informed consent, with less informed consent required in some situations and greater informed consent in others. By this conceptualization, greater informed consent would be required incrementally in situations in which there are an increasing number of the following variables present: no emergency, no patient waiver, a competent patient, provision of information not potentially harmful, invasive procedure, experimental procedure, high risk/benefit ratio, patient objects, acceptable medical alternatives available, physician approaches patient, known physician, demanding patient *(27)*. Greater informed consent might be promoted better through the process model of implementation, whereas less explicit informed consent might be satisfied through the event model. In both cases it is also appropriate to respect a patient's wish for less information and less decision-making responsibility. Cultural factors as well as individual preferences can influence a patient's desire for information *(29,47–50)*.

Much has been written about striking the "right" balance between respecting a patient's autonomy and respecting a physician's influence on behalf of a patient's health *(51)*. This struggle between the values of a patient and physician in the physician–patient relationship can shape the implementation of informed consent. The Emanuels *(51)* have outlined four models of the physician–patient relationship: the paternalistic, the informative, the interpretive, and the deliberative models. They advocate the deliberative model as the most ideal one to aspire to because it more fully recognizes a patient's autonomy. In this kind of relationship, physicians discuss information about the patient's clinical condition, then help elucidate the values embodied in the available options. The deliberative physician does not paternalistically impose values upon a patient. Instead, this physician tries to persuade the patient of the worthiness of certain ones. This physician helps the patient engage in moral deliberation and dialogue about which course of action would be best. In this manner, patient autonomy is more fully realized. A patient can critically assess values and preferences, his own and those of his physician, determine which ones are desirable, and then pursue a course of action that realizes them *(51)*.

Quill and Brody *(52)* describe an ideal physician–patient relationship similar to the one advocated by the Emanuels *(51)*. They envision two medical decision models, the enhanced autonomy model and the independent choice model. In the independent choice model, the physician's primary role in medical decision making is to inform patients about their options and the odds of success. Patients are encouraged to make decisions without the influence of the physician. In the enhanced autonomy model, which they endorse, a patient's autonomous choice is enhanced, rather than undermined, by the support of the physician *(52)*. Like the Emanuels' deliberative model, patients consider their values and those of their physicians to arrive at an enhanced, but autonomous, medical decision.

Both the deliberative model and the enhanced autonomy model of the physician-patient relationship fit well with the process model of implementing informed consent. These approaches to informed consent are also supported by the President's Commission for the Study of Ethical Problems in Medicine and Biomedical and Behavioral Research *(51–54)*.

Standards: "How Much Do I Disclose?"

When implementing informed consent, a practical question that physicians face is: "How much do I disclose?" Two legal standards of disclosure have emerged: the professional standard and the reasonable person standard. Under the professional standard, physicians ought to disclose information that expert physicians practicing in the same or in a similar community would customarily disclose in the patient's best interest. Under the reasonable person standard, physicians ought to disclose information that a hypothetical reasonable person would need to know in order to make an informed decision. Those who support the reasonable person standard believe that the obligation to respect patient autonomy requires that the information disclosed ought to be determined more from the patient's perspective than the physician's. This makes it morally preferable to the professional practice standard *(27,55,56)*.

Content: "What Do I Say?"

Another practical question physicians face is: "What do I say?" Legal standards of disclosure set guidelines rather than explicitly state which facts ought to be disclosed. Chan and Sulmasy conducted a study to determine the facts about PSA screening that physicians and patients believe ought to be disclosed in an informed consent discussion. Their findings can form the basis of discussions that follow either the event or process models of informed consent *(57)*.

To find out what men ought to know about PSA screening, Chan and Sulmasy first collected primary data by two qualitative methods, the Delphi method and the Nominal Group Technique (58). Because the reasonable person standard presupposes that the information disclosed depends on what a hypothetical reasonable person ought to know, Chan and Sulmasy asked several types of people for their point of view. They asked 12 experts and 24 couples what key facts men ought to know. Using the Delphi method, they asked two types of experts: urologists and nonurologists. Using the nominal group technique to run six focus groups of couples, Chan and Sulmasy asked two types of couples: those with men who had already undergone PSA screening and those who had not. The Delphi method and nominal group technique can run in tandem. Both methods help a group of people generate ideas in response to a question and then prune them to a core set of ideas that all agree upon *(57)*.

Chan and Sulmasy then compared what each group had to say. They compared the views of experts with couples, the views of urologists with nonurologists, and the views of couples with screened and unscreened men. Finally, they convened a multidisciplinary focus group to help interpret this information and to define what a reasonable person ought to know before consenting to PSA screening (57).

To apply the Delphi method, Chan and Sulmasy convened a panel of 12 nationally known experts in prostate cancer screening from across the country. They recruited six urologists and six nonurologists, two each from Internal Medicine, Family Medicine, and Oncology. By the end of the Delphi process, an iterative series of questionnaires and feedback reports, panelists had voted and agreed upon the top 10 key facts that men ought to know (57).

Experts said that men ought to know that false-positive and false-negative PSA results are possible, that regular PSA screening is controversial, and that it is not clear whether it will reduce the mortality from prostate cancer even though it can detect cancer sooner than the digital rectal exam alone. Experts also said that men should understand the natural history of prostate cancer and its potential for slow growth. This makes screening with the PSA and digital rectal exam most appropriate for men with a greater than a 10-yr life expectancy. Men ought to understand the treatment options and that there is uncertainty about the benefits of treating early, localized prostate cancer. Experts also said that after weighing the risks and benefits, men should make their own decision about whether to undergo PSA screening (57).

Using nominal group technique, Chan and Sulmasy asked African-American and Caucasian couples with screened and unscreened men what facts men ought to know about PSA screening. They asked couples rather than men alone because health promotion programs recommend targeting women in order to reach the men in their lives (59,60). Wives often provide information about prostate cancer screening to their husbands as well as schedule their screening appointments (59–61). Furthermore, prostate cancer treatments can affect the quality of life of both partners when a potential complication such as erectile dysfunction occurs (33).

After viewing a videotape about PSA screening designed by members of the Prostate Patient Outcomes Research Team (62) and engaging in a focus group discussion, couples arrived at the key facts that they believed men ought to know. Focus groups of couples with men who had already been screened would disclose the natural history of prostate cancer and how the PSA test can detect cancer sooner than the digital rectal exam. Focus groups of couples with unscreened men would disclose that PSA testing is controversial and that complications can occur with prostate cancer treatment. All couples agreed that it is important to disclose that the PSA test is a blood test with false-positive or false-negative test results, that it is unclear whether PSA screening reduces the mortality from prostate cancer, and that taking the test may lead to anxiety over what a test result means *(57)*.

Chan and Sulmasy's results show that physicians and patients can agree upon key facts that men ought to know about PSA screening. However, they also show that physicians fail to emphasize some facts that patients find important. None of the experts included 'what a PSA test is' among their top 10 facts to disclose. Moreover, physicians may underestimate the potential for patient anxiety over what an elevated PSA result means *(57)*.

To help further interpret the primary data collected by the Delphi method and by nominal group technique, a multidisciplinary group of couples, experts, ethicists, and a lawyer was convened. Group members viewed the same videotape that the couples had seen and reviewed the key facts that experts and couples had selected. Then, they proposed what they thought a reasonable person ought to know before giving informed consent for PSA screening *(57)*.

The group consensus was that men ideally ought to know *all* of the facts shown in Table 1. They agreed with all other study participants (experts and couples) that at the minimum, men ought to know that false-positive and false-negative PSA results are possible and that it is not clear whether PSA screening reduces the mortality from prostate cancer. However, they noted that physicians may not have the time to disclose everything and that patients may feel overwhelmed. Therefore, the group recommended that physicians disclose some of the most important facts during a conversation and the rest in a brochure *(57)*.

A limitation of the study is that the responses Chan and Sulmasy found may not have been representative of physicians and patients in general because their use of qualitative methods limited the number of participants. Additionally, although the PSA videotape gave each focus group participant core knowledge about PSA screening so that each could engage in group discussions, the videotape may have introduced nonverbal cues highlighting some facts over others. Notably, in spite of such potential limitations, Chan and Sulmasy found that experts and couples consistently mentioned three key facts that patients, at a minimum, ought to know: (1) Nobody knows whether regular PSA screening will reduce the number of deaths from prostate cancer. (2) False-positive PSA test results can occur. (3) False-negative PSA test results and false-negative biopsies of the prostate can occur. Physicians disclosing any less would be imparting less importance to patient autonomy *(57)*.

Table 1
Proposed Content for Informed Consent for PSA Screening

I. Basic Minimum

1. False positive PSA test results can occur.
2. False negative PSA test results and false negative biopsies of the prostate can occur.
3. Nobody knows whether regular PSA screening will reduce the number of deaths from prostate cancer.

II. Conversation

4. The PSA test is a blood test for prostate cancer.
5. Done together, the digital rectal exam and the PSA test can screen for prostate cancer.
6. The PSA screening test can detect prostate cancer sooner than the digital rectal exam alone.
7. An elevated PSA test result may lead to other tests to see whether prostate cancer is present.
8. The risk of getting prostate cancer is higher is a man who:
   is older
   has a family history of it
   is African-American
9. Prostate cancer may grow slowly and not cause any symptoms. That is why prostate cancer may not kill older men. They may outlive this cancer and die from something else.
10. A man over age 70 is less likely to die from prostate cancer even though he is at higher risk to have it.

III. Brochure

11. The PSA screening test is controversial.
12. There are advantages and disadvantages to taking the PSA test. One disadvantage is that a man could end up worrying about what an elevated PSA test result means.
13. Done together, the PSA and digital rectal exam, are most appropriate for men who have more than 10 years left to live.
14. A man with early prostate cancer can choose one of these options:
   watchful waiting
   radical prostatectomy
   radiation therapy
15. There are side effects from prostate cancer treatment such as:
   impotence
   incontinence
   narrowing of the urethra, strictures
   trouble urinating and rectal scarring
16. Nobody knows whether treating prostate cancer early is helpful or whether one treatment is better than another.
17. Although a man thinking about taking the PSA test can consult a doctor, he should make the final decision himself.

Reprinted with permission *(57)*.

In their entirety, the facts that Chan and Sulmasy found can form the basis of a one-on-one discussion between a physician and patient in the clinic setting to facilitate the process model of informed consent. For example, a physician who believes that PSA screening may be beneficial for some patients may begin a conversation with facts that Chan and Sulmasy found and then indicate the manner in which PSA screening may be beneficial for that particular patient. Consistent with the process model of informed consent, this physician could disclose his own values, his own reasons for supporting PSA screening for a particular patient, and encourage the patient to choose between those values and the patient's own. In contrast, at a mass-screening event, the event model of informed consent might be more practical. Facts could be incorporated into a brochure or consent form to facilitate patient decision making *(57)*.

Understanding and Consent: "Did the Patient Understand?"

Although there is no consensus on the nature of understanding and more research is needed to determine how to promote and evaluate it, patients need to be able to indicate that they understood the facts discussed in order to make a decision about screening *(55)*. Physicians can assess patient understanding by asking open-ended questions *(63)*. One common myth is that patients cannot give informed consent because they cannot understand complex information. However, patients do not need to understand information in exactly the same way and to the same extent as a physician. They just need to be able to understand their options, the potential risks, the benefits of these options and then make a decision consistent with the values they choose *(44)*.

RISK COMMUNICATION

In their study about what men ought to know about PSA screening, Chan and Sulmasy found that even though couples desired information about their risk factors and the incidence and prevalence of prostate cancer, their experts did not mention these among their key facts to disclose. It may have been a limitation of the Delphi method that although their experts believed such facts are important to disclose, the experts were not able to reach a consensus on whether, or how, such population-based information could be disclosed in a meaningful way to individual patients *(57)*. Therefore, physicians can begin with the facts that Chan and Sulmasy found and elaborate upon them with information about personal risk as they consider the circumstances of each individual patient.

In a review of the literature, Rothman and Kiviniemi *(64)* described two general approaches to communicating health risk information: a numerical probability-based approach and a contextualized approach. Lay perceptions of risk are affected not only by probability information but also by a richer set of cognitive and affective beliefs that include knowledge about the antecedents (e.g., "Is it controllable?") and consequences of a problem *(64)*.

With a probability-based approach, a physician would present numerical information about the probability of a given risk occurring. This could be done by framing the information in terms of how frequently someone will die as a result of a risk or by presenting the risk information in such a way that its magnitude can be compared to that of other risks. The main challenge is that although a statistical number offers people precise information, many people have difficulty accurately interpreting and using numerical probabilities *(64)*.

With a contextualized approach, a physician provides an informational context with which to help a patient understand and interpret the relevance of a risk. Examples of this would include information about what causes prostate cancer, the severity of the consequences, and what can be done to prevent or treat it. One main challenge in this area is that people may selectively attend to the information presented in order to maintain a favorable impression of their health status *(64)*.

Additionally, there are five basic dimensions of risk that a physician may discuss with a patient: identity, permanence, timing, probability (quantitative frequency), and value (subjective "badness"). A physician can help a patient identify the pertinent unwanted outcomes of an intervention, assess how permanent the unwanted outcome will be, when it will occur, the likelihood it will happen, and whether it will matter to the patient *(65)*.

Much research is needed to determine the optimal way to communicate cancer risk to patients of different socioeconomic, educational, and cultural backgrounds. In 1999, the National Cancer Institute sponsored a conference on "Cancer Risk Communication: What We Know and What We Need to Learn." Papers presented at that conference appear as a monograph in the *Journal of the National Cancer Institute* and describe the challenges that confront individual health professionals, institutions, and mass media communicating cancer risk *(65)*.

DECISION AIDS

Decision support interventions known as "decision aids" or "shared-decision-making programs" are being developed in cancer screening programs as adjuncts to physician counseling. They are designed to help patients understand the benefits and risks of options, to consider the values they place on those benefits and risks, and to participate actively in the decision-making process with their physician. They may be administered with various media such as interactive videodiscs, audiotapes, personal computers, audio-guided workbooks, pamphlets, and group presentations *(67)*. They have the potential to promote informed decision making in busy clinics *(68,69)* and to tailor information to the specific needs of individual patients *(67)*.

O'Connor and colleagues reviewed the evidence about the efficacy of decision aids focused on cancer outcomes and found that, in many cases, decision aids are superior to usual care in improving knowledge and in creating realistic expectations. They found that decision aids are better than usual care at moderating patients' exaggerated perceptions of risk of disease and exaggerated perceptions of the benefits of interventions *(67)*.

Few studies have been done to evaluate decision aids specifically designed for PSA screening and to determine how they might be incorporated in a busy clinic practice to promote informed consent. Two trials using a videotape about PSA screening produced by the Prostate Patient Outcomes Research Team (PORT) have shown that this kind of decision aid can improve knowledge about PSA screening over usual care, but by itself does not necessarily clarify patients' values *(70,71)*.

Studies are also needed to determine how information is framed affects patient knowledge and decision making in different ethnic groups. A study using the PORT videotape found that a group of predominantly Caucasian men receiving the intervention were less likely to be interested in PSA screening *(57)*. Similarly, another trial comparing a scripted informational intervention with facts about PSA screening to a single sentence about PSA screening found that men receiving the intervention were less likely to be interested in PSA screening *(72)*. However, in a trial involving a tailored behavioral intervention with facts about PSA screening, Myers and colleagues found that African-American men receiving the intervention were more likely to adhere to PSA screening *(73)*. Notably, none of the interventions in the three trials mentioned *(72,73)* or highlighted *(70)* the potential risk for patient anxiety over what an elevated PSA result means, a key finding that experts and couples believed men ought to know in Chan and Sulmasy's study *(57)*.

CONCLUSION

Just as our concept of informed consent has expanded beyond a single event to a process of shared decision making, our concept of health care has expanded beyond the traditional biomedical model with its focus on disease to the outcomes model with its focus on quality of life. Because the biomedical model is directed toward diagnosing and treating conditions, success occurs when diseases have been accurately diagnosed and treated. Because the outcomes model is directed toward maximizing quality-adjusted life expectancy, success occurs when patients have made a decision that improves the quality of their lives. This model encourages shared decision making about PSA screening *(74)*. In shared decision making, physicians must communicate medical uncertainty and help patients identify values that form the basis for preferred outcomes *(74)*. Until randomized clinical trials clarify the role of PSA screening, physicians should adhere to the maxim *Primum non nocere*, respect patient autonomy, and engage patients in informed consent.

REFERENCES

1. Mettlin C, Jones G, Averett H, et al. (1993) Defining and updating the American Cancer Society guidelines for the cancer-related checkup. CA: *Cancer Clin J* 43:42–46.
2. American Urological Association, Inc. (1992) Early detection of prostate cancer. American Urological Association Executive Committee Report. Baltimore, MD.
3. Eschenbach AV, Ho R, Murphy GP, Cunningham M, Lins N. (1997) American Cancer Society Guideline for the Early Detection of Prostate Cancer: Update 1997. *CA Cancer J Clin* 47:261–264.
4. American Urological Association, Inc. (1997) Early detection of prostate cancer. *American Urological Association Executive Committee Report*. Baltimore, MD.
5. U.S. Preventive Services Task Force. (1996) *Guide to Clinical Preventive Services*. 2nd ed., Baltimore, MD: Williams & Wilkins.
6. Physician Data Query (computer database). (1996) Prostate Cancer Screening State-of-the-Art Statement. Bethesda, MD: National Cancer Institute.
7. Gohagan JK, Prorok PC, Kramer BS, Cornett JE. (1994) Prostate cancer screening in the prostate, lung, colorectal and ovarian cancer screening trial of the National Cancer Institute. *J Urol* 152:1905–1909.
8. Kramer BS, Gohagan J, Prorok PC, Smart C. (1993) A National Cancer Institute sponsored screening trial for prostatic, lung, colorectal, and ovarian cancers. *Cancer* 71(2):589–593.
9. Woolf SH. (1995) Screening for prostate cancer with prostate-specific antigen. An examination of the evidence. *N Engl J Med* 333(21):1401–1405.
10. The Prostate Cancer Research Stamp Act of 1997, H.R. 2545. 105th Congress, 1997.
11. Woloshin S, Schwartz LM. (1999) The U.S. postal service and cancer screening—stamps of approval? *N Engl J Med* 340(11):884–887.
12. Friedrich MJ. (1999) Issues in prostate cancer screening. *JAMA* 281(17):1573–1575.
13. Hicks RJ, Hamm RM, Bemben DA. (1995) Prostate cancer screening: what family physicians believe is best. *Arch Fam Med* 4:317–322.
14. Catalona WJ (1999) The postal service and cancer screening. *N Engl J Med* 341(7):542.

15. Middleton RG. (1997) Prostate cancer: are we screening and treating too much? *Ann Intern Med* 126:465–467.

16. American Academy of Family Physicians. (1999) Summary of recommendations for periodic health examination. Available at www.aafp.org/exam/app-d_c.html. Accessed December 3, 1999.

17. Coley CM, Barry MJ, Mulley AG. (1997) Clinical Guideline: Part III. Screening for prostate cancer. *Ann Intern Med* 126:480–484.

18. Glode LM. (1994) Prostate cancer screening: a place for informed consent? *Hosp Pract* 29:8–12.

19. Brett AS. (1995) The mammography and prostate-specific antigen controversies: implication for patient-physician encounters and public policy. *J Gen Intern Med* 10:266–270.

20. Kramer BS, Brown ML, Prorok PC, Potosky AL, Gohagan JK. (1993) Prostate cancer screening: what we know and what we need to know. *Ann Intern Med* 119(9):914–922.

21. Beauchamp TL, Childress JF. (1994) Nonmaleficence In: *Principles of Biomedical Ethics*. 4th ed., Oxford University Press, pp. 189–258.

22. Malm HM. (1999) Medical screening and value of early detection. When unwarranted faith leads to unethical recommendations. *Hastings Center Report* 29(1):26–37.

23. Barry MJ. (1997) Is there an easier way to determine whether early detection of prostate cancer reduces mortality? *J Gen Intern Med* 12(10):657–658.

24. McKnight JT, Tietze PH, Adcock BB, Maxwell AJ, Smith WO, Nagy MC. (1996) Screening for prostate cancer: a comparison of urologists and primary care physicians. *Southern Med J* 89(9):885–888.

25. Williams RB, Boles M, Johnson RE. (1995) Use of prostate-specific antigen for prostate cancer screening in primary care practice. *Arch Fam Med* 4:311–315.

26. Hoffman RM, Blume P, Gilliland F. (1998) Prostate-specific antigen testing practices and outcomes. *J Gen Intern Med* 13:106–110.

27. Sprung CL, Winick BJ. (1989) Informed consent in theory and practice: legal and medical perspectives on the informed consent doctrine and a proposed reconceptualization. *Crit Care Med* 17(12):1346–1354.

28. Hollander RD. (1984) Changes in the concept of informed consent in medical encounters. *J Med Educ* 59:783–788.

29. Diem SJ. (1997) How and when should physicians discuss clinical decisions with patients? *J Gen Intern Med* 12(6):397–398.

30. Lidz CW, Appelbaum PS, Meisel A. (1988) Two models of implementing informed consent. *Arch Intern Med* 148:1385–1389.

31. Diefenbach PN, Ganz PA, Pawlow AJ, Guthrie D. (1996) Screening by the prostate-specific antigen test: What do the patients know? *J Cancer Educ* 11:39–44.

32. Federman DG, Goyal S, Kamina A, Peduzzi P, Concato J. (1999) Informed consent for PSA screening: Does it happen? *Effective Clin Practice* 2(4):152–157.

33. Mainous AG III, Hagen MD. (1994) Public awareness of prostate cancer and the prostate-specific antigen test. *Cancer Pract* 2(3):217-221.

34. O'Dell KJ, Volk RJ, Cass AR, Spann SJ. (1999) Screening for prostate cancer with the prostate-specific antigen test. Are patients making informed decisions? *J Fam Pract* 48:682–688.

35. Demark-Wahnefried W, Catoe KE, Paskett E, Robertson CN, Rimer BK. (1993) Characteristics of men reporting for prostate cancer screening. *Urology* 42(3):269–275.

36. Landis SH, Murray T, Bolden S, Wingo PA. (1999) Cancer Statistics, 1999. CA *Cancer J Clin* 49(1): 8–31.

37. Powell IJ. (1997) Prostate cancer and African-American men. *Oncology* 11(5):599–605.

38. Brawn PN, Johnson EH, Kuhl DI., Riggs MW, Speights VO, Johnson CF, et al. (1993) Stage at presentation and survival of white and black patients with prostate carcinoma. *Cancer* 72:2569–2573.

39. Natarajan N, Murphy GP, Mettlin C. (1989) Prostate cancer in blacks: an update from the American College of Surgeons' patterns of care studies. *J Surg Oncol* 40:232–236.

40. Weinrich SP, Weinrich MC, Boyd MD, Atkinson C. (1998) The impact of prostate cancer knowledge on cancer screening. *Oncol Nurs Forum* 25(3):527–534.

41. Barber KR, Shaw R, Folts M, Taylor DK, Ryan A, Hughes M, et al. (1998) Differences between African-American and Caucasian men participating in a community-based prostate cancer screening program. *J Community Health* 23(6):441–451.

42. Smith GE, DeHaven MJ, Grundig JP, Wilson GR. (1997) African-American males and prostate cancer: assessing knowledge levels in the community. *J Natl Med Assoc* 89(6):387–391.

43. Demark-Wahnefried W, Strigo T, Catoe K, Conaway M, Brunetti M, Rimer BK, et al. (1995) Knowledge, beliefs, and prior screening behavior among blacks and whites reporting for prostate cancer screening. *Urology* 46(3):346–351.

44. Meisel A, Kuczewski M. (1996) Legal and ethical myths about informed consent. *Arch Intern Med* 156:2521–2526.

45. Geller G, Botkin JR, Green MJ, Press N, Biesecker BB, Wilfond B, et al. (1997) Genetic testing for susceptibility to adult-onset cancer. The process and content of informed consent. *JAMA* 277(18):1467–1474.

46. Volk RJ, Cantor SB, Spann SJ, Cass AR, Cardenas MP, Warren MM. (1997) Preferences of husbands and wives for prostate cancer screening. *Arch Fam Med* 6:72–76.

47. Tobias JS, Souhami RL. (1993) Fully informed consent can be needlessly cruel. *Br Med J* 307(6913:1199–1201.

48. Blackhall LJ, Murphy ST, Frank G, Michel V, Azen S. (1995) Ethnicity and attitudes toward patient autonomy. *JAMA* 274:820–825.

49. Carrese JA, Rhodes LA. (1995) Western bioethics on the Navajo reservation: benefit or harm? *JAMA* 274(10):826–829.

50. Gostin LO. (1995) Informed consent, cultural sensitivity, and respect for persons. *JAMA* 274(10): 844–845.

51. Emanuel EJ, Emanuel LL. (1992) Four models of the physician-patient relationship. *JAMA* 267(16):2221–2226.

52. Quill TE, Brody H. (1996) Physician recommendations and patient autonomy: finding a balance between physician power and patient choice. *Ann Intern Med* 125(9):763–769.

53. *President's Commission for the Study of Ethical Problems in Medicine and Biomedical Research: Making Health Care Decisions*. Washington, DC: Government Printing Office, 1982 Vol. 1.

54. Forrow L, Wartman SA, Brock DW. (1988) Science, ethics and the making of clinical decisions. Implications for risk factor intervention. *JAMA* 259(21):3161–3167.

55. Beauchamp TL, Childress JF. (1994) , Respect for Autonomy. In: *Principles of Biomedical Ethics*. 4th ed., Oxford University Press, pp. 120–188.
56. Faden RR, Beauchamp TL. (1986) *A History and Theory of Informed Consent*. New York: Oxford University Press.
57. Chan ECY, Sulmasy DP. (1998) What should men know about prostate-specific antigen screening before giving informed consent? *Am J Med* 105:266–274.
58. Delbecq AL, Van de Ven AH, Gustafson DH. (1986) Group Techniques for Program Planning: A Guide to Nominal Group and Delphi Processes. Middleton, WI: Green Briar Press.
59. AARP. (1994) Health Promotion for Men 50+. Washington, DC: American Association of Retired Persons.
60. Rubenstein L. (1994) Strategies to overcome barriers to early detection of cancer among older adults. *Cancer* 74:2190–2193.
61. Stair J. (1992) Public awareness of screening programs. *Oncol Nurs Forum* 19:93–94.
62. Foundation for Informed Medical Decision Making. (1995) The PSA decision: what YOU need to know. Videotape. Hanover, NH: Foundation for Informed Medical Decision Making.
63. Searight HR, Barbarash RA. (1994) Informed Consent: clinical and legal issues in family practice. *Fam Med* 26:244–249.
64. Rothman AJ, Kiviniemi MT. (1999) Treating people with information: an analysis and review of approaches to communicating health risk information. *J Natl Cancer Inst Monogr* 25:44–51.
65. Bogardus ST, Holmboe E, Jekel JF. (1999) Perils, pitfalls, and possibilities in talking about medical risk. *JAMA* 281(11):1037–1041.
66. National Cancer Institute, (1999) Monogr Natl Cancer Inst. No. 25.
67. O'Connor AM, Fiset V, DeGrasse C, Graham ID, Evans W, Stacey D, et al. (1999) Decision aids for patients considering options affecting cancer outcomes: evidence of efficacy and policy implications. *Natl Cancer Inst Monogr* 25:67–80.
68. Taylor HA. (1999) Barriers to informed consent. *Semin Oncol Nurs* 15(2):89–95.
69. Braddock CH III, Fihn SD, Levinson W, Jonsen AR, Pearlman RA. (1997) How doctors and patients discuss routine clinical decisions. *J Gen Intern Med* 12:339–345.
70. Volk RJ, Cass AR, Spann SJ. (1999) A randomized controlled trial of shared decision making for prostate cancer screening. *Arch Fam Med* 8:333–340.
71. Flood AB, Wennberg JE, Nease RF, Fowler FJ, Ding J, Hynes LM. (1996) Members of the Prostate Patient Outcomes Research Team. *J Gen Intern Med* 11:342–349.
72. Wolf A, Nasser JF, Wolf AM, Schorling JB. (1996) The impact of informed consent on patient interest in prostate-specific antigen screening. *Arch Intern Med* 156:1333–1336.
73. Myers RE, Chodak GW, Wolf TA, Burgh DY, McGrory GT, Marcus SM, et al. (1999) Adherence by African-American men to prostate cancer education and early detection. *Cancer* 86:88–104.
74. Kaplan RM. (1999) Shared medical decision-making: a new paradigm for behavioral medicine—1997 presidential address. *Ann Behav Med* 21(1):3–11.

16 Experience of Prostate Cancer Awareness Week

Zinelabidine Abouelfadel, MD
and E. David Crawford, MD

CONTENTS

INTRODUCTION
THE PHENOMENAL GROWTH OF PCAW
PCAW AND THE INTERNET
RESULTS OF THE LONGITUDINAL STUDY
SPECIAL STUDIES
OUTLOOK
REFERENCES

INTRODUCTION

Prostate cancer is now the most commonly diagnosed cancer and the second leading cause of death among men, surpassing lung cancer. It is estimated that 179,300 new cases will be diagnosed in the United States in 1999, and approx 37,000 men will die from this disease. In the past 12 yr, the incidence has increased 50%, but recently it is starting to decline *(1)*.

Since the late 1980s, it has been evident that prostate cancer was soon to become a major health issue. At that time, most cases diagnosed were either locally advanced or metastatic disease. Disease mortality was inevitable unless death from competing causes occurred first. The lack of public awareness and the absence of any large effort toward early detection were largely responsible for this grim picture.

From: *Current Clinical Urology: Prostate Cancer Screening*
Edited by: I. M. Thompson, M. I. Resnick, and E. A. Klein
© Humana Press Inc., Totowa, NJ

Table 1
Prostate Cancer Education Council

E. David Crawford, MD
  Chairman; University of
  Colorado Health Sciences
  Center, Denver, CO
	Diane S. Blum, MSW
	  Cancer Care, Inc., New York

E. Roy Berger, MD
  Memorial Sloan Kettering,
  New York
	Thomas M. Bruckman
	  American Foundation of Urologic
	  Disease; Baltimore, MD

Wendy Poage, M.H.A
  Director of PCEC; Denver, CO
	Mario Eisenberger. MD
	  John Hopkins University,
	  Baltimore, MD

Frank E. Staggers, MD
  National Medical Association,
  Oakland, CA
	David G. McLeod, MD
	  Walter Reed Army Medical Center,
	  Washington, DC

Robert Lipuma, PhD
  Project Coordinator, Denver, CO
	Nelson Stone, MD
	  Mount Sinai School of Medicine,
	  New York

	Turner C. Lisle
	  Clinical Research Director,
	  Denver, CO

As a result of the high incidence and mortality from this disease, in 1988, we contacted several organizations to initiate a public awareness campaign for the early detection of prostate cancer. Only one organization, Schering Plough, was interested in supporting this effort.

Initiation of the Prostate Cancer Education Council (PCEC) was the first step to creating awareness of the benefits of early detection of this disease. This council is a consortium of members from different disciplines and backgrounds encompassing urology, oncology, clinical and behavioral research, and representatives from prostate cancer patient advocates and minority groups. The current composition of the Prostate Cancer Education Council is listed in Table 1.

The second step in the process was initiating a large health survey, which began in March 1989, to assess the status of public knowledge, attitudes, and health practices regarding prostate cancer. This survey discovered that only 50% of men older than age 40 were having physical examinations, and only half of those men who had physical examinations received a digital rectal examination (DRE).

Despite being the most common cancer in men, in 1989, prostate cancer ranked only eighth in health issues discussed between patient and physician. Prostate cancer research received fewer funds than other programs such as breast cancer and AIDS research. This data demonstrated the discrepancy between public awareness and the magnitude of the problem. It also showed that prostate cancer was simply an ignored disease. The PCEC set as a goal to educate men and women about this deadly disease and to urge men to be screened yearly for it.

At the time, there was no clear screening protocol defined and the usefulness of the prostate-specific antigen (PSA) test was not clearly understood. Although many well-known men were diagnosed with this disease, it was difficult to find a national spokesman to support this cause. Finally, we were able to secure the assistance of football star Rocky Blyer. He had a family member diagnosed with prostate cancer and had been informed on many issues regarding this disease.

A mass-media campaign was initiated and a press conference was held in New York during the summer of 1989. The third week of September was designated as National Prostate Cancer Awareness Week (PCAW). Members involved with the promotion of breast cancer awareness month and the Great American Smoke-out offered their support to this campaign. Effort was initiated in metropolitan centers and at the national level. The first year 15,000 men were screened at 91 participating institutions nationwide. PSA testing was introduced that same year *(2)*.

This massive campaign brought the issue of prostate cancer to the nation's attention. Since then, the diagnosis of many nationally and internationally well-known men with prostate cancer has stressed the importance of screening and early detection. Unfortunately, the death of some of these celebrities has also focused attention on this disease.

THE PHENOMENAL GROWTH OF PCAW

PCAW has become the largest cancer screening program in the United States. Because of its outstanding success, a decision was made to continue this effort. In the 1990s, there were as many as 2400 screening centers participating in the campaign. The number of participants has surpassed more than 3 million, and more than 6000 urologists have dedicated themselves to this effort by offering free prostate examinations.

The PCEC established the standards for screening by defining the guidelines and instituting data collection and reporting procedures. Since 1993, the department of public relations at the University of Colorado Health Sciences Center (UCHSC) has assumed the responsibility of sustaining the national media effort. Dr. David McLeod at Walter Reed Army Medical Center in Washington, DC. was able to secure our most effective spokesman, retired General *Norman Schwarz-*

kopf. He appeared on numerous television shows and was on the cover of *Time* in 1996 promoting the benefits of early detection of this disease. His involvement generated enormous national media attention and increased public awareness of prostate cancer.

A full-time director of PCAW, a data manager, and a biostatistician were appointed. In 1992, the Prostate Cancer Educational Council brought the PCAW under its auspices and started a longitudinal study to collect demographic and clinical data. In order to standardize the screening process, a single method of PSA determination was necessary. The Abbott IMX test was chosen and is now used exclusively. A goal of approx 12,000 participants is targeted for the longitudinal study. At least one-third to one-half of the men were expected to continue with annual screening, which would provide a large enough cohort to examine several variables.

The screening centers provide educational and media support and set up a hotline to schedule appointments. The PCEC provides additional support by informing patients that the screening process does not provide absolute diagnosis of cancer and that abnormal findings warrant further evaluation. Follow-up centers were established for participants with abnormal test results. In 1993, some centers established their own screening calendars and schedules, independent of PCAW, to meet local needs. This accounted for the drop in the number of men participating in the screening; others did not take part because of the cost associated with PSA testing.

In 1994, the PCEC allowed screening centers to charge men a nominal fee for PSA testing: $10 for on-site testing and $20 for off-site testing, which bolstered accrual. In the early stages of the detection effort, the policy was not to charge participants in PCAW for the DRE or the PSA test.

During PCAW, technical assistance was offered to participating centers and a comprehensive guide with step-by-step instructions for running a PCAW screening center was prepared. Patient educational materials were developed and distributed to centers as were summaries of research findings, media materials, and advertisement posters—all of which were provided at no charge.

The PCAW is now under the auspices of the American Foundation for Urological Diseases (AFUD). The annual reports are created with the advice and guidance of its Prostate Health Council. This evolution was the result of the pioneering efforts of Dr. Gene Carlton, Dr. Daracott Vaughan, Dr. Peter Scardino, Dr. Logan Holtgrewe, Dr. William Turner, and AFUD Director Dr. Tom Bruckman.

One of the major disappointments during the early years of PCAW development was finding spokesmen for ethnic minority groups, especially African-Americans. This was especially important because this is a high-risk population for developing prostate cancer. African-Americans are two and a half times more likely to get the disease than any other ethnic group. Recent estimates suggest that one in every eight African-American men will develop this disease in his lifetime. The reason for this high incidence is still unknown although research has shown that they develop the disease earlier than Caucasian men, but are diagnosed later; this tends to make their mortality higher. Nearly 3 million men have been screened in PCAW since it started in 1989, yet only 5.8% were African-American (*see* Fig. 1).

The involvement of some celebrities, such as actor *Danny Glover* in 1996 and *Harry Belafonte,* who was treated for prostate cancer and became the spokesman in 1997, has emphasized the importance of screening and encouraged African-Americans to get tested for the disease.

The Council recognizes that the long-term benefits of screening remain controversial. The discovery of latent cancers and the diagnosis of prostate cancer in patients that would otherwise die of other competing diseases can lead to a dilemma regarding treatment options. Nevertheless, the PCEC believes that men diagnosed early in the course of the disease are in a much better position to evaluate all their treatment options.

PCAW AND THE INTERNET

Many patients turn to the Internet for information. Although the Internet does provide a vast array of information, it is largely unstructured and can be difficult for the layman to navigate. Also, it is important that patients receive reliable information. Our website http://www.pcaw. com provides valuable information on prostate cancer such as the anatomy and physiology of the gland, incidence of disease, risk factors, early disease symptoms, methods of detection, and current available treatments. The information provided stresses the importance of the screening program, sets the program guidelines, and defines the criteria of eligibility for PCAW screening centers. It also provides links to other reliable websites.

RESULTS OF THE LONGITUDINAL STUDY

The majority of participants are between 60 and 70 yr of age. The remaining participants were either below age 40, above age 80, or did not report age or birth date (Fig. 2).

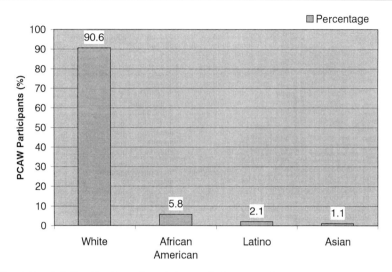

Fig. 1. Racial distribution of participants in Prostate Cancer Awareness Week.

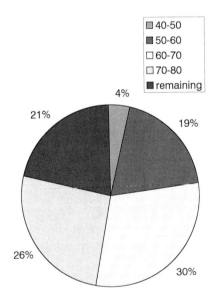

Fig. 2. Age breakdown of participants in longitudinal study.

The longitudinal study has also provided data on variability of average PSA in different ethnic groups, and the screening test values by age range (Table 2 and 3, respectively).

For DRE, we chose these references as a guideline: normal = 1, enlarged benign prostate hyperplasia (BPH) = 2, abnormal—not suspicious = 3, abnormal—suspicious = 4, patient refused = 5.

Table 2
Average PSA by Ethnic Group

Ethnic group	Average PSA
White	1.84
African-American	2.47
Latino-American	1.56
Oriental/Asian	1.74
Other	1.75
Unidentified	1.8

Table 3
Average Screening Test Values
(PSA+DRE) by Age Range

Age (yr)	PSA	DRE
40–50	0.77	1.36
50–60	1.13	1.74
60–70	1.74	2.01
70–80	2.34	2.13

The Efficacy of PSA and DRE in Screening When Using 4.0 ng/mL and Age-Related PSAReference Range as the Cutoff for Abnormal PSA

Between 1992 and 1995, 116,073 men 40–79 yr old were screened during PCAW. Using 4.0 ng/mL and age-specific reference ranges (ASRR) as the abnormal PSA cutoff value, 22,014 and 17,561 men respectively had either abnormal PSA, abnormal DRE, or both *(3)*. When using a 4.0 ng/mL cutoff PSA value, the positive predictive value (PPV) of abnormal PSA alone, abnormal DRE alone, and combined abnormal PSA and DRE are depicted in Fig. 3.

When using ASRR, the cutoff PSA value of the PPV, sensitivity, and specificity of each category were as illustrated in Fig. 4.

The PPV of PSA, DRE, and the combined tests when using an ASRR were higher than those when using a 4.0 ng/mL without statistical significance (all $p > 0.05$). The sensitivity of PSA when using an ASRR was lower than when using 4.0 ng/ml. The significantly higher PPV indicated that the combination of PSA and DRE testing was necessary in screening. Although higher PPVs when using an ASRR cutoff PSA

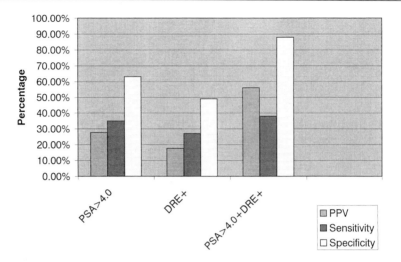

Fig. 3. Sensitivity, specificity, and positive predictive value of PSA, DRE and PSA+DRE using 0.4 ng/ml PSA as the cutoff.

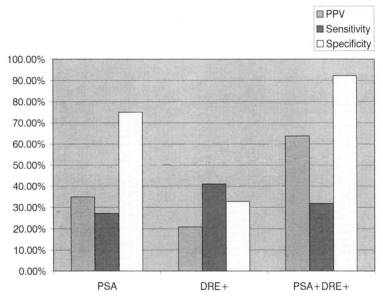

Fig. 4. Sensitivity, specificity, and positive predictive value of PSA, DRE, and PSA+DRE using ASRR as the cutoff.

value suggested fewer unnecessary biopsies, lower sensitivities resulted in fewer cancers detected. Therefore, a PSA value of 4.0 ng/mL is used in the majority of screening programs.

Table 4
Age- Specific Reference Range

Age (yr)	Number screened	Normal PSA range
40–49	2530	0–2.5
50–59	2531	0–3.5
60–69	2532	0–4.5
70–79	2533	0–6.5

Age-related PSA Differences

Since 1989, when PCAW began and only 400 patients had PSA levels checked, it was noted that there was a link between age and PSA level. These data were presented at the American Urological Association meeting in 1991. In 1993, we reported on age-specific reference ranges in 53,000 men. The results are reported in Table 4.

The enrollment of 50,000 additional participants in the longitudinal study and the determination of their PSA levels has led to the development of our current age specific reference ranges shown in Fig. 5.

The retrospective comparison of age-specific reference ranges to the standard reference point of 4.0 ng/mL in predicting prostate cancer has shown that ASRR does increase sensitivity among younger men (less than 60 yr) and specificity among older men (more than 60 yr). These reference ranges included a large cross section of the United States and encompassed several different races. However, 90% of participants were Caucasians.

The upper normal limit was determined as 4.0 ng/mL by Hybritech Company. This was based on level studies in 860 men without prostate cancer (4). It has been noted that age specific reference ranges for African-Americans are different from those for Caucasians. However, ASRR has not been widely accepted as a screening tool. Concerns have been raised about changes in sensitivity and specificity of testing when these reference ranges are being used.

Investigators have reported that the relative risk of developing prostate cancer in younger men increases substantially when the PSA level is more than 1.0 ng/mL. For this category of men, the 4.0-ng/mL value may not be appropriate. If a level less than 4.0 ng/mL is chosen, the sensitivity increases. However, this results in a dramatic reduction in test specificity. Some of those who treat prostate cancer tend to favor sensitivity over specificity because clinically important organ-confined disease is detected by sensitivity testing. ASRR seems to perform best in lower age groups, but it sacrifices sensitivity in the older age groups.

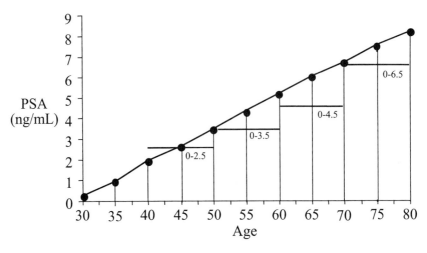

Fig. 5. Age-specific PSA reference ranges, ages 30–80. (From Ref. *11.*)

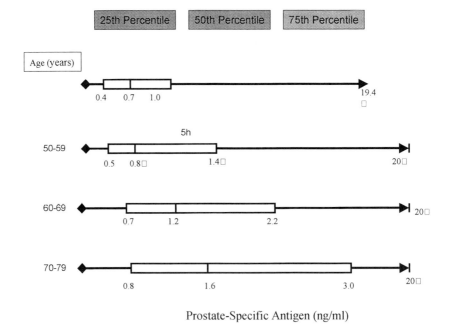

Prostate-Specific Antigen (ng/ml)

Fig. 6. Variability of PSA level with age.

Results have shown that men in their seventies show a greater variability in PSA levels than do men in their fifties (Fig. 6). This is obviously associated with the increasing incidence of BPH, prostate cancer, and other physiologic factors.

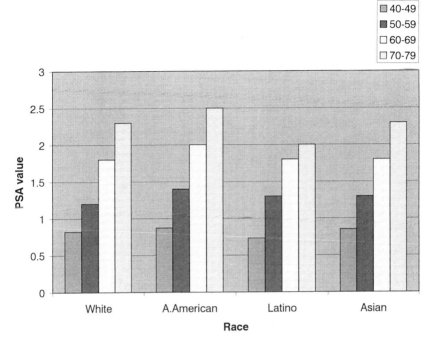

Fig. 7. Mean PSA values in ethnic groups by age.

Race-Related PSA

A retrospective study was performed that included the records of 77,700 men aged 40–79 yr, between 1993 and 1994, that analyzed the relationship of age and race to PSA level. Significant differences in mean PSA by race were found *(5)* (Fig. 7). Differences in age-specific PSA references were found between Caucasians and African-American, Caucasians and Latinos, African-American and Asians, and Asians and Latinos (Table 5).

Still, the clinical significance of race-specific PSA reference is yet to be defined. More studies in this area are warranted.

Yearly PSA Screening in Men
with Initial Normal PSA and Normal DRE

To evaluate the usefulness of yearly follow-up in patients with normal PSA and normal DRE, 6804 men who participated in the PCAW from 1992 to 1995 who had both a normal PSA and normal DRE were categorized into three groups according to their PSA levels: 0–1 ng/mL, 1.1–2 ng/mL, or 2.1–4 ng/mL. The risk of developing an abnormal PSA>4.0 ng/ mL was studied among these cohorts over a period of 3 yr (Table 6).

Table 5
Age-Specific PSA Reference Ranges by Race.

Age	Caucasian	African-American	Latino	Asian
40–49	0–2.3	0–2.7	0–2.1	0–2.0
50–59	0–3.8	0–4.4	0–4.3	0–4.5
60–69	0–5.6	0–6.7	0–6.0	0–4.5
70–79	0–6.9	0–7.7	0–6.6	0–6.8

Table 6
Risk of Developing Abnormal PSA (>4.0 ng/mL)

Initial PSA (ng/ml)	Number screened	Risk of developing abnormal PSA (>4.0 ng/ml)
0–1.0	4013	38 (0.9%)
1–1.2	1844	77 (4.1%)
2.1–4	947	320 (33.8%)

The risk of developing an abnormal PSA in men with an initial PSA of 2.1–4 ng/mL when compared to men with an initial PSA of 0–1 ng/mL or 1.1–2 ng/mL was 35.68 (95% CI = 25.51, 49.95, $p < 0.0001$) and 8.09 (95%CI = 6.40 and 10.23, $p < 0.0001$), respectively.

This study concluded that men with a PSA of 2 ng/mL or less and an initial normal DRE had very little risk of developing an abnormal PSA within the subsequent 3-yr period. Therefore, annual monitoring of the PSA in this group of men may not be necessary for the subsequent 3-yr period. In contrast, the data suggest that men with an initial PSA of 2.1–4 ng/mL should have annual monitoring of their PSA levels for the early detection of prostate cancer.

The Stage of Prostate Cancer vs the Number of Times Screened

Figure 8 represents a comparison of stages seen at the initial screening and during the second-, third-, and fourth-year follow-up periods.

A decrease in the risk of developing advanced prostate cancer, especially stage M+(D2), was seen in patients who had at least two negative screenings. However, it was not eliminated in all men who underwent yearly screening examinations. The number of men with M+ disease seems to increase between years 3 and 4, (Fig. 9). Men with previous

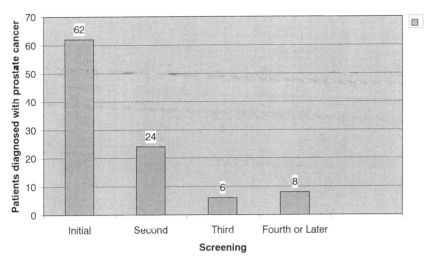

Fig. 8. Prostate cancer detection by years screened.

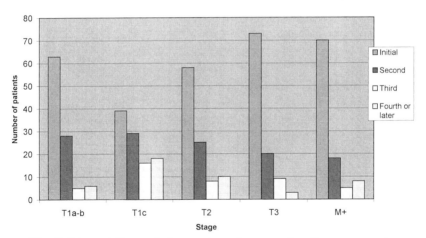

Fig. 9. Stage at diagnosis by number of consecutive times screened.

abnormalities who were not evaluated might account for these results. It also has been noted that there were a few men with near-normal PSA who were seen a year later with metastatic disease. Locally advanced and metastatic disease was markedly reduced with screening support, but the value of early detection was not useful for this group of men.

From 1992 to 1996, in our longitudinal study, more than 60% of the cancers were found in the first year, most of the remaining cancers were detected in the second year.

Table 7
Positive Predictive Value of Screening Tests for Prostate Cancer
by Number of Consecutive Times Screened

Test	1	2	3	>4	Overall
DRE	31.4	20.4	16.5	18.6	25.6
PSA	42.1	26.7	23.3	29.9	35.1
PSA or DRE	26.6	19.5	16.9	21.3	23.2
PSA and DRE	60.6	38.7	34.0	37.5	52.5
Number	91,000	72,000	24,000	29,000	

The PPV of Screening Test
the Number of Consecutive Times Screened

The PPV of screening tests decreases with the number of consecutive times screened. The PPV is highest the first year of screening and rapidly drops with each successive screening (Table 7).

One implication of these findings is that new assays and methods for detecting prostate cancer may not be performing well in men who have undergone serial screening.

Prostate Cancer and Vasectomy

Some studies have found a relationship between prostate cancer and men who have had a vasectomy (6). Between 1993 and 1995, the records of 95,000 men were examined; 28% of these men had undergone a vasectomy. Two-thousand five hundred thirty men who had abnormal PSA levels or abnormal DREs had undergone biopsies; 36% of these biopsies were positive. We did not find any established link between vasectomy and prostate cancer regardless of how much time had elapsed since the vasectomy. It was determined that age, not length of time since the vasectomy, was associated with prostate cancer.

SPECIAL STUDIES
DRE and PSA

Stamey was the first to report that digital rectal examination increases the serum PSA (7). We conducted a clinical trial in five centers that included 2754 men to determine whether or not a DRE performed in a screening setting would alter the levels of PSA. PSA levels were determined before and after DRE, and no statistically significant difference between the level of PSA before and after the examination could be found. However, men with a higher baseline PSA did experience an elevation of their PSA (8).

Ejaculation

During PCAW 1996 at the University of Colorado, Denver, more than 750 participants volunteered to have their PSA levels evaluated before and after ejaculation. The PSA was drawn with at least 3 d of abstinence from ejaculation. When stratified by every 3 h of time elapsed after ejaculation, a significant change was noted: Closer to the ejaculation the change is negative, then becomes positive; after 12 h, the serum level tends to return to baseline. However, none of these changes were statistically significant. The higher the baseline, the greater the magnitude of change. Therefore, caution must be taken for those with an elevated PSA. This study concluded that ejaculation has no clinically significant effect on serum PSA levels *(9)*. However, for men with abnormal levels, the PSA increased after ejaculation. Because this physiologic condition does not effect the sensitivity of PSA for screening trials, men should not be asked to abstain from sexual activity before PSA screening for prostate cancer.

The Effect of Bicycle Riding on PSA Levels

PSA levels were measured in 260 volunteers before a 250-mile bicycle ride and after a 4-d race through the Colorado mountains. Prerace and postrace PSA levels were compared and there was no statistically or clinically significant increase in PSA. A few participants with initial elevated PSA had an increase after bicycle riding *(10)*.

Overall, the findings of these studies show that rectal examination, ejaculation, and bicycle riding do not significantly alter the PSA level in men with normal PSA. Therefore, men in mass-screening settings should not be asked about these activities.

OUTLOOK

Prostate Cancer Awareness Week has become a recognized national event with one of the largest databases in the world. The majority of cancers detected currently are localized and, therefore, potentially curable. Only 7% have been advanced cases of the disease and these were usually diagnosed during the first year of screening.

Our primary goal remains education and early detection. We are also looking at improving the sensitivity and specificity of our testing and joint collaboration to assess the outcome. To date, these studies have yielded valuable research results, including PPVs of DRE, PSA, and the benefit of using both to screen for prostate cancer. We believe that a baseline assessment of PSA is indicated at age 35 in the high-risk group. Similarly, a baseline PSA and DRE at age 45 is indicated for men at normal risk.

We have collaborated with many other organizations including the American Urological Association. Our database, under the auspices of Dr. Brian Miles of Baylor University, was involved in an outcome analysis for local therapies.

The promotion of public education and early detection has had a positive impact on the detection of prostate cancer. Highlighted by the involvement of media and other organizations like the U.S. Postal Service, which issued the first PCAW stamp this year, countries throughout the world have emulated PCAW and efforts to develop a worldwide campaign are ongoing. Although the amount of research dollars earmarked to prostate cancer has tripled, the amount of money allocated is still not matching the scale of this problem. We need action through either local community fundraising or by getting support from congressional representatives at the national level to meet the challenge.

REFERENCES

1. Parkin DM, Pisani, Ferlay J. (1999) Global prostate cancer statistics. *CA Cancer J Clin* 49:33–64.
2. Crawford ED: Prostate cancer awareness week: September 22 to 28, 1997. *CA Cancer J Clin* 47:288–296, 1997.
3. Crawford ED, Leewarsantong S, Goktais S, et al. (1999) The efficiency of prostate specific antigen and digital rectal examination in screening using 4.0 ng/mL and age specific reference range as a cutoff for abnormal PSA. *Prostate* 38(4): 296–230.
4. Myrtle JF, Klimley PG, Ivor LP, et al. (1986) Clinical utility of prostate specific antigen (PSA) in the management of prostate cancer. Advance in Cancer Diagnostics, Hybritech Inc., 1986.
5. Deantoni EP, Crawford ED, Oesterling JE, Ross CA, Berger ER, Mcleod DG. (1993) Age and race specific references ranges for prostate specific antigen from a large community based study. *Urology* 48:234–239, 1996.
6. Hayes RB, Pottern LM, Greenberg R, et al. (1993) Vasectomy and prostate cancer in US black and whites. Am J Epidemiology 137:263–269.
7. Samey TA, Yang N, Hay AR, et al. (1987) A prostate-specific Antigen as a serum marker for adenocarcinoma of prostate. *N Engl J Med* 317:909–916, 1987.
8. Crawford ED, Shutz MJ, Clejan S, et al. (1992) The effect of digital rectal examination on rostate-specific antigen level. *JAMA* 267:2227–2228.
9. Stenner J, Kolthaus K, Mackenzie SH, Crawford ED. (1998) The effect of ejaculation on prostate-specific-antigen in a prostate cancer screening population. *Urology* 51:455–459.
10. Crawford Ed, Mackenzie SH, Safford HR III, Capriola M. (1996) The effect of bicycle riding on serum prostate specific antigen levels. *J Am Med Assoc* 276:1309–1315.
11. Oesterling JE, Jacobsen SJ, Chute CG, et al. (1993) Serum prostate-specific antigen in a community-based population of healthy men. *JAMA* 270:860–864.

17 The Laval University Screening Trial Results

Fernand Labrie, Bernard Candas,
Lionel Cusan, and Jose-luis Gomez

CONTENTS

INTRODUCTION
SUBJECT AND METHODS
RESULTS
IMPACT ON SURVIVAL
DISCUSSION
REFERENCES

INTRODUCTION

It is clear that if prostate cancer is not treated at a localized stage, this cancer will remain the second cause of cancer death in men *(1)*. In fact, it was predicted that 37,800 men would die from prostate cancer in the United States in 1999, whereas 43,700 or only 15.6% more deaths were estimated for breast cancer during the same time period. At the present rate, it is estimated that prostate cancer will kill more than 3 million men among the male population currently living in the United States. Thus, prostate cancer is a major medical and social problem in urgent need of a significant improvement in diagnosis and treatment.

Because prostate cancer usually develops insidiously for many years without signs or symptoms until it reaches the noncurable stage of metastases in the bones, screening in asymptomatic men is essential. Despite this logic, the acceptance of screening for prostate cancer has long been delayed by the absence of clinical trials showing that treat-

From: *Current Clinical Urology: Prostate Cancer Screening*
Edited by: I. M. Thompson, M. I. Resnick, and E. A. Klein
© Humana Press Inc., Totowa, NJ

ment of localized disease prolongs life *(2,3)*. The absence of data show-ing the efficacy of early treatment was erroneously interpreted as being equivalent to negative results. Most fortunately, four prospective ran-domized trials have recently demonstrated for the first time that prolon-gation of life is achieved in patients with localized prostate cancer treated with androgen blockade. A particularly important landmark is the EORTC (European Organization for Research and Treatment of Can-cer) trial performed in stage T_3 patients where overall survival at 5 yr was increased from 62% in the group of patients who received radiation therapy alone to 79% (45% relative difference) in those who received androgen blockade for 3 yr in association with radiotherapy *(4)*. Most important, in that study, death from prostate cancer was decreased by 77% by androgen blockade. A 20% improvement in overall survival at 5 yr has also been found in RTOG (Radiation Therapy Oncology Group) trial 08351 in the subgroup of high Gleason score patients who received androgen blockade indefinitely or until progression *(5)* .

Following a long controversy, a large prospective and randomized clinical trial performed by the Medical Research Council Prostate Can-cer Working Party Investigators Group has shown the benefits of early androgen blockade in locally advanced or asymptomatic metastatic disease *(6)*. A 21% decrease in cancer-specific death was observed in patients who had androgen blockade at time of diagnosis. It can be added that the 69% decrease in the incidence of death from prostate cancer observed during the first 8 yr of our randomized study on prostate can-cer screening can only be the result of the treatment used and its early application. Most important, it should be remembered that no prospec-tive study on the effect of early treatment of prostate cancer has ever shown negative results, whereas, as mentioned earlier, all the studies performed so far have shown positive results. Consequently, no valid reason remains to doubt that treatment of clinically localized prostate cancer prolongs survival, thus automatically demonstrating the major importance of early diagnosis or screening.

The essential objective of screening for prostate cancer is the detec-tion of the cancer at a localized and thus curable stage before the cancer reaches the bones, where the success of treatment is limited and tempo-rary. In order to be useful and applicable in the general population, the screening tests used must be simple, noninvasive, reliable, efficient, and low cost. It thus becomes particularly important to obtain precise infor-mation on the performance of the two tests most currently available for screening, namely prostate-specific antigen (PSA) and digital rectal examination (DRE). It is clear that such information can only be obtained from large-scale studies. The interest in this area is particularly high following the decision of the European Randomized Study Screening for Prostate Cancer not to use DRE for screening when PSA is normal (3.0 ng/mL) *(7)*. It will also be of interest to compare the results obtained in the groups of men invited and not invited for screening.

SUBJECTS AND METHODS

As part of the prospective, randomized, and controlled Laval University Prostate Cancer Detection Program (LUPCDP), men aged 45–80 yr were randomly selected for screening tests from the electoral rolls of Québec City and its vicinity. Men in the control group not invited for screening were followed according to current medical practice for diagnosis and treatment of prostate cancer and were identified during follow-up in the Quebec Cancer Death Registry, and the men selected for screening were invited to participate by letter and were followed by annual visits at the prostate cancer clinic. To minimize bias, no public announcement was made through the media. From November 1988 to December 1998, a total of 7195 men (>99% Caucasians) in the invited group of the electoral rolls were examined at first visit; and 30,891 follow-up visits were performed. The number of men selected in each age group was proportional to that in the general male population. Other men (4616) not invited for screening as part of the LUPC-DP received the same screening tests at first visit, whereas 15,860 follow-up visits were performed in this group of not invited men. Those men were not part of the analysis on the impact of screening on survival *(3)*.

Participants completed a questionnaire on familial incidence of prostate cancer and provided information on genitourinary history and present symptomatology. Then, they had measurement of serum PSA and underwent DRE. The PSA and DRE tests were performed independently. Transrectal ultrasonagraphy (TRUS) was performed only in cases with positive PSA and/or DRE, except for the first 1002 men, who all had the three procedures, as previously reported *(8)*. At follow-up visits, TRUS was done if serum PSA already above 3.0 ng/mL had increased by more than 20% compared with the value measured 1 yr earlier (the interassay coefficient of variation [cv] being 9.6%, we accepted 10% as a possible increase attributable to the interassay [cv]), leaving a 10% increase attributable to changes in PSA secretion, or if the measured PSA was increased by more than 20% above the predicted PSA *(9–11)*. Serum samples were taken before the DRE for measurement of PSA by immunoradiometric assay (Tandem-R PSA, Hybritech, Inc. or its equivalent).

RESULTS

Because the population of invited men was exclusively composed of previously unscreened men, we had the opportunity to obtain information specific for each visit and thus compare the findings at first visit with those obtained at annual follow-up visits. As shown in Table 1, Part A, 15.5% of the 7195 men invited for screening and examined at first visit had serum PSA above 3.0 ng/mL, the optimal cutoff value previously determined by receiver– operator curve analysis (8). Comparable results were obtained in the 4616 not invited men where 18.3% of men had serum PSA above 3.0 ng/mL and were thus candidates for TRUS at their first visits.

On the other hand, at 30,891 follow-up visits in the invited group, 15.1% of men had serum PSA above 3.0 ng/mL. Comparable results were obtained in the 15,860 follow-up visits in the group of men not invited for screening where 16.5% had serum PSA above the cutoff value of 3.0 ng/mL (Table 1, Part B).

The group of not invited men included men listed in the electoral rolls and who were originally part of the control group of our randomized screening study as well as men from outside the metropolitan area of Québec City who came to our clinic on their own without being invited by letter. When all the data were pooled (Table 1), 16.6% of 11,811 men at first visit had abnormal PSA whereas, at 46,751 follow-up visits, PSA was abnormal in 15.6% of cases. Thus, at first (11,811) and follow-up (46,751) visits, 83.4% and 84.4%, respectively, of men had serum PSA within normal limits or below 3.0 ng/mL. Serum PSA was at or below 2.0 ng/mL in 72.5% of men at first visits and 73.6% of them at follow-up visits.

The most significant changes observed between first and annual follow-up visits of invited men were seen at serum PSA values above 20 ng/mL, where a 6.7-fold reduction was seen at follow-up visits in the percentage of men having a serum PSA above 20 ng/mL, the incidence rate decreasing from 0.60% at first visit to 0.09% at follow-up visits of invited men. Similarly, in the group of not invited men, there was a 5.4-fold reduction in the number of men who had serum PSA above 20 ng/mL at follow-up compared to first visits.

Because a major concern about screening is a potential increase in the number of clinically not significant cancers detected, it is important to see in Table 1 and Fig. 1 that only 128 cancers were found at 30,891 follow-up visits in invited men for an incidence of 0.41% compared to a prevalence of 2.93% (211 cancers in 7195 men) at first visit. The

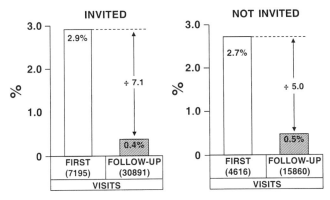

Fig. 1. Percentage of men diagnosed with prostate cancer at first and follow-up visits.

percentage of men found as having prostate cancer at follow-up visits is thus 7.1 times lower at follow-up compared to first visits. In the not invited men, 126 cancers were found at 4616 first visits for a prevalence of 2.73% whereas at 15,860 follow-up visits, 87 cancers were found, for an incidence of 0.55%. The percentage of not invited men diagnosed with prostate cancer is thus 5.0 times lower at follow-up compared to first visits.

A particularly important finding (illustrated in Fig. 2) is that the percentage of men showing serum PSA above 3.0 ng/mL who were found as having prostate cancer decreased from 17.0% at first visits (1118) to 2.7% at follow-up visits (4664) in the group of invited men. Thus, there was a 6.3-fold decrease in the incidence of diagnosed prostate cancer at follow-up compared to first visits in men having abnormal PSA. In other words, prostate cancer was found in 1 out of 5.9 men having serum PSA above 3.0 ng/mL at first visits compared to only 1 out of 37 men having similar PSA levels at follow-up visits. In the group of not invited men having an abnormal PSA at first visits (>3.0 ng/mL), 110 cancers were diagnosed in 845 men with abnormal PSA for an incidence rate of 13.0% and cancer was thus found in 1 out of 7.7 men. At follow-up visits, on the other hand, the percentage of men with abnormal PSA found with cancer decreased to 3.1% (80 cancers in 2618 men with abnormal PSA). A cancer was thus found in 1 out of 33 not invited men having abnormal PSA at follow-up visits, showing a 4.3-fold decrease compared to first visits.

Table 2 describes the relative sensitivity of serum PSA and DRE to detect prostate cancer at first visits and at annual follow-up visits.

Table 1
Correlation Between Serum PSA Levels and the Presence of Detectable Prostate Cancer in 45- to 80-yr Old Invited Men at 7195 First Visits (A) and 30,891 Follow-up Visits (B)

A. First visit

PSA (ng/ml)	Not invited				Invited				All subjects			
	No. Visits	% Total	No. CaP	% CaP	No. Visits	% Total	No. CaP	% CaP	No. Visits	% Total	# CaP	% CaP
0.0–1.0	2090	45.3%	5	0.24%	3086	42.9%	3	0.10%	5176	43.8%	8	0.15%
1.1–2.0	1236	26.8%	3	0.24%	2153	29.9%	6	0.28%	3389	28.7%	9	0.27%
2.1–3.0	445	9.6%	8	1.80%	838	11.7%	12	1.43%	1283	10.9%	20	1.56%
3.1–4.0	259	5.6%	12	4.63%	427	5.9%	29	6.79%	686	5.8%	41	5.98%
4.1–5.0	162	3.5%	13	8.02%	212	3.0%	18	8.49%	374	3.2%	31	8.29%
5.1–7.0	184	4.0%	19	10.33%	218	3.0%	37	16.97%	402	3.4%	56	13.93%
7.1–10.0	111	2.4%	23	20.72%	120	1.7%	29	24.17%	231	2.0%	52	22.51%
10.1–20.0	90	2.0%	18	20.00%	98	1.4%	41	41.84%	188	1.6%	59	31.38%
>20.1	39	0.8%	25	64.10%	43	0.6%	36	83.72%	82	0.7%	61	74.39%
Total	4616	100%	126	2.73%	7195	100%	211	2.93%	11811	100%	337	2.85%

B. Follow-up Visits

	Not invited				Invited				All subjects			
0.0–1.0	7554	47.6%	1	0.01%	14490	46.9%	1	0.01%	22044	47.2%	2	0.01%
1.1–2.0	4016	25.3%	2	0.05%	8345	27.0%	1	0.01%	12361	26.4%	3	0.02%
2.1–3.0	1672	10.5%	4	0.24%	3392	11.0%	1	0.03%	5064	10.8%	5	0.10%
3.1–4.0	909	5.7%	12	1.32%	1847	6.0%	31	1.68%	2756	5.9%	43	1.56%
4.1–5.0	536	3.4%	16	2.99%	1023	3.3%	19	1.86%	1559	3.3%	35	2.25%
5.1–7.0	609	3.8%	21	3.45%	1042	3.4%	33	3.17%	1651	3.5%	54	3.27%
7.1–10.0	346	2.2%	22	6.36%	467	1.5%	20	4.28%	813	1.7%	42	5.17%
10.1–20.0	193	1.2%	9	4.66%	257	0.8%	18	7.00%	450	1.0%	27	6.00%
>20.1	25	0.2%	0	0.00%	28	0.1%	4	14.29%	53	0.1%	4	7.55%
Total	15860	100%	87	0.55%	30891	100%	128	0.41%	46751	100%	215	0.46%

Note: Similar data are presented for 4,616 first visits and 15,860 follow-up visits in a similar population of uninvited men.

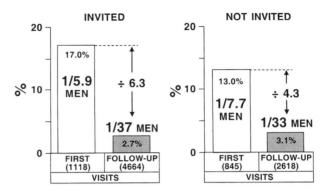

Fig. 2. Percentage of invited and not invited men with abnormal PSA (>3.0 ng/mL) diagnosed with prostate cancer at first and follow-up visits.

Because DRE was eliminated from follow-up visits in January 1993, the data are presented only for the visits where both PSA and DRE were performed. These data do not include the cancers found by TRUS in the presence of normal PSA and DRE in the early phase of the detection program (first 1002 men [8]). At first visit of the invited men, 53 of the 168 (31.5%) cancers were both PSA$^+$ and DRE$^+$; 99 of 168 (58.9%) cancers were PSA$^+$ and DRE–; only 16 cancers (9.2%) were PSA$^-$ and DRE$^+$. At follow-up visits, 8 of the 40 cancers (20.0%) were PSA$^+$ and DRE$^+$; 30 (75.0%) were PSA$^+$ and DRE$^-$; only 2 (5.0%) were PSA$^-$ and DRE$^+$. Thus, 152 of the 168 cancers (90.5%) detected at the first visits were PSA$^+$ whereas 69 (41.1%) were DRE$^+$ (Fig. 3). At the follow-up visits, 38 of the 40 cancers (95.0%) were PSA$^+$, but only 10 (25.0%) cancers were DRE+. Combining all 11,970 visits, 190 of the 208 cancers (91.3%) were PSA$^+$ and 79 (38.0%) were DRE$^+$, thus showing that PSA has a 2.4-fold higher sensitivity than DRE at first visit. At first visits, PSA detects 2.2 times more cancers than DRE, whereas at follow-up visits, 3.8 times more cancers are PSA$^+$ than DRE$^+$.

It is important to mention that of the 40 prostate cancers diagnosed at follow-up visits in invited men who had DRE and PSA at all visits, 38 were PSA$^+$ and only 2 (5.0%) were missed by PSA and found by DRE, thus demonstrating the unique importance of serum PSA to detect prostate cancer, especially at annual follow-up screening visits (Table 2, Part B). On the other hand, at first visits, 90.5% of cancers in invited men were PSA$^+$, 9.5% were found by DRE in the presence of normal PSA (Table 2, Part A) (Fig. 3).

Similar results were obtained in the group of not invited men where 44 of the 114 cancers (38.6%) at first visit were both PSA$^+$ and DRE$^+$;

Table 2

Number of TRUS-Guided Biopsies and Positive Biopsies According to Serum PSA and DRE in Men Who Had Both Exams at All Visits at First (A) and Follow-up (B) Visits

A — First Visit

PSA	DRE	Uninvited Visits #	TRUS #	TRUS % Visits	Biopsies #	Biopsies % TRUS	CaP #	CaP % Biopsies	Invited Visits #	TRUS #	TRUS % Visits	Biopsies #	Biopsies % TRUS	CaP #	CaP % Biopsies	All Subjects Visits #	TRUS #	TRUS % Visits	Biopsies #	Biopsies % TRUS	CaP #	CaP % Biopsies
		2951							4330							7281						
-	-	172	158	91.9%	85	54.8%	11	12.9%	232	223	96.1%	161	72.2%	16	9.9%	404	381	94.3%	246	64.6%	27	11.0%
+	-	620	576	92.9%	210	36.5%	59	28.1%	759	722	95.1%	284	39.3%	99	34.9%	1379	1298	94.1%	494	38.1%	158	32.0%
-	+	125	115	92.0%	85	73.9%	44	51.8%	107	105	98.1%	88	83.8%	53	60.2%	232	220	94.3%	173	76.6%	97	56.1%
Total		3868	849	21.9%	380	44.8%	114	30.0%	5428	1050	19.3%	533	50.8%	168	31.5%	9296	1899	20.4%	913	48.1%	282	30.9%

B — Follow-up Visits

PSA	DRE	Uninvited Visits #	TRUS #	TRUS % Visits	Biopsies #	Biopsies % TRUS	CaP #	CaP % Biopsies	Invited Visits #	TRUS #	TRUS % Visits	Biopsies #	Biopsies % TRUS	CaP #	CaP % Biopsies	All Subjects Visits #	TRUS #	TRUS % Visits	Biopsies #	Biopsies % TRUS	CaP #	CaP % Biopsies
-	-	2296	20	0.9%	5	25.0%	1	20.0%	5378	25	0.5%	10	40.0%	0	0.0%	7674	45	0.6?	15	33.3%	1	6.7%
+	-	80	53	66.3%	30	56.5%	3	10.0%	109	62	56.9%	29	46.8%	2	6.9%	189	115	60.8%	59	51.3%	5	8.5%
-	+	641	218	34.0%	89	40.8%	23	25.8%	1021	366	35.8%	135	36.9%	30	22.2%	1662	584	35.1%	224	38.4%	53	23.7%
+	+	34	22	64.7%	19	86.4%	7	36.8%	34	21	61.8%	13	61.9%	8	61.5%	68	43	63.2%	32	74.4%	15	46.9%
Total		3051	313	10.3%	143	45.7%	34	23.8%	6542	474	7.2%	187	39.5%	40	21.4%	9593	787	8.2%	330	41.9%	74	22.4%

263

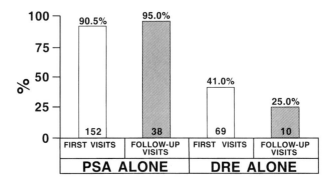

Fig. 3. Percentage of prostate cancer diagnosed by PSA or DRE alone at first and follow-up visits.

59 cancers (51.8%) were PSA$^+$ and DRE$^-$ and only 11 cancers (9.6%) were PSA$^-$ and DRE$^+$. At follow-up visits in the not invited group of men, 7 of the 34 cancers (20.6%) were PSA$^+$ and DRE$^+$; 67.6% (23 of 34 cancers) were PSA$^+$ and DRE$^-$. On the other hand, only three cancers (8.8%) were PSA$^-$ and DRE$^+$. Thus, whereas at first visit, 90.4% of the cancers were PSA$^+$, PSA was positive in 95% of the cancers at follow-up visits of not invited men. When combining all data of first and follow-up visits, 133 out of 148 cancers (89.9%) were PSA$^+$ whereas 43.9% of cancers (65 out of 148 cancers) were DRE$^+$ and 9.5% of cancers were DRE$^+$ in the presence of normal PSA.

Based on the above-described data, it seems appropriate to combine the results obtained in the invited and not invited men. It can be seen in Table 2 that the major difference between first and follow-up visits is the decrease in the percentage of both PSA$^+$ and DRE$^+$ cancers from 34.4% at first visit to 20.3% at follow-up visits with a corresponding increase in the percentage of PSA$^+$ and DRE$^-$ cancers from 56.0% at first visit to 71.6% at follow-up visits. DRE$^+$ PSA$^-$ cancers, on the other hand, decreased from 9.6% at first visit to 6.8% at follow-up visits. The percentage of PSA$^+$ DRE$^+$ in the total population decreased from 2.45% at first visit to 0.71% at follow-up visits. The percentage of PSA$^+$ DRE$^-$, on the other hand, increased from 14.8% to 17.3%. All cancers with both negative PSA and DRE, at first visit, were removed from the present calculations. In fact, 78.3% of men at first visit and 80.0% of men at follow-up visits had both normal PSA ($\leq$3.0 ng/mL) and normal DRE.

It then becomes of interest to calculate the number of DREs and PSA measurements required to find one case of prostate cancer at first and follow-up visits in men who had both PSA and DRE at all visits. As can be seen in Table 2 , Part A, 27 (9.6%) of the 282 cancers diagnosed at

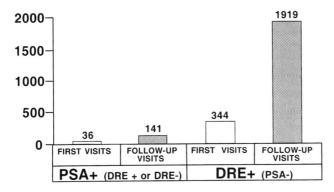

Fig. 4. Number of PSAs and DREs required to diagnose one prostate cancer at first and follow-up visits.

all first visits (9296) were found by DRE⁺ in PSA⁻ patients. At follow-up visits (9593), on the other hand, 5 (6.8%) of 74 cancers were diagnosed in PSA⁻ and DRE⁺ patients. Thus, 344 DREs are required to find 1 case of prostate cancer at first visit, whereas 1919 DREs are required at follow-up visits (Fig. 4). On the other hand, 36 and 141 PSA measurements are required at first and follow-up visits to diagnose 1 case of prostate cancer.

If only PSA above 3.0 ng/mL had been used to identify the population of men at high risk and selected for TRUS, 27 cancers (9.6%) would have been missed at first visit and 5 (6.6%) cancers would have been missed at follow-up. On the other hand, if only DRE had been used, 158 cancers (56.0%) would have been missed at first visit and 53 (71.6%) at follow-up. Combining all visits, 32 cancers (9.0%) would have been missed using serum PSA alone, but 211 (59.3%) would have been missed using DRE alone, for a 6.6-fold higher sensitivity of PSA compared to DRE. On the other hand, when all data are combined at first visit, 90.4% (255 out of 282) of the cancers were diagnosed with PSA⁺ at first visit; only 44.0% (124) were DRE⁺. At follow-up visits, 91.9% (68 of 74) of the cancers diagnosed were PSA⁺; only 27.0% (20) were DRE⁺.

The most important finding is that only two out of 215 (1.0%) cancers diagnosed at follow-up visits were metastatic compared with 6.7% at first visit (Fig. 5). Stage C_2 prostate cancers, on the other hand, decreased from 10.7% at first visit to only 2.4% at follow-ups. Stages B_0, on the other hand, increased from 6.1% at first visit to 18.4% at follow-up visits, whereas stage B_1 disease increased from 35.5% to 51.9% and stage B_2 cancers, on the other hand, decreased from 29.1% to 18.4%.

As part of the assessment of feasibility, cost-effectiveness, and acceptability of detection of early-stage prostate cancer, it is important

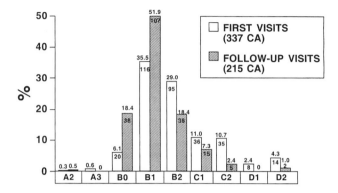

Fig. 5. Distribution of clinical stages of 337 and 215 (327 and 206 staged) prostate cancers diagnosed at first and follow-up screening visits, respectively. Data are expressed as percentage of total number of staged cancers in each group to facilitate comparison.

to consider the number of TRUSs and biopsies required to detect cancer in men having serum PSA above 3.0 ng/mL and/or positive DRE. In our study, in invited men (Table 2, Part A), TRUS was done in 19.3% of men at first visit and biopsies in 50.8% of those undergoing echography, for a percentage of positive biopsies of 31.5%. At follow-up, on the other hand, 474 TRUS were performed for 6542 visits (7.2% of visits). Biopsies were done in 39.5% of the 474 men having TRUS, and cancer was found in 21.4% of biopsies. Of the 11,970 visits, 1524 (12.7%) TRUS and 720 biopsies were done, and 208 cancers were detected, for an overall 28.9% of biopsies positive for prostate cancer.

The particularly large size of the population studied, the random selection of a large proportion of the subjects, as well as the similarity of the results obtained in a population of subjects presenting themselves for screening provide the basis for a valid estimate of the costs associated with the detection of early-stage prostate cancer in the general population. Despite the close similarity of the results, however, the cost calculations will be made with the population of men invited for screening. It is somewhat obvious that all three techniques presently available for detection of prostate cancer, namely, PSA, DRE, and TRUS, although permitting the diagnosis of the largest number of prostate cancers, cannot be used together as a first-line approach in the general population.

As clearly suggested in our previous report (8) and well demonstrated by the present update and extension of the previous data, the most cost-effective strategy is the measurement of serum PSA as a first-line approach, as recently concluded by Schröder et al. *(7)* in another large-scale screening study. In fact, PSA is free of subjective assessment, is a procedure easily acceptable by the general population, and requires minimal health professional personnel. Following this strategy, the cost for finding one case of prostate cancer at first visit is estimated at $2,418.75 (Table 3).

Such costs include measurement of serum PSA in 36 men for every cancer diagnosed (at $25.00 each, for a subtotal of $900.00), followed by TRUS at $200.00 per man in an average of 5.5 men found to have serum PSA above 3.0 ng/mL for a second subtotal of $1100.00. These 5.5 men will also have DREs at $25.00 per subject for a subtotal of $137.50 (Table 3). Because more than 50% of men having serum PSA above 3.0 ng/mL have benign prostatic hyperplasia, which accounts for the elevated serum PSA (predicted PSA), biopsies will be performed in an average of 2.25 men having high serum PSA (2.25 × $125.00 = $281.25). The total cost for finding one case of prostate cancer using this approach is thus estimated at $2,418.75.

If, as a second cost-effective approach (Table 3), DRE is added routinely at the first visit, as we have done in the present study, 32 instead of 36 men will need to be examined to find 1 case of prostate cancer. The costs of serum PSA are thus reduced from $900.00 to $800.00, while the costs of DREs increased from $137.50 to $800.00. The number of men at risk following the addition of a DRE is increased to 6.5 men. The costs of TRUS are thus increased to $1,300.00. It is also likely that the man having DRE$^+$ PSA$^-$ will have a biopsy, for a total number of 3.3 biopsies, thus increasing the cost to $412.50, for a total of $3,312.50. On the other hand, if PSA, DRE, and TRUS are all performed at the first visit, we have previously estimated the costs for finding one cancer at $6,125.00 *(12)*.

If follow-up visits are performed annually, 172 serum PSA measurements (× $25.00) must be performed in order to find 1 case of prostate cancer, for a total cost for PSA of $4,300.00 (Table 4). Among the 28 men at high risk, 10.3 will have a DRE, and TRUS and biopsy will be performed in an average of 3.9 men, for a total estimated cost of $7,105.00 to identify 1 case of prostate cancer. If a DRE is added to a PSA at each follow-up visit, 163 men will need to be examined, thus increasing the costs of the DRE from $257.50 to $4,075.00. The number of men considered at risk will increase from 28 to 29, while increasing the number of TRUS to 11.2 and the number of biopsies to 4.4, for a total estimated cost of $10,940.00.

Table 3
Estimated Costs for Finding One Prostate Cancer in a Randomly Selected Population of Men Aged Between 45–80 yr Using PSA Alone, PSA + DRE or PSA + DRE + TRUS as First Approach at First Visit

Strategy	No. of Men	At high risk No. of Men	%	Costs PSA ($25.00)	DRE ($25.00)	TRUS ($200.00)	Biopsy–histo-pathology ($125.00)	Total
PSA alone followed by DRE and TRUS	36	5.5	15.2	$900.00	$137.50	$1,100.00	$281.25	$2,418.75
PSA followed by TRUS	32	6.5	20.2	$800.00	$800.00	$1,300.00	$412.50	$3,312.50

Table 4
Estimated Costs for Finding One Prostate Cancer at Follow-up Annual Visits in a Randomly Selected Population of Men Aged 45–80 yr Using PSA Alone or PSA + DRE as First Approach at Follow-up

Strategy	No. of Men	At high risk No. of Men	%	Costs PSA ($25.00)	DRE ($25.00)	TRUS ($200.00)	Biopsy–histo-pathology ($125.00)	Total
PSA alone followed by DRE and TRUS	172	28	16.1	$4,300.00	$257.50	$2,060.00	$487.50	$7,105.00
PSA followed by TRUS	163	29	17.8	$4,075.00	$4,075.00	$2,240.00	$550.00	$10,940.00

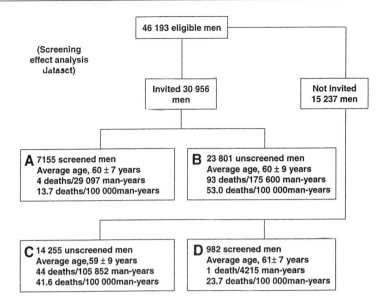

Fig. 6. Trial profile of the Laval University Prostate Cancer Screening Program (November 15, 1988 to December 31, 1996).

IMPACT ON SURVIVAL

Of the 46,193 eligible men between 45 and 80 yr of age included in the study started in 1988, 30,956 were invited by letter to be screened for prostate cancer and 15,237 were allocated to the control unscreened group. Figure 6 shows the breakdown of these numbers according to original randomization and participation in screening. In the invited group, 7155 (23.1%) eligible men were screened at our prostate clinic from November 15, 1988 to December 31, 1996. On the other hand, 982 men (6.5% of the initial control group of 15,237 men) presented themselves at the clinic for screening, despite not being invited by letter, and had to be withdrawn from the original control group. The age distribution of the men in the four subgroups is the same. The mean age ranges from 59 to 61 yr and the standard deviations from 7 to 9 yr (Table 5).

Four out of the 7155 men who responded to the invitation for screening (Group A) died from prostate cancer and 44 men died among the 14,255 unscreened men of the initial control group (Group C). The exposures in the screened and unscreened control groups are 29,097 and 105,852 man-years, respectively. Thus, over the 8-yr period, the annual cause-specific death rate incidences are 13.7 and 41.6 per 100,000 man-years in the screened and control unscreened groups, respectively ($p = 0.02$). Thus the

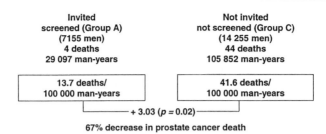

Fig. 7. Effect of screening on the incidence of death. Comparison is made between 7155 men invited for screening and screened and 14,255 men not invited for screening and not screened (controls).

prostate cancer death rate incidence is 67.1% lower in men of the screened group (Fig. 7).

Several other tests were performed on the basis of the eligible cases in order to assess any possible lack of homogeneity that might be related to the lack of compliance to initial randomization. The men who were invited but did not come to our clinic for screening were first compared to the unscreened controls (Fig. 6, Group B vs Group C). Ninety-three prostate cancer deaths were recorded in the 23,801 men (Group B) who did not respond to the invitation, for a total number 175,600 man-years. This translates into an annual death rate of 53.0/100,000 man-years compared to 41.6/100,000 man-years in the unscreened men who were not invited (Group B) ($p = 0.22$). Thus, among men who were not screened, no difference in prostate cancer death can be detected between the group of men who were not invited for screening (original control group, Group C) and were not screened and the group of men who were invited for screening but were not screened (Group B).

On the other hand, among the originally invited men, comparison of the incidence rates of death between the screened (Fig. 6, Group A) and the unscreened (Fig. 6, Group B) men reveals a highly significant effect of screening (odds ratio = 3.85, $p < 0.01$). Finally, the odds ratio of the two 2 × 2 tables of men who complied with initial randomization (Fig. 6, Groups A and C) and those who did not (Fig. 6, Groups B and D) are not statistically different ($p = 0.57$). Thus, it can be concluded that there is no significant relationship between the randomly assigned invitation and the observed incidence rates of death from prostate cancer, screening being the only significant determinant factor of the outcome.

According to the results of the above-described analyses, the subpopulations of screened (Fig. 6, Groups A and D) and unscreened (Fig. 6, Groups B and C) men can be pooled, regardless of the initial treatment allocation (Fig. 8). Among the 38,056 men who were not screened, 137 deaths from prostate cancer occurred for an annual death rate of 48.7/

Table 5
Treatment Received by 339 Patients (92%) out of the 367 Men Diagnosed
with Prostate Cancer Between November 15, 1988, and December 31, 1996
(others were treated elsewhere)

	Radical Prostatectomy	Radiotherapy	Hormonal Treatment	Total No.	%
No CAB	49	25	25 (delayed)	99	29.2
Hormonal monotherapy	–	1	–	1	0.3
CAB	106	83	50	239	70.5
Total	155	109	75	339	

100,000 man-years, whereas only 5 deaths were found in the 8137 men enrolled in the screening program for an annual incidence rate of 15.0/100,000 man-years. Thus the death rate is 3.25-fold lower in the screened men ($p < 0.01$). In the total population, screening led to a 69% decrease in prostate cancer death.

Because a limitation of screening studies is the high percentage of men who do not respond to the invitation to be screened, it was also of interest to analyze the data on an intent-to-screen basis (3). The intent-to-screen analysis with 23.1% of men actually screened shows a 6% decrease of the prostate cancer death rate in favor of the group of men who were initially invited to be screened. This 6% difference is obtained despite a noncompliance of 76.9% and a contamination of the noninvited men of 6.6%. When the difference observed between the randomization groups is adjusted for such noncompliance and contamination, the effect of screening is estimated to reduce death from prostate cancer by 54% and 100%, respectively. The analysis, presented above, of a 69% benefit associated with screening is well supported by the results of the intent-to-screen analysis.

DISCUSSION

This first randomized and prospective study on prostate cancer screening shows a 69% decrease in the incidence of deaths as a result of prostate cancer in the screened compared to the unscreened populations. Ten years after the start of this screening study, the present data clearly demonstrate the efficacy, reliability, feasibility, and acceptability of diagnosis and treatment of localized prostate cancer in the general population. The data obtained in this study permit, for the first time, to inform men of the estimated risk of death from prostate cancer if not screened and not treated early. Knowing the medical benefits of a screening pro-

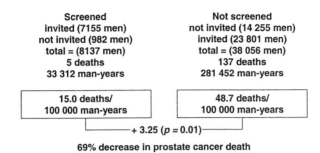

Fig. 8. Effect of screening in the total population of screened (8137) and not screened (38,056) men following the demonstration of lack of influence of compliance to the original invitation.

gram, it is now a matter of medical policy and ethics to create the appropriate conditions that will allow the general population of men to benefit from this new information. Thus it seems appropriate to briefly comment on the algorithm of prostate cancer screening recommended for the general population.

We would like to insist that the upper limit of normal serum PSA should be 3.0 ng/mL and not 4.0 ng/mL (as measured by the Hybritech assay or its equivalent). It should be remembered that the cutoff value of 3.0 ng/mL is the only value scientifically demonstrated to provide optimal sensitivity and specificity to the PSA test *(8,13)*. In fact, the still commonly used value of 4.0 ng/mL suggested by the manufacturer is empirical and not scientifically based. It should be remembered that 11% and 18% of the smaller and potentially most curable prostate cancers are missed when a cutoff value of 4.0 ng/mL is used instead of 3.0 ng/mL at first and follow-up visits, respectively *(14)*. It should be mentioned that the same cutoff value of 3.0 ng/mL has been adopted in the European screening study *(7)*.

With 11,811 first visits and 46,751 follow-up annual visits extending up to 11 yr, the present study clearly demonstrates the high level of efficacy of a low-cost strategy that can be easily, efficiently, and successfully applied in the general population for screening and diagnosis of prostate cancer at a localized and curable stage. In fact, as demonstrated before and confirmed by the present study, the diagnosis of metastatic prostate cancer can practically be eliminated by screening (ref. *14* and the present data), thus offering a unique opportunity to use curative therapies and successfully decrease death from prostate cancer. If every man simply follows the recommendations of the American Cancer Society *(15)* and of the American Urological Association *(16)*, namely, annual screening starting at the age of 50 yr in the general population and at 40 yr for men at high risk, the proportion of localized or potentially curable prostate cancer can be increased from approx. 40% in the absence of screening *(17,18)* to close to 100% (ref. *14* and the present data).

As shown in this study, only 2 out of 215 cancers (1%) diagnosed at follow-up visits were metastatic, thus permitting 99% of patients to be diagnosed at a localized stage and be candidates for curative therapy. Similarly, in the screening program of the American Cancer Society National Prostate Cancer Detection Program (ACS-NPCDP), only 1 of a total of 73 cancers diagnosed at follow-up visits was at a clinically advanced stage (C1 to D2) *(19)*. It is thus reasonable to suggest that if one starts screening at the age of 50 yr, all subsequent visits should be equivalent to the follow-up visits of the present study, thus practically eliminating the diagnosis of metastatic prostate cancer.

Screening for prostate cancer is accepted as a health care policy by prestigious organizations, but other disagree *(15,16,20)*. Nobody can argue, however, that the high mortality and morbidity rates associated with prostate cancer very strongly support the need for screening *(21–23)*. Knowing that the possibility of a cure cannot be offered to patients diagnosed at the metastatic stage *(24–29)*, it is logical that many recent studies have focused on the detection of prostate cancer confined to the prostate and still potentially curable. A main issue in deciding the best screening strategy is the relative value of PSA and DRE.

PSA was first purified in 1979 *(30)* and identified in the blood in 1980 *(31)*. PSA measurement in blood *(32)* was then rapidly used to monitor prostate cancer *(33)*. In today's practice, the majority of prostate cancers are diagnosed by abnormal PSA in the presence of normal DRE *(34,35)*. However, although diagnosis with PSA permits the diagnosis of prostate cancer earlier *(22)*, only 60% of the cancers detectable by PSA are organ confined at radical prostatectomy *(36)*. When DRE is added to PSA, only 60% of the newly diagnosed tumors are clinically localized *(34,35,37)*. Such data presented in the recent review on PSA by Polascik et al. *(34)* indicate, as expected, that although DRE added to PSA can increase the number of prostate cancers detected compared to PSA alone, the percentage of cancers organ confined or curable by surgery is lower by adding DRE, thus confirming the lower sensitivity of DRE to diagnose organ-confined prostate cancer.

A recent study offers very important support for the unique role of PSA in prostate cancer diagnosis: 75% of prostate cancers that were diagnosed during the 4 yr following the first PSA measurement had abnormal PSA at the start of study *(38)*. Most importantly, men having a serum PSA between 3.01 and 4.0 ng/mL had a 8.6-fold increased risk of being diagnosed with prostate cancer, whereas men having a serum PSA between 4.01 and 10.0 ng/mL had a 22.2-fold increased risk compared to those having a serum PSA below 1.0 ng/mL. These risk values are much higher than any other risk factor so-far described for prostate cancer *(39)* or any other type of cancer. In agreement with those data, the present study shows that men who had an abnormal PSA (3.0 ng/mL) and were not diagnosed with prostate cancer at first visit had a six-fold higher risk of being diagnosed with prostate cancer at follow-up visits than those with normal PSA at first visit.

It is also important to indicate that the present study confirms that screening does not detect an important proportion of small cancers *(12,40)*. Following surgical staging, Catalona et al. *(22)* have found microscopically focal and well-differentiated cancer in 2.5% (1/40) of patients referred to the clinic, 2.9% of men screened for the first time and 7.8% of men at follow-up screening. It is important to mention that all cancers detected by the present approach have an average diameter larger than 0.7 cm (0.33 cm^3) *(41)* and, thus, cannot be considered cancers of no significance to the future health and life of the patients, unlike tumors with average diameter less than 0.7 cm, which could be regarded as less aggressive *(42)*. Of the autopsy cancers and those diagnosed in a series of cytoprostatectomies for pathological conditions of the bladder *(43–45)*, only 3% had extracapsular extension and nondemonstrated positive surgical margins, seminal vesicle invasion, or positive lymph nodes (reviewed in ref. *46*).

Prostate cancer has resulted in high individual and social costs *(47–49)*. The positive economic impact of such an approach on health care costs has been previously discussed *(12,50–52)*. The calculations then performed leave little doubt that this strategy, based on efficient screening, could play a key role in a successful fight against prostate cancer while decreasing the costs for the health care system and society *(53,54)*.

As mentioned earlier, no curative therapy exists for advanced prostate cancer. Unfortunately, such a cure is unlikely to be available in the foreseeable future, thus illustrating the absolute requirement to diagnose and treat prostate cancer at a localized stage. Reports from cancer registries in all the states followed by the SEER program of the NCI indicate that prostate cancer incidence rates have begun to fall *(55)*. In Olmsted County, a 22% decline in prostate cancer death has been observed between 1980 and 1997 after PSA screening was introduced *(56)*. Part of the success could be attributed to the early treatment applied at the Mayo Clinic, a major treatment site in Olmsted County. This finding parallels a 6.3% decrease in prostate cancer death nationwide in the United States *(57)*. In Canada, the death rate from prostate cancer has decreased by 9.6% between 1992 and 1996 whereas, in the province of Quebec, prostate cancer death has decreased by 23% (58). It is reasonable to assume that the recently observed decrease in deaths from prostate cancer is the result of earlier diagnosis with serum PSA (8,14,59) and transrectal echography of the prostate (60) coupled with improved treatment of localized disease by surgery, radiotherapy, brachytherapy, and endocrine therapy (4,41,61–65).

Although screening of prostate cancer is a controversial issue, it remains that the diagnosis of prostate cancer at a localized stage is the only foreseeable possibility for reducing the high death rate from this disease. In fact, the remarkable progress recently achieved in the screening procedures (8,12,62,66–68) have made detection of localized prostate cancer a realistic objective. Moreover, recent data provide extremely convincing evidence for the need to detect and treat prostate cancer at a localized stage (3–6,38,56,69–73). It seems reasonable to suggest that the use of the presently available technology for diagnostic and treatment of localized prostate cancer could lead to a dramatic decrease in the death rate from prostate cancer. In fact, the data of our randomized screening study have shown a 69% decrease in prostate cancer death in the period 1988–1996 in the group of men screened compared to a randomized control group of men followed by standard medical practice (3).

REFERENCES

1. Landis SH, Murray T, Bolden S, Wingo PA. (1999) Cancer statistics. *CA Cancer J Clin* 49:8–31.
2. Kolata G. (1987) Prostate cancer consensus hampered by lack of data. *Science* 236:1626–1627.
3. Labrie F, Candas B, Dupont A, Cusan L, Gomez JL, Suburu RE, et al. (1999) Screening decreases prostate cancer death: first analysis of the 1988 Quebec prospective randomized controlled trial. *Prostate* 38:83–91.
4. Bolla M, Gonzalez D, Warde P, Dubois JB, Mirimanoff RO, Storme G, et al. (1997) Improved survival in patients with locally advanced prostate cancer treated with radiotherapy and goserelin. *N Engl J Med* 337:295–300.
5. Pilepich MV, Caplan R, Byhardt RW, Lawton CA, Gallagher MJ, Mesic JB, et al. (1997) Phase III trial of androgen suppression using Goserelin in unfavorable prognosis carcinoma of the prostate treated with definitive radiotherapy: report of Radiation Therapy Oncology Group protocol 85-31. *J Clin Oncol* 15:1013–1021.
6. The Medical Research Council Prostate Cancer Working Party Investigators Group. (1997) Immediate versus deferred treatment for advanced prostatic cancer: initial results of the Medical Research Council trial. *Br J Urol* 79:235–246.
7. Schröder FH, van der Maas P, Beemsterboer P, Kruger AB, Hoedemaeker R, Rietbergen J, et al. (1998) Evaluation of the digital rectal examination as a screening test for prostate cancer. *J Natl Cancer Inst* 90:1817–1823.
8. Labrie F, Dupont A, Suburu R, Cusan L, Tremblay M, Gomez JL, et al. (1992) Serum prostatic specific antigen (PSA) as prescreening test for prostate cancer. *J Urol* 147:846–851.

9. Lee F, Littrup PJ, Loft-Christensen L, Kelly Jr BS, McHugh TA, Siders DB, et al. (1992)Predicted prostate specific antigen results using transrectal ultrasound gland volume. Differentiation of benign prostatic hyperplasia and prostate cancer. *Cancer*, 70(Suppl.):211–220 .

10. Littrup PJ, Williams, CR Egglin, TK, Kane, RA. (1991) Determination of prostate volume by transrectal US for cancer screening. Part II. Clinical utility of transrectal accuracy of in vivo and in vitro techniques. *Radiology* 179:45–53 .

11. Myschetzky PS, Suburu RE, Kelly BSJ, Wilson ML, Chen SC, Lee F. (1991) Determination of prostate gland volume by transrectal ultrasound: correlation with radical prostatectomy specimens. *Scand J Urol Nephrol* 137(Suppl):107–111 .

12. Labrie F, Dupont A, Suburu R, Cusan L, Gomez JL, Koutsilieris M, et al. (1993) Optimized strategy for detection of early stage, curable prostate cancer: role of prescreening with prostatic-specific antigen. *Clin Invest Med* 16:425–439.

13. Littrup PJ, Goodman AC, Mettlin CJ. (1993) The benefit and cost of prostate cancer early detection. The Investivators of the American Cancer Society-National Prostate Cancer Detection Project. *CA: Cancer J Clin* 43:143–149.

14. Labrie F, Candas B, Cusan L, Gomez JL, Diamond P, Suburu R, et al. (1996) Diagnosis of advanced or noncurable prostate cancer can be practically eliminated by prostate-specific antigen. *Urology* 47:212–217.

15. American Cancer Society. (1993) *Guidelines for the Cancer-Related Checkup*: an update. Atlanta, GA: American Cancer Society.

16. American Urological Association (1992) Executive Committee report. Baltimore, MD: American Urological Association.

17. Murphy GP, Natarajan N, Pontes JE, Schmitz RL, Smart CR, Schmidt JD, et al. (1982) The national survey of prostate cancer in the United States by the American College of Surgeons. *J Urol* 127:928–934.

18. Schmidt JD, Mettlin CJ, Natarajan N, Peace, BB, Beart Jr RW, Winchester DP, et al. (1986) Trends in patterns of care for prostatic cancer, 1974–1983: results of surveys by the American College of Surgeons. *J Urol* 136:416–421.

19. Mettlin C, Murphy GP, Lee F, Littrup PJ, Chesley A, Babaian R, et al. (1993) Characteristics of prostate cancers deteted in a multimodality early detection program. The Investigators of the American Cancer Society–National Prostate Cancer Detection Project. *Cancer* 72:1701–1708.

20. Adami HO, Baron JA, Rothman KJ. (1994) Ethics of a prostate cancer screening trial. *Lancet* 343:958-960.

21. Andriole GL Catalona WJ. (1993) Usine PSA to screen for prostate cancer. *Urol Clinics North Am* 20:647–651.

22. Catalona WJ, Smith DS, Ratliff TL, Basler JW. (1993) Detection of organ-confined prostate cancer is increased through prostate-specific antigen-based screening. *JAMA* 270:948–954.

23. Slawin KM, Ohori M, Dillioglugil O, Scardino PT. (1995) Screening for prostate cancer: an analysis of the early experience. *CA: Cancer J Clin* 45:134–147.

24. Labrie F, Dupont A, Bélanger A, Cusan L, Lacourcière Y, Monfette G, et al. (1982) New hormonal therapy in prostatic carcinoma: combined treatment with an LHRH agonist and an antiandrogen. *Clin Invest Med* 5:267–275.

25. Labrie F. (1991) Endocrine therapy for prostate cancer. *Endocrinol Metab Clin North Am,* 20:845–872.

26. Crawford ED, Eisenberger MA, McLeod DG, Spaulding JT, Benson R, Dorr FA, et al. (1989) A controlled trial of leuprolide with and without flutamide in prostatic carcinoma. *N Engl J Med* 321:419–424.

27. Denis L, Carnelro de Moura JL, Bono A, Sylvester R, Whelan R, Newling D, et al. (1993) Goserelin acetate and flutamide vs bilateral orchiectomy: a phase III

EORTC trial (30853). EORTC GU Group and EORTC Data Center. *Urology* 42:119–129.

28. Janknegt RA, Abbou CC, Bartoletti R, Bernstein-Hahn L, Bracken B, Brisset JM, et al. (1993) Orchiectomy and nilutamide or placebo as treatment of metastatic prostatic cancer in a multinational double-blind randomized trial. *J Urol* 149:77–83.

29. Dijkman GA, Janknegt RA, Dereijke TM, Debruyne FMJ. (1997) Long-term efficacy and safety of nilutamide plus castration in advanced prostate-cancer, and the significance of early prostate specific antigen normalization. *J Urol* 158:160–163.

30. Wang MC, Valenzuela LA, Murphy GP, Chu TM. (1979) Purification of human prostate specific antigen. *Invest Urol* 17:159–163.

31. Papsidero LD, Wang MC, Valenzuela LA, Murphy GP, Chu TM. (1980) A prostate antigen in sera of prostatic cancer patients. *Cancer Res* 40:2428–2432.

32. Kuriyama M, Wang MC, Papsidero LD, Killian CS, Chu TM. (1980) Quantitation of prostate-specific antigen in serum by a sensitive enzyme immunoassay. *Cancer Res* 40:4658–4662.

33. Kuriyama M, Wang MC, Lee CL, Papsidero LD, Killian CS, Inaji H, et al. (1981) Use of human prostate-specific antigen in monitoring prostate cancer. *Cancer Res* 41:3874–3876.

34. Polascik TJ, Oesterling JE, Partin AW. (1999) Prostate specific antigen: a decade of discovery—what we have learned and where we are going. *J Urol* 162:293–306.

35. Pound CR, Partin AW, Epstein JI, Walsh PC. (1997) Prostate-specific antigen after anatomic radical retropubic prostatectomy. Patterns of recurrence and cancer control. *Urol Clin North Am* 24:395–406.

36. Partin AW, Kattan MW, Subong EN, Walsh PC, Wojno KJ, Oesterling JE, et al. (1997) Combination of prostate-specific antigen, clinical stage, and Gleason score to predict pathological stage of localized prostate cancer. A multi-institutional update (see comments). *JAMA* 277:1445–1451, erratum: *JAMA* 278(2):118(1997).

37. Parker SL, Tong T, Bolden S, Wingo PA. (1996) Cancer statistics, 1996 (see comments). *CA Cancer J Clin* 46:5–27.

38. Gann PH, Hennekens CH, Stampfer MJ. (1995) A prospective evaluation of plasma prostate-specific antigen for detection of prostatic cancer. *JAMA* 273:289–294.

39. Narod S, Dupon, A, Cusan L, Diamond P, Gomez JL, Suburu RE, et al. (1995) The impact of family history on early detection of prostate cancer. *Nat Med* 1:99–101.

40. Catalona WJ(1994) Management of cancer of the prostate. *N Engl J Med* 331:996–1004.

41. Labrie F, Cusan L, Gomez JL, Diamond P, Suburu R, Lemay M, et al. (1994) Down-staging of early stage prostate cancer before radical prostatectomy: the first randomized trial of neoadjuvant combination therapy with Flutamide and a luteinizing hormone-releasing hormone agonist. *Urology* 44:29–37.

42. Bostwick DG. (1992) Anatomy of the prostate: histopathology of cancer and BPH. In: *7th International Symposium: Transrectal Ultrasound in the Diagnosis and Management of BPH and Prostate Cancer* Chicago: American Institute of Ultrasound and Medicine pp. 1–13.

43. Franks LM. (1954) Latent carcinoma of the prostate. *J Pathol Bacteriol*, 68:603–616.

44. Montie JE, Wood DP Jr, Pontes JE, Boyett JM, Levin HS. (1989) Adenocarcinoma of the prostate in cystoprotatectomy specimens removed for bladder cancer. *Cancer* 63:381–385.

45. Kabalin JN, McNeal JE, Price HM, Freiha FS, Stamey TA. (1989) Unsuspected adenocarcinoma of the prostate in patients undergoing cystoprostatectomy for

other causes: incidence, histology and morphometric observations. *J Urol* 141:1091–1094.

46. Reitbergen JB, Hoedemaeker RF, Kruger AE, Kirkels WJ, Schroder FH. (1999) The changing pattern of prostate cancer at the time of diagnosis: characteristics of screen detected prostate cancer in a population-based screening study. *J Urol* 161:1192–1198.

47. Ellison LF, Stokes J, Gibbons L, Lindsay J, Levy I, Morrison H. (1998) Monograph series on aging-related diseases. X. Prostate cancer. *Chronic Dis Can* 19:1–18.

48. Litwin MS, Pasta DJ, Stoddard ML, Henning JM, Carroll PR (1998) Epidemiological trends and financial outcomes in radical prostatectomy among Medicare beneficiaries, 1991 to 1993. *J Urol* 160:445–448; erratum: *J Urol* 160 (6 Pt 1):2164.

49. Borre M, Nerstrom B, Overgaard J. (1997) The dilemna of prostate cancer—a growing human and economic burden irrespective of treatment strategies. *Acta Oncol* 36:681–687.

50. Labrie F, Dupont A, Cusan L, Gomez JL, Diamond P, Koutsilieris M, et al. (1993) Downstaging of localized prostate cancer by neoadjuvant therapy with flutamide and lupron: the first controlled and randomized trial. *Clin Invest Med* 16:499–509.

51. Littrup PJ, Kane RA, Mettlin CJ, Murphy GP, Lee F, Toi A, et al. (1994) Cost-effective prostate-cancer detection. Reduction of low-field biopsies. *Cancer* 74:3146–3158.

52. Aus G, Hugosson J, Norlén L. (1995) Long-term survival and mortality in prostate cancer treated with noncurative intent. *J Urol* 154:460–465.

53. Labrie F. (1994) Intracrinology and cancer therapy. *Science Watch* 5:3–8.

54. Labrie F, Cusan L, Gomez JL, Diamond P, Candas B. (1995) Combination of screening and preoperative endocrine therapy: the potential for an important decrease in prostate cancer mortality. *J Clin Endocrinol Metab* 80:2002–2013.

55. Merrill, RM, Potosky, AL, Feuer, EJ. (1996) Changing trends in U.S. prostate cancer incidence rates. J Natl Cancer Inst, 88:1683-1685.

56. Roberts RO, Bergstralh EJ, Katusic SK, Lieber MM, Jacobsen SJ. (1999) Decline in prostate cancer mortality from 1980 to 1997, and an update on incidence trends in Olmsted County, Minnesota. *J Urol* 161:529–533.

57. Hoeksema MJ Law C. (1996) Cancer mortality rates fall: a turning point for the nation. *J Natl Cancer Inst* 88:1706–1707.

58. Meyer F, Moore L, Bairati I, Fradet Y. (1999) Downward trend in prostate cancer mortality in Quebec and Canada. *J Urol* 161;1189–1191.

59. Killian CS, Emrich LJ, Vargas FP, Yang N, Wang MC, Priore RL, et al. (1986) Relative reliability of five serially measured markers for prognosis of progression in prostate cancer. *J Natl Cancer Inst* 76:179–185.

60. Lee F, Torp-Pedersen ST, Siders DB, Littrup PJ, McLeary RD. (1989) Transrectal ultrasound in the diagnosis and staging of prostatic carcinoma. *Radiology* 170:609–615.

61. Hanks GE, Asbell SO, Krall JM, Perez CA, Doggett S, Rubin P, et al. (1991) Outcome for lymph node dissection negative T-1b, T-2 (A-2,B) prostate cancer treated with external beam radiation therapy in RTOG 77-06. *Int J Radiat Oncol Biol Phys* 21:1099–1103.

62. Cooner WH, Mosley BR, Rutherford Jr CL, Beard JH, Pond HS, Terry WJ, et al. (1990) Prostate cancer detection in a clinical urological practice by ultrasonography, digital rectal examination and prostate-specific antigen. *Urology* 143:1146–1154.

63. Laverdiere J, Gomez JL, Cusan L, Suburu R, Diamond P, Lemay M, et al. (1997) Beneficial effect of combination therapy administered prior and following external beam radiation therapy in localized prostate cancer. *Int J Radiat Oncol Biol Phys* 37:247–252.

64. Pilepich MV, Krall JM, Al-Saffaf M, John MJ, Dogget RL, Sause WT, et al. (1995) Androgen deprivation with radiation therapy compared with radiation therapy alone for locally advanced prostatic carcinoma: a randomized comparative trial of the Radiation Therapy Oncology Group. *Urology* 45:616–623.

65. Blasko JC, Ragde H, Luse RW, Sylvester JE, Cavanagh W, Grimm PD. (1996) Should brachytherapy be considered a therapeutic option in localized prostate cancer? *Urol Clin North Am* 23:633–649.

66. Lee F, Torp-Pedersen ST, Siders DB. (1989) Use of transrectal ultrasound in diagnosis, guided biopsy, staging, and screening of prostate cancer. *Urology* 33 (suppl):7–12.

67. Catalona WJ, Smith DS, Ratliff TL, Dodds KM, Coplen DE, Yuan JJ, et al. (1991) Measurement of prostate-specific antigen in serum as a screening test for prostate cancer. *New Engl J Med* 324:1156–1161.

68. Mettlin C. (1993) Early detection of prostate cancer following repeated examinations by multiple modalities: results of the American Cancer Society National Prostate Cancer Detection Project. *Clin Invest Med* 16:440–447.

69. Aus G, Bergdahl S, Hugosson J, Lodding P, Norlén L. (1994) Influence of benign prostatic hyperplasia, testosterone and age on serum levels of prostate-specific antigen. *Scand J Urol Nephrol* 28:379–384.

70. Hugosson J, Aus G, Bergdahl C, Bergdahl S. (1995) Prostate cancer mortality in patients surviving more than 10 yr after diagnosis. *J Urol* 154:2115–2117.

71. Krongrad A, Lai H, Lamm SH, Lai S. (1996) Mortality in prostate cancer. *J Urol* 156:1084–1091.

72. Lu-Yao GL, Yao SL. (1997) Population-based study of long-term survival in patients with clinically localised prostate cancer. *Lancet* 349:906–910.

73. Brasso K, Friis S, Juel K, Jorgensen T, Iversen P. (1999) Mortality of patients with clinically localized prostate cancer treated with observation for 10 yr or longer: a population based registry study. *J Urol* 161:524–528.

18 Cancer of the Prostate Risk Index Test and Software (CAPRI)

Scott A. Optenberg, PhD,
Atanacio C. Guillen, MS, John P. Campbell, MS,
and Ian M. Thompson, MD

CONTENTS

INTRODUCTION TO CAPRI MODEL DEVELOPMENT
SUMMARY OF CAPRI MODEL DEVELOPMENT
THE CAPRI SOFTWARE PROGRAM DEVELOPMENT
CAPRI TEST AND SOFTWARE DEVELOPMENT SUMMARY
REFERENCES

INTRODUCTION TO CAPRI MODEL DEVELOPMENT

The significance of prostate cancer and its impact on the world's population is well recognized. It is currently estimated by the American Cancer Society (ACS) that at least 180,400 new cases of prostate cancer will be diagnosed that in the year 2000 and that approx 31,900 men will die of the disease *(1)*.

Historically, the digital rectal examination (DRE) has been used for early detection of prostate cancer, but its predictive value, particularly in view of the increased use of the prostate specific antegen (PSA) as a screening tool has been questioned *(2,3)*. The impact of ethnicity has also been well documented in the literature, with the historical emphasis on how blacks experience increased incidence, tumor progression, and mortality when compared to white populations *(4)*.

From: *Current Clinical Urology: Prostate Cancer Screening*
Edited by: I. M. Thompson, M. I. Resnick, and E. A. Klein
© Humana Press Inc., Totowa, NJ

Moreover, what further complicates clinical assessment and treatment planning are DRE, PSA, and racial background, the relative influence of these predictors are confounded by patient age, which is also a known risk factor. Finally, the situation facing the clinician is only going to become more complicated with genetic and environmental risk factors, and even patterns of dietary intake are hypothesized as having a role in the overall etiology and prognosis of prostate cancer (5,6).

It was within this clinical and scientific backdrop that an effort was undertaken to develop an easily implemented test, based on a sound mathematical model, to provide a simple and reliable clinical prediction for an individual patient's risk of disease. The second objective was to develop a software program, providing that prerequisite research supported such development, that would be easily implemented, regardless of the clinical setting. The priorities during both the model and the software development were to make the test intuitive, collect the necessary information, calculate an accurate risk of prostate cancer, and display this risk in a visually appealing and intuitive manner. Finally it was the objective of the authors to use a model-building and software development process that would be able to efficiently incorporate changes, modifications, and additions of additional prognostic factors as the research continues in this area.

SUMMARY OF CAPRI MODEL DEVELOPMENT

Because the test development is covered in significant detail in other publications, only a summary will be provided (7). Data were collected from 1991 and 1995 from a model population. The model was tested for validity and generalizability using a completely independent patient population from an external and geographically separate region of the country. All patients were screened to determine whether a prebiopsy-detectable serum PSA and DRE were conducted. The DRE was considered abnormal if there were one or more of the following clinical findings: (1) asymmetry, (2) induration, (3) nodularity, or (4) firmness upon palpation of the gland. Actual PSA was determined using the Tosoh assay and reported as a continuous variable in nanograms per milliliter (ng/mL). Patient age was recorded as age on the date of prostate biopsy and was computed in whole years. Patient race was categorized into white (non-Hispanic), black, Hispanic, or other. However, because of small-sample limitations, only white and black patients were used to compute model estimates.

Analysis demonstrated that each of the four factors—(1) total PSA, (2) DRE, (3) race, and (4) age—contributed significantly to the predictive value of the test. Overall, the predictive capability of the CAPRI test was high within both the model population (receiver–operator characteristic [ROC] = 80.8%) and when applied to the external population (ROC = 76.1%). Even more important, the predictive quality of the CAPRI test performed equally well in both model and external populations throughout the risk spectrum.

Increasing levels of PSA were highly predictive of prostate cancer. It was noteworthy that the research clearly demonstrated that a "PSA-only" model was not adequate for use as a stand-alone screening tool for estimating the risk of prostate cancer. The contribution of the additional factors of DRE, race, and age were clearly demonstrated to assist not only in the level of overall predictive quality but also to significantly improved model fit and generalizability to external populations.

One of the most intriguing findings resulting from the development phase of the overall effort was that when placed in the overall model, the four factors; (1) PSA, (2) DRE, (3) race, and (4) age, were not only statistically significant but also demonstrated a substantial impact. When controlling for PSA, patients demonstrating an abnormal DRE had an overall 255% increase in the probability of cancer at biopsy, and blacks exhibited an overall 89% increase in risk as compared to whites when controlling for both PSA and DRE. Finally, even when controlling for PSA, DRE, and race, the patient age at biopsy remained statistically significant in predicting the presence of cancer in both the model and external populations. However, an important finding made during the model development was the differential risk of an abnormal DRE and being black is not constant because of a clear nonlinear relationship that both PSA and patient age exhibited with risk of cancer at biopsy. The highest magnitude of differential risk impact of both DRE findings and race was seen between PSA levels of 5.0 and 10.0 ng/mL. Moreover, the CAPRI test demonstrated no significant lack of fit in either the model or the external population, indicating that the test predicted equally well throughout the risk spectrum. In fact, it should be emphasized that throughout the model-building and validation process, substantial effort was directed toward deriving a predictive model that demonstrated equivalent predictive power across the spectrum of patient risk.

One of the primary observations drawn from the model development research was that not only was there compelling evidence that PSA, DRE, race, and age all contribute significantly and independently to the prediction of prostate cancer in an individual patient, but these factors worked well together within a combined model. It was therefore concluded that the CAPRI test protocol was likely to be attractive to both the patient and clinician in the clinical setting. This conclusion was based on the fact that the test could depict individual risk (with confidence intervals if desired) in an easily-understood, visually provocative manner, allowing both clinician and patient to more easily reach the decision as to whether biopsy is appropriate as well as to educate the patient in general.

THE CAPRI SOFTWARE PROGRAM DEVELOPMENT

Because of the success achieved in CAPRI test development and validation, a software program was developed. The goal of this development was to directly assist physicians and patients in treatment planning to enable the research results to be applied in the clinical setting through the use of a simple easy-to-use patient-tracking and prostate predictive program. Based on the model research four prognostic variables are included in the current test version: (1) overall PSA, (2) DRE, (3) patient race, and (4) patient age at biopsy. The software program is divided into three major software modules.

CAPRI Software Physician Module

The Physician Module contains information about attending physicians. This information is used to tie the patient to a particular physician. The module contains the following information on physicians involved in the care of any given patient:

1. Full name of the physician
2. Physician address (street, city, state, and zip code)
3. Physician office name (if applicable)
4. Physician's phone/Fax number "(nnn) nnn-nnnn"

Figure 1 demonstrates how this information would typically be displayed.

CAPRI Software Patient Module

The CAPRI Software Patient Module provides information about the patients treated within any given practice setting. This module consists of several submodules. First, *Patient Information* provides demographic data about the patient. Next, *Family History* provides information about relatives of the patient and to what extent prostate cancer is present in the family tree of the patient. Finally, *Medication Information* provides data as to what medications the patient is currently taking as well as medication history of the patient. Patient information collected include the following data:

1. Patient full name
2. Patient address (street, city, state, and zip code)
3. Patient phone/Fax number "(nnn) nnn-nnnn"
4. Patient SSN

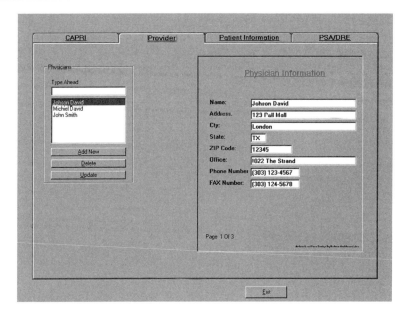

Fig. 1. CAPRI physician information display.

5. Patient birth date ("dd/mm/yyyy") and age (computed)
6. Patient race
7. Physician referral data

Figure 2 demonstrates how this Patient Information sub-module of the Patient Module would typically be displayed.

Family History provides information about other members of the patient's family. Information is collected on both the number of relatives, as well as the number of those relatives that tested positive for either prostate cancer if the relative was a male, or breast cancer if the relative was female.

Figure 3 demonstrates how this Family History sub-module would be displayed.

Finally, the Medication Information sub-module displayed in Fig. 4 provides information about the medications prescribed for the patient and uses a preprogrammed formulary supplied with the software.

Current Risk of Prostate Cancer

The risk of prostate cancer employs the predictive algorithms developed and published by Optenberg et al *(8)*, and predicts the patient's current risk of prostate cancer. The module collects and displays the following information concerning the clinical history of the following:

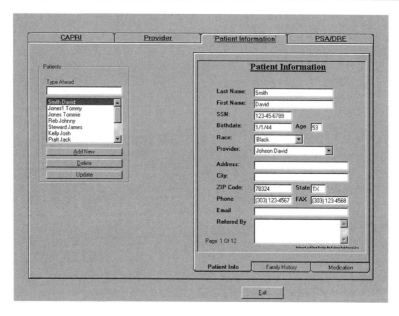

Fig. 2. Patient Information submodule display.

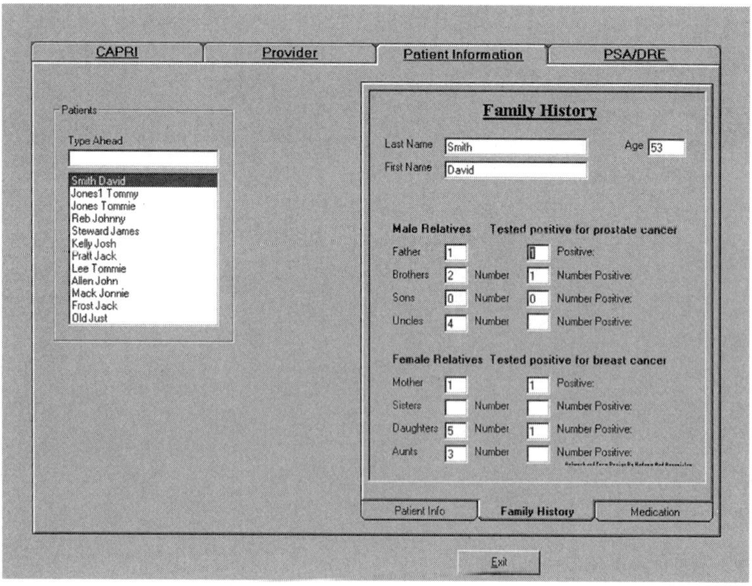

Fig. 3. Family History submodule display.

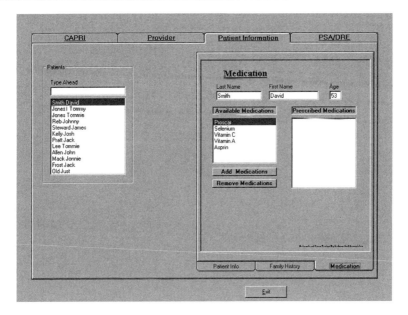

Fig. 4. Patient Medication submodule.

1. Prostate-specific antigen (PSA) date
2. PSA results
3. Digital rectal examination (DRE) date
4. DRE findings
5. Biopsy date
6. Biopsy results
7. Gleason score (if applicable, computed 1–5)

When a new patient is registered and PSA results and the DRE findings are entered, the current risk is calculated and the graph showing the calculated risk is displayed. Whenever the PSA results or the DRE findings are changed through subsequent screening, the risk is recalculated and the graph is redisplayed. Because the risk is a predictive calculated risk, the risk is presented as a range. Figure 5 displays how this risk would be presented to the physician or patient. Figure 5. CAPRI Computed Risk of Prostate Cancer

CAPRI TEST
AND SOFTWARE DEVELOPMENT SUMMARY

The CAPRI research was conducted and the software was developed with the primary objective of assisting the clinician to provide the highest quality of service to the patient. Since its development, the CAPRI

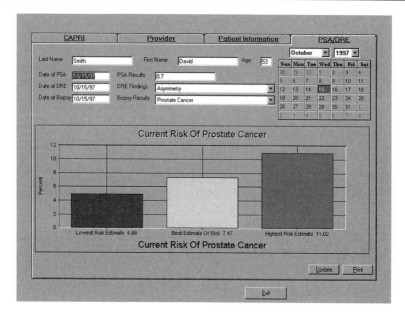

Fig. 5. Current Risk of Prostate Cancer screen.

test software has been tested and implemented in numerous clinical settings over an extended period of time. Obviously, the CAPRI software is NOT intended as a substitute for the provider–patient treatment process, but rather to augment and facilitate this existing process. Periodic follow-up of those clinicians using the CAPRI V1.0 software on a prototype basis has demonstrated a high level of satisfaction and perceived value. In particular, clinicians have singled out one particular benefit of the software. Clinicians have felt that the software has assisted them to better translate a very complex set of clinical decisions imposed on the patient into terms better grasped by the patient.

As part of this volume, a CD is included. This CD contains (1) an installation utility, (2) CAPRI V1.0, (3) CAPRI user's manual, and (4) reprint of the original article by Optenberg et al. If the install utility is executed, it will install the above four components to C:\CAPRI, or as specified by the user. The software is provided free of charge with purchase of this volume. The software is configured to run within any Pentium-based Windows 95/98/NT software architecture. Installation of the software constitutes the user's agreement to the data use agreement and conditions contained in the Introduction of the CAPRI *user's manual*.

Currently, CAPRI Version 2.0 is scheduled for release in the Fall, 2000. Several important enhancements will include explicit enumeration of Hispanic and family history risks, inclusion of free serum PSA, and the ability to compute risk in the absence of complete clinical data. Contact CAPRI@texas.net for information requests concerning release V2.0.

Note: If the CD is missing from the book contact CAPRI@texasnet via e-mail to obtain a certified copy.

REFERENCES

1 Anon. (2000) Prostate Cancer: can we reduce deaths and preserve quality of life? at-a-glance 2000. Atlanta, GA: Centers for Disease Control and Prevention, National Center for Chronic Disease Prevention and Health Promotion.
2. Kramer BS, Brown ML, Prorok PC, Potosky AL, Gohagan JK. (1993) Prostate cancer screening: what we know and what we need to know. *Ann Intern Med* 119:914–923.
3. US Preventive Services Task Force. (1995) *Guide to Clinical Preventive Services*, 2nd ed. Baltimore, MD: Williams & Wilkins, pp. 119–134.
4. Optenberg SA, Thompson IM, Friedrichs P, Wojcik B, Stein CR, Kramer B. (1995) Race, treatment, and long-term survival from prostate cancer in an equal-access medical care delivery system. *JAMA* 274:1599–1605.
5. Blair A, Fraumeni JF Jr. (1978) Geographic patterns of prostate cancer in the United States. *J Natl Cancer Inst* 61:1379–1384.
6. Whittemore AS, Kolonel LN, Wu AH, John EM, Gallagher RP, Howe GR, et al. (1995) Prostate cancer in relation to diet, physical activity, and body size in blacks, whites, and Asians in the United States and Canada. *J Natl Cancer Inst* 87:652–661.
7. Optenberg SA, Clark CY, Brawer MK, Thompson IM, Stein CR, Friedrichs P. (1995) Development of a decision-making tool to predict risk of prostate cancer: the Cancer of the Prostate Risk Index (CAPRI) Test, *Urology* 50: 665–672.

19 The European Randomized Study of Screening for Prostate Cancer (ERSPC)

*Fritz H. Schröder, MD
and Ingrid van der Cruijsen-Koeter, MD
for the ERSPC Study Group*

CONTENTS

INTRODUCTION
BACKGROUND
PURPOSE OF THE STUDY
THE STRUCTURE OF ERSPC AND THE CONDITIONS OF
    PARTICIPATION
PRELIMINARY DATA
REFERENCES

INTRODUCTION

In this chapter an attempt is made to describe the ongoing European Randomized Study of Screening for Prostate Cancer (ERSPC). This randomized study represents a very large clinical research effort in which at this time, June 2000, eight European countries are involved. This summary is given on behalf of the whole European research group. All names are listed at the end of this contribution. This chapter includes a summary description of the background on which the study was initiated, the rules and regulations for participation, the study group and some of the differences per country, the purpose of the study, and preliminary results obtained. Unless interim evaluations show a significant

From: *Current Clinical Urology: Prostate Cancer Screening*
Edited by: I. M. Thompson, M. I. Resnick, and E. A. Klein
© Humana Press Inc., Totowa, NJ

difference that might lead to the discontinuation of the study, a final analysis is expected to be carried out during the year 2008. This time period seems agonizingly long in the face of a situation where increasing indirect evidence accumulates that may indicate that prostate cancer mortality can be reduced by screening.

BACKGROUND

The idea of conducting ERSPC originated independently in the centers Antwerp, Belgium and Rotterdam, The Netherlands, during the years 1990–1991. A first grant financing international cooperation was obtained from Europe against Cancer (EaC) in 1992 by L. Denis. It soon became clear that considering the enormous sample size necessary, this large trial could not be run in Belgium and The Netherlands alone. Early contacts with the early detection and prevention branch of the National Cancer Institute (USA) during the late 1980s had been useful to develop ideas on the setup of this study.

From the beginning, the undertaking was controversial to the extreme. Extreme views were encountered in private and public discussions. The strength of the study group has been and is still derived from the conviction that at this moment an effect of screening on prostate cancer mortality is unproven (1,2). In this situation, some experts felt that it was unethical to screen and even to carry out a randomized screening study (3) and clarification in public was necessary (4–6). Others felt that the contrary was the case, and evidence was sufficient to even apply screening as a health-care policy. The latter was the case in Germany. Views did not only differ per person and investigator but also per country between these extremes. Fortunately a sufficient number of centers and countries could be convinced to participate in a very large randomized clinical trial of screening, which turned out to be an effective minimal unifying denominator. The first pilot studies in Belgium and The Netherlands were carried out between 1991 and 1994 (7–12) and other pilot studies followed. The pilot studies were feasibility studies, which included different schemes of randomization, different biopsy indications, the study of participation rates and all the logistics that would then have to be applied to a very large study. Some of the logistics were subject to an independent process evaluation (13,14). It is fortunate that the idea and the plan of a close and coherent international cooperation as well as the first available scientific results of pilot studies apparently produced sufficient attraction for others to join. The study was formally initiated on July 1, 1994 in Belgium and The Netherlands. During the year of 1994, four more countries joined (Finland, Sweden, Italy, and Portugal). Based on the capability to carry out pilot studies, estimates of numbers to be recruited per country seemed to be realistic and approached the numbers needed according to an initial sample size calculation.

PURPOSE OF THE STUDY

The main purpose of the study is to show or to exclude a prostate cancer mortality reduction through screening and early treatment. This task is dealt with in a large randomized clinical trial in which screening is offered to the intervention group while the control group is managed according to regional health care routines. The initial sample size calculation amounts to 132,000 participants, 66,000 per arm. The calculation took into account the possibility of a 20% mortality reduction and aimed at a power of 90%. The 20% estimate was made in absence of prospective randomized treatment studies comparing watchful waiting to either radical prostatectomy or radiotherapy based on retrospective data available in the literature (15). The sample size was later adjusted to 190,000 randomized men, 85,000 per treatment arm, because of "contamination" of the control arm by opportunistic Prostate-specific antigen (PSA)-based screening. In some of the participating countries, the use of PSA-based testing was carefully studied, especially in the control arm population. In The Netherlands it amounted to 8% and later rose to 13%, much lower rates were found in Spain (16). Obviously, a further increase in contamination could jeopardize the study. A plan for common evaluation of the European study with the prostate arm of the PLCO study (Prostate, Lung, Colon, and Ovary screening study of the US National Cancer Institute) provides some extra buffer in terms of recruitment. Common evaluation of both studies is an option. A prospective common evaluation plan has been established and agreed upon (17). If necessary, power can be made greater by increasing recruitment or by the number of screens. Both options are kept open within the European study.

The status of recruitment per country is shown in Table 1. Note that in Finland randomization is 1:2 with respect to screening:control. In most counties the second round of screening has started; it has been completed in Sweden. Clearly, the expected sample size of 190,000 randomized men is within reach. Further details will be given in a following section.

QUALITY OF LIFE

While prostate cancer mortality reduction is considered the primary end point of ERSPC, the evaluation of quality of life within the screen-

Table 1
Progress of the ERSPC Per Center (November 1999)

Country	Expected Contribution	No. of men Randomized (11/99)	No. of men in the Control Arm (11/99)	No. of men in the Screening Arm (11/99)
Netherlands	40,000	42,333	21,140	21,193
Belgium	17,500	8,381	4,167	4,214
Italy	14,000	12,220	6,107	6,113
Spain	10,000	4,278	1,862	2,416
Finland	67,000	78,861	48,458	30,403
Sweden	20,000	19,950	9,976	9,974
Portugal	10,000	3,307	1,682	1,625
Switzerland	42,000	930	808	122
France*	26,500			
Total	205,000	169,330	93,392	75,938

*Candidate Center

ing and the control groups has been considered to be essential from the beginning. Such evaluations are carried out in two of the participating countries (The Netherlands and Finland). In addition to mortality reduction, quality adjusted life years (QUALYs) will be calculated. Initial results have been published (18,19); other publications are in preparation. In close connection with these studies, cost effectiveness will be evaluated. Appropriate data collections are already being carried out.

TEST PROCEDURES AND SIDE STUDIES

Screening for prostate cancer leads at least initially to an increase in prostate cancer incidence with respect to control populations where diagnostic procedures are applied according to existing clinical routines (20,21). While it may be expected that with repeated screening incidence will decrease over time, at this moment it is unknown which balance will be reached between the screening and control arm incidence within ERSPC and in screen populations vs nonscreen populations in general (22). Figure 1 gives an illustration of the hypothetical development. Obviously, the future balance with repeated screening depends on rescreening intervals, lead time, biopsy techniques, the sensitivity of the screening tests, age, and other factors. Clearly, overdiagnosis of which a proper definition is lacking at this time, occurs to an unknown extent. In the future, screening strategies must be adjusted to the proper "window of opportunity." This will have to be achieved by

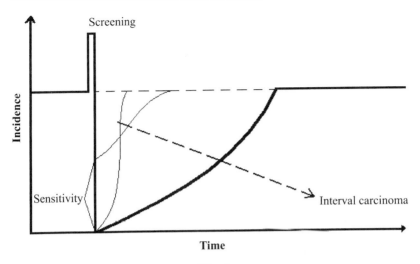

Fig. 1.

focusing on those cases in whom "cure is necessary and possible" and by avoiding those cases in whom "cure may be possible but not necessary" *(23)*. With this background, an evaluation of test procedures is an essential part of ERSPC. Prior to initiation of the study, it was agreed that screening procedures would be adjusted one time if necessary. While improvements in sensitivity (finding all relevant cancers) and specificity (avoiding unnecessary biopsies) are major goals of these side studies, obviously "selectivity" for lesions in whom "cure is possible and necessary" will be of crucial importance in avoiding overdiagnosis if screening is ever to become a health care policy. This latter goal can only be achieved by comparing findings in the screening and control arm. The PSA history of those men who underwent opportunistic screening in the control arm may be of crucial importance in this respect.

Next to the study and improvement of screening procedures, the following issues have been and are still subject to evaluation: the study of tumor characteristics in relation to pretreatment parameters, the medical complications of the screening procedure and of treatment *(24,25,26)*, quality control procedures with respect to the PSA test *(27,28)* and modeling of the screening process *(29)*. Modeling of outcomes is a continuous process within ERSPC Rotterdam with the use of the *MISCAN* model system. In addition, an international consortium is tackling the issue of the improvement of serum-based testing with respect to sensitivity, specificity, and selectivity for aggressive lesions *(30,31)*.

THE STRUCTURE OF ERSPC
AND THE CONDITIONS OF PARTICIPATION

ERSPC is conducted in a decentralized fashion. This is necessary because of the relative autonomy of the segments of ERSPC within the individual European countries. Also, in setting up ERSPC, financing was an extreme limitation. Randomized screening studies are very expensive; the European Union was generous in financing the European coordination (Europe Against Cancer: SOC95 35109, SOC 96 2018869 05F02, SOC 97 201329, and SOC 98 32241) but could not finance individual countries. Financing in the participating countries was variable, but in general very limited. The group decided that ERSPC had to be run on the basis of mutual written commitments on participation and continued participation, which would also cover publication policies and evaluation policies. Furthermore, a centralized data collection by an independent center, which does not participate in the screening study itself, was agreed. The Central Database is located in Edinburgh and is in the hands of Professor Freda Alexander, an epidemiologist. ERSPC is run and controlled by the following committees:

Scientific Committee:
1. Netherlands
   Prof. Dr. F.H. Schröder (chairman)
   Dr. W.J. Kirkels
2. Belgium:
   Prof. Dr. L. Denis
   Dr. V. Nelen
3. Sweden:
   Prof. Dr. J. Hugosson
   Dr. P.A. Lodding
4. Italy:
   Dr. S. Ciatto
   Dr. M. Zappa
5. Portugal:
   Dr. F. Calais da Silva
   Dr. H. Monteiro
6. Finland:
   Prof. Dr. T. Tammela
   Prof. Dr. A. Auvinen
7. Spain:
   Dr. A. Berenguer
   Dr. A. Paez

8. Switzerland
    Dr. F. Recker
    Dr. M. Kwiatkowsky
9. France (candidate center)
    Dr. A. Villers
    To be determined
Noncenter members
10. Prof. Dr. F.E. Alexander (EC)
11. Dr. P. Smith (DMC)
Epidemiology Committee
    Dr. F.E. Alexander (Chairman)
    Prof. Dr. P. Maas/Dr. de Koning
    Dr. V. Nelen
    Dr. F. Figueiredo
    Prof. A. Auvinen
    Prof. Dr. M. Hakama
Ad hoc advisors:
    Drs. R. Damhuis/Dr. M. Wildhagen
Advising Urologists:
    Prof. Dr. F. Schröder/Dr. W. Kirkels
Data Monitoring Committee
(not affiliated with a center)
    Mr. P. Smith (chairman)
    Prof. Dr. I. de Beaufort
    Prof. Chamberlain
    Dr. H.J. de Koning (secretary)
    Prof. Dr. T. Hakulinen
Quality Control Committee
    Dr. Ciatto (chairman)
    Dr. M. Wildhagen
    Dr. H.J. de Koning
    Dr. W.J. Kirkels
    Dr. V. Nelen
    Dr. J. Hugosson
    Dr. F. Calais da Silva
    Dr. A. Auvinen
    Prof. Dr. T. Tammela
    Dr. A. Berenguer
    Prof. Dr. F.E. Alexander
Causes of Death Committee
    Dr. H.J. de Koning (chairman)
    Dr. J.H.M. Blom
    Dr. J.W. Merkelbach

Prof. Dr. Denis
Dr. V. Neelen
Dr. P. Lodding
Dr. S. Ciatto
Dr. R. Bonardi
Dr. F. Calais da Silva
Prof. Dr. T. Tammela
Dr. A. Berenguer
Dr. A. Paez
Prof. L. Teppo
Dr. J. Aro
Dr. V. Lindstroöm
PSA standardization Committee
Dr. B.G. Blijenberg (chairman)
Dr. H. Neels
Prof. Dr. H. Lilja
Dr. U.H. Stenman
Pathology Committee
Prof. Dr. Th.H. van der Kwast
Dr. Neetens
Dr. Pihl
Dr. S. di Lollo
Prof. Dr. C. Lopes
Prof. Dr. L. Teppo
Dr. P. Fernandez-Segoviano

The Scientific Committee is the governing body of the study; all important decisions are taken by this group, which consists of two representatives of each center. The Central Database, the Quality Control Committee, and the Data Monitoring Committee work together in producing semiannual updates of the study and in applying quality control and ethical control procedures to this process. The group has agreed to provide data according to a minimal dataset of which an outline is given in Table 2. Conditions for participation and continuous participation have been established and are supervised by the Epidemiology Committee, the Quality Control Committee, the Data Monitoring Committee in cooperation with the Central Database. All participants have accepted by signature the essential basic rules of ERSPC, which also include the acceptance of the authority of the Quality Control and Data Monitoring Committees.

PRELIMINARY DATA

This section will be limited to data coming from the Rotterdam center of ERSPC. A summary of the European study as a whole will shortly

Table 2
Minimal Dataset for Common Analysis European Randomized Study
of Screening for Prostate Cancer (ERSPC)

1.   All Study Subjects
1.1   Baseline Information
1.2   Follow-up Information
      Required
      – Type of follow-up (active/passive)
      Vital status
         * Alive
         * Dead
         * Lost of follow-up (emigrated / no contact)
      – Date of last contact/record linkage
      – Date of death
      – Causes of death
      – Exclusion after randomization
2.   Screening Arm Only
      Required
      – Dates of attendance
      – Screening test(s) performed
      – Diagnostic test(s) performed
      – Severe complications of test, e.g. fever, bleeding, following biopsy
      – Final diagnosis and further procedures e.g. intensive/normal
        follow-up
3.   All prostate Cancer Cases in Both Arms (Incl. Non-compliers if Feasible)
      – Stage at diagnosis
      – Tumor grade
      – Primary treatment
      – Side effects and complications of treatment
      – Progression/relapse
4.   Information on Aggregate Level
      Data on contamination levels (i.e. prevalence of screening test in control
      arm) for each screening tests at baseline and during the trial at least from
      a sample of the population

appear in the literature *(32)*. This paper gives a summary on the status
of ERSPC as a whole and on the performance per center. The status of
recruitment is indicated in Table 1. For better understanding of the
following information, Fig. 2 indicates the flow sheet of ERSPC
Rotterdam. About 42,000 men have been randomized by May 2000.
Consent to randomize was given by 49.6% of all invited men. In
Rotterdam, contrary to other centers, the age group 70–74 is included.
Age distribution is one of the agreed and permitted heterogeneity's within

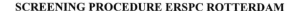

SCREENING PROCEDURE ERSPC ROTTERDAM

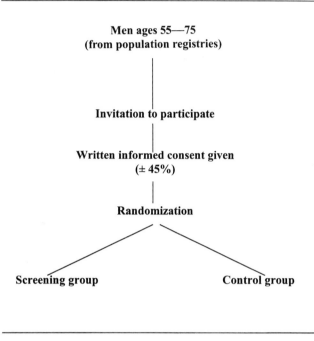

Men ages 55—75
(from population registries)

Invitation to participate

Written informed consent given
(± 45%)

Randomization

Screening group   Control group

Re-screening after 4 yr

Fig. 2.

ERSPC. The core age groups on which power is calculated is 55–69 yr. Obviously, data relating to prostate cancer mortality cannot be given at this time. This is restricted information collected centrally within the central database and made available only to the Data Monitoring Committee, the ethical watchdog of the study. A complete evaluation of ERSPC is carried out every 2 yr. If no significant differences occur and if no reason to discontinue ERSPC occurs before that date, the final evaluation is expected in 2008.

Test Performance and Selectiveness of Screening

As already mentioned earlier, the performance of the screening procedures applied within ERSPC has been a major concern from the beginning. Evidence of overdiagnosis and overtreatment of an unknown degree, uncertainty about the relative sensitivity and selectiveness of the procedure, as well as a large proportion of false positive

Table 3
PSA Screening—Biopsy at PSA = 3,
No DRE and TRUS with PSA < 3.0 ng/mL

Impact (based on logistic regression)		
	Old	New
DRE + TRUS	100%	20%
Detection rate	4.8%	4.7%
Biopsied	23.7%	19.8%
False positives	19.6%	15.1%
Clin. Confined	78%	76%
Path. Confined	60%	56%
Negative margins	72%	68%
% Grade 3	12%	15%

Source: ERSPC Rotterdam, 1997.

biopsy indications led to the decision to evaluate test performance during the early phase of ERSPC mainly in Rotterdam and Sweden. The group furthermore agreed that according to the results of such an evaluation screening tests should be changed ONE time during the recruitment phase to the prevalence screen. This evaluation has been completed, and the resulting information has been or is in the process of being reported *(33–44)*. The issue of overdiagnosis is a major concern to the group. Preliminary definitions and estimates are offered on the basis of the pilot study's results conducted in Italy *(45)*. At this time it remains unknown which cancers will contribute to the potential decrease of prostate cancer mortality, it is most likely that overdiagnosis will be somehow related to those cases that present with minimal disease at the time of screening. Surrogacy for prognostic parameters as T-category and grade of differentiation can by no means be considered to be established. These parameters have been carefully studied within ERSPC and will become more useful as the study proceeds and correlations with the major end points become possible. In the meantime, there is clear evidence that the pattern of aggressiveness of prostate cancers detected in the prevalence screens shows an important stage reduction and differs from established health care patterns in the same areas *(46)*. A comparison of the prevalence of metastatic disease between ERSPC Rotterdam and the preceding 5-yr period within the Amsterdam Cancer Registry shows, for example, a 12-fold higher prevalence of metastatic disease. In spite of the uncertainty about defining tumor aggressiveness stage and grade distributions were considered in revising the screening policy within ERSPC *(43,47,48)*.

Table 4
Screening Tests, Biopsy Results and Cancer Detection
—Old (PSA 4.0, DRE$^+$, TRUS$^+$) and New (PSA $\geq$ 3.0, No DRE/TRUS)

		Biopsy Indication		
		Old, N (%) (95% Cl) p-value	New, N (%) (95% Cl) p-value	
A	Screened	8.612	8.726	
B	DRE + TRUS	8.612 (100%) (15.6–17.2)	1.302 (16.4%)	p = 0.001
C	PSA 3–3.9	642 (7.5% of A) (6.9–8.0)	534 (6.7%) (6.1–7.3)	p = 0.001
D	Biopsies PSA 3–3.9	160 (1.8% of A) 1.6–2.2)	446 (5.6%) (5.1–6.1)	p = 0.001
E	Biopsy done (overall)	2250 (26.1% of A) (25.1–22.6)	1.302 (16.4%) (15.6-17.2)	p = 0.001
F	Cancers PSA 3–3.9	41 (6.4% of C) (4.6–8.6)	96 (18%) (14.8–21.5)	p = 0.32
G	Cancers* (detection rate)	430 (5.0% of A) (4.5–5.5)	377 (4.7%) (4.3–5.2)	p = 0.47
H	Cancers/biopsy % (-PPV, G/D)	19.1 (17.5–20.8)	29.0 (26.5–31.5)	p = 0.001
I	False-positive biopsy indication	80.9% (79.2–82.5)	75.7% (68.5–73.5)	p = 0.001

(E-F)/F(%)

By extrapolation from 183 men biopsied with PSA 0–0.9 to 3045 men in the same PSA range without DRE + TRUS, 5 cancers and 327 biopsies were added. DRE and TRUS was discontinued for PSA 0–0.9 ng/mL in January 1996. Modified from (51).

Tumor characteristics were in fact decisive for the major change in biopsy indications, which was implemented within ERSPC in 1997. Based on a logistic regression analysis, it was predicted that about 66% of sextant biopsy detectable cancers were missed in the PSA range 0–4 ng/mL, this translated into an overall figure of 33% (49). These data related to the age group 55–74. Based on knowledge of tumor charac-teristics of cancers detected in the PSA range 3–3.9 ng/mL (43,47) and on cancers detected by rectal examination with lower PSA values (50), it was decided to omit rectal examination and transrectal ultrasound entirely and to biopsy all participants with a PSA value of ≥3 ng/mL. Table 3 shows the predictions of the effect of this change with respect to the previous regimen where a PSA ≥ 4 ng/mL and/or a suspicious rectal examination and/or transrectal ultrasonography (TRUS) indicated

Table 5
Characteristics of Cancers "Missed" and "Gained"
by Omitting DRE and TRUS

Biopsy Indications (DRE and/or TRUS positive, old protocol 5–9)
PSA ≤ 2.9 ng/mL   PSA 3–3.9 ng/mL   PSA ≥ 4.0 ng/mL

	N	(%)	N	(%)	N	(%)
No. cancers	79	(16.7)	44	(9.3)	474	(100)
No. RP	32	(40.5)	18	(40.5)	166	(35.0)
Gleason ≥ 7	15	(46.9)	9	(50.0)	65	(39.2)
PT ≤ 2	26	(81.3)	16	(88.9)	102	(61.4)
Volume ≥ 0.5 mL	8	(25.0)	9	(50.0)	88	(75.9)
Minimal	16	(50.0)	5	(27.8)	34	(20.5)
Advanced	6	(18.8)	1	(5.5)	44	(26.5)

Modified from *(51)*

a biopsy. This policy was subsequently validated in a prospective fashion; 10,450 men screened with the old regimen were compared to the results of 8,726 men screened by means of PSA only. The results of this validation experiment are summarized in Table 4. The data show that with the new screening regimen digital rectal examination (DRE) and TRUS are unnecessary in more than 80% of men. While the PSA distribution within old and new was shown to be comparable, the detection rate for PSA 3–3.9 ng/mL is almost threefold higher without DRE. The overall false positive biopsy rate is reduced from 4 in 5 to 3 in 4. The overall detection rate remains virtually unchanged.

In Table 5, the characteristics of cancers, which are potentially missed and gained by omitting DRE and TRUS, and biopsying all men with a PSA of 3–3.9 ng/mL are given. The data based on 166 radical prostatectomies all recruited from the prevalence screen of ERSPC Rotterdam. Cancers with PSA values ≥2.9 ng/mL have very favorable prognostic factors, 50% are classified as minimal; however, 18.8% seemed too advanced for cure. The fact that 81% are classified as ≥pT2 and still 47% were reported as Gleason 7 shows that this group contains a large proportion of potentially aggressive and curable cancers. Probably biopsy indications will have to be brought down even further to lower total PSA ranges. Before this can be done, however, the specificity of testing in this range needs to be improved. Obviously, with no increase in biopsy rates, the group of men diagnosed in the PSA range 3–3.9 ng/mL show patterns that make their inclusion into a screening study desirable.

The group realizes that a risk of missing important cancers in the lower PSA range is taken. Especially with the background of a long screening interval (4 yr in most centers) it would be desirable to include cases in lower PSA ranges. Feasibility studies to this effect have been planned.

Contamination

Contamination, the use of screening tests prior to or after randomization in the control arm, has a very strong impact on the power of a randomized screening study. Contamination enters the sample size calculation as an exponential function. All countries have accepted the obligation to study contamination. The sample size was adjusted to accommodate a contamination of 10%. Obviously, an effect of contamination on power depends on following up abnormal screening tests by biopsy and the diagnosis of cancer. Studies of all elements are in process in Rotterdam. Preliminary results are in press *(52)*. At the time of an interim evaluation in 1998 (27,533 men randomized, ages 55–69), PSA use was detected in 13% prior to randomization. After randomization, PSA testing was used in 3.3% in the screening and 7.7% in the control group. When detection rates were analyzed in those men who had been using PSA and/or DRE prior to randomization, no differences were found. The detection rate without prior PSA testing was 4.8%, and with prior PSA testing, it was 5.4%. A study evaluating the rate of biopsy and cancer diagnosis in the "contamination sample" is in progress.

Intermediate End Points

Intermediate end points such as the distribution of T-categories, pT-categories, metastatic disease, and grade of differentiation require validation. Table 6, which is based on 33,557 men randomized to either screening or control in ERSPC Rotterdam, gives an interim evaluation of potential intermediate end points obtained during 1999. It is evident that the distribution of potentially prognostically relevant parameters is more favorable in the screening group. This is especially true for the presence of metastatic disease, which was 14 times higher in the control group. However, these percentages, which demonstrate a significant stage migration, cannot be considered decisive for outcome. Absolute numbers may be more important in determining prostate cancer mortality. If one would assume that stage T3–4 prostate cancer is noncurable and will kill, then already at this time prostate cancer mortality would have to be assumed to be higher in the screening arm than in the control group. This short section on "intermediate end points" comparing the screening and control group data is meant mainly to discourage the use of these parameters to predict screening results. At this moment, no parameter can replace the outcome data with respect to prostate cancer mortality which will eventually result from this large trial.

Table 6
Intermediate Endpoints—Screening vs Control

	Screening		Control	
	n	(%)	n	(%)
Population	16.859		16.698	
Cancers	706		131	
Prevalence/det.rate	4.44		0.78	
Grade 3 PC	63	(8.9)*	28	(21.4)*
T3-4 PC	157	(22.2)*	39	(29.8)*
M+PC	4	(0.6)*	11	(8.4)*
PSA >10	161	(22.8)*	70	(53.4)*

*$p < 0.001$
ERSPC Rotterdam 1999

Interval Cancers

Most centers within ERSPC have chosen a rescreen interval of 4 yr. This was based on estimates of lead time, which were in the range of 6–10 yr (53,54). Both calculations are based on cancers diagnosed in clinical routine. It may therefore be assumed that lead time in a screen-detected population is even longer. Still, the group awaits confirmation of this assumption by a complete study of interval cancers, which at this moment has not yet been carried out. Table 7 shows the results of an interim analysis conducted over the years 1994–1998 when 13,704 men age 55–74 were randomized to control and 13,558 to screening. The total number of cancers diagnosed in the screening group during the 4-yr interval (the fourth year is not yet complete) was 13, or 13.4% of the 97 cancers found during the same time period in the control group. However, four of these cancers must be classified as incidental findings at TUR or cystoprostatectomy. Four were detected at screening, two had refused biopsy within ERSPC, and two were symptomatic. The classification is given in Table 7. A clear definition of interval cancers is lacking at this moment. The low proportion of interval cancers found, however, seems to confirm the correctness of the choice of a long rescreening interval.

Ethical Concerns

Indirect evidence is increasing, which is interpreted as pointing in the direction of effectiveness of screening for prostate cancer in terms of mortality reduction (20,55,56,57). These data, which are based on cancer registry information and geographical comparisons, all show a

Table 7
Interval Cancers ERSPC Rotterdam 1994–1998
(Control Group = 13.704, Screening Group = 13.558)

Year	Control group prostate cancer	Interval cancers Incidental (T1a-c)*	Interval cancers T2-T4**	Interval prostate cancer total
	N	N	N	N
1	44	3	4	7
2	24	2	–	2
3	20	2	1	3
4	9	1	–	1
Total	97	8	5	13

*Diagnosis: TUR (3), cystoprostatectomy (1), biopsy prior to screening (2), GP screening (2).

**Diagnosis: symptoms (2), biopsy prior to screening (1), refused biopsy (2).

decrease of prostate cancer mortality from 1992 on. This decrease is preceded by an increase in incidence owing to PSA screening. However, a similar decrease in prostate cancer mortality is also seen in areas where opportunistic screening is not prevalent *(58)*. The data so far present indirect and therefore unreliable evidence. The continuation of randomized studies so far seems to be justified and mandatory. Information on mortality available so far is indirect and does not have the level of certainty, which is necessary to introduce screening for prostate cancer as a health care policy.

REFERENCES

1. Schröder FH. (1993) Prostate cancer: to screen or not to screen? *BMJ* 1993; 306:407–408.
2. Schröder FH, Boyle P. (1993) Screening for prostate cancer - necessity or nonsense? *Eur J Cancer* 993;29A(5):656–661.
3. Adami HO, Baron JA, Rothman KJ. (1994) Ethics of a prostate cancer screening trial. *Lancet* 343: 958–960.
4. Schröder FH. (1993) Screening for prostate cancer (letter to the editor). *Lancet* 343:1438–1439.
5. Schröder FH. (1995) Detection of prostate cancer, screening the whole population has not yet been shown to be worth while (letter to the editor). *BMJ* 310:140–141.
6. Denis L, Standaert B. (1995) Contributors Chapter Prostate Cancer. (Döbrössy L ed.) Prevention in Primary Care. Recommendations for Promoting Good Practice. Copenhagen, SHO Regional Office for Europe; pp. 139–145.
7. Schröder FH, Denis LJ, Kirkels WJ, De Koning HJ, Standaert B. (1995) European randomized study of screening for prostate cancer, progress report of Antwerp and Rotterdam pilot studies. *Cancer* 76(1):129–134.

8. Schröder FH, Damhuis RAM, Kirkels WJ, De Koning HJ, Kranse R, Nijs HGT, Blijenberg BG (1996) European randomized study of screening for prostate cancer—The Rotterdam pilot studies. *Intern J Cancer* 65:145–151.

9. Ciatto S, Bonardi R, Mazzotta A, Lombardi C, Santoni R, Cardini S, Zappa M. (1995) Comparing two modalities of screening for prostate cancer: digital rectal examination and transrectal ultrasonography vs. prostate specific antigen. *Tumori* 81:225–229.

10. Auvinen A, Tammela T, Stenman U-H, et al. (1996) Screening for prostate cancer using serum prostate specific antigen: a randomized, population-based pilot study in Finland. Br J Cancer. *Br J Cancer* 74:568–572.

11. Herrero A, Paez A, Sanchez E, Berenguer A. (1996) Screening del cancer de prostata: estudio en una poblacion espanola. *Archivos Esp Urol* 49:595–606.

12. Martin E, Lujan M, Sanchez E, Herrero A, Paez A, Berenguer A. (1999) Final results of a screening campaign for prostate cancer. *European Urol* 35:26–31.

13. Nijs HGT, Tordoir DMR, Schuurman JH, Kirkels WJ, Schröder FH. (1993) Evaluatie van de vroege opsporing van prostaatkanker. *Tijdschr Soc Gezondheidszorg* 78:31A.

14. Nijs HTG, Tordoir DMR, Schuurman JH, Kirkels WJ, Schröder FH. (1997) Randomized trials of prostate cancer screening in the Netherlands: assessment of acceptance and motives for attendance. *J Med Screening* 4:102–106.

15. Adolfsson J, Steineck G, Whitmore WF Jr. (1993) Recent results of management of palpable clinically localized prostatic cancer: a review and commentary. *Cancer* 72:310–322.

16. Lujan M, Paëz A. (1999) Contamination in the Spanish arm of ERSPC (personal communication).

17. Auvinen A, Rietbergen JBW, Denis LJ, Schröder FH, Prorok PC. (1996) Prospective evaluation plan for randomized trials of prostate cancer screening. *J Med Screening* 3(2):97–104.

18. Essink-Bot ML, De Koning HJ, Nijs HGT, Kirkels WJ, Van der Maas PJ, Schröder FH. (1998) Population based screening for prostate cancer on Health-Related Quality of Life. *JNCI* 12:925–931.

19. Beemsterboer PMM, De Koning HJ, Birnie E, Blom FHM, Van der Maas PJ, Schröder FH.. (1999) Advanced disease in prostate cancer, course, care and cost implications. *Prostate* 40:97–104.

20. Sanford JL, Stephenson RA, Coyle LM, et al. (1998) Prostate cancer trends 1973–1995. SEER program. NIH publication, Bethesda, MD: National Cancer Institute. 1998, www.seer.img.nci.nih.gov.

21. Zappa M, Ciatto S, Bonardi R, Mazzotta A. (1998) Overdiagnosis of prostate carcinoma by screening: an estimate based on the results of the Florence screening pilot study. *Ann Oncol* 9:1297–1301.

22. Schröder FH, Alexander FE, Bangma CH, Hugosson J, Smith DS. (2000) Screening and early detection of prostate cancer. *The Prostate*, in press.

23. Whitmore Jr WF. (1988) Overview: historical and contemporary. *NCI Monograph* 7:7–11.

24. Rietbergen JBW, Boeken Kruger AE, Kranse R, Schröder FH. (1997) Complications of transrectal ultrasound-guided systematic sextant biopsies of the prostate: evaluation of complication rates and risk factors within a population-based screening program. *Urology* 49(6):875–880.

25. Aus G, Ahlgren G, Bergdahl S, Hugossson J. (1996) Infection after transrectal core biopsies of the prostate - risk factors and antibiotic prophylaxis. *Br J Urol* 77:851–855.

26. Davidson PJT, Van den Ouden D, Schröder FH. (1994) Radical Prostatectomy: prostective assessment of mortality and morbidity. *Eur Urol* 29;168–173.
27. Blijenberg BG (1994) De standaardisatie van de PSA-bepaling. *Tijdschr Klin Chemie.*
28. Blijenberg BG, Kranse R, Eman I, Schröder FH. (1996) Some Analytical considerations on the measurement of prostate-specific antigen. *Eur J Clin Chem Clin Biochem* 34:817–821.
29. Kranse R, Beemsterboer PMM, Rietbergen JBW, Habbema D, Hugosson J, Schröder FH. (1999) Predictors for Biopsy Outcome in the European Randomized Study of Screening for Prostate Cancer (Rotterdam region). *Prostate* 39:316–322.
30. Becker C, Piironen T, Pettersson K, Hugosson J, Lilja H. (2000) Clinical value of human glandular kallikrein 2 and free and total prostate-specific antigen in serum from a population of men with prostate-specific antigen levels 3.0 ng/mL or greater. *Urology* 2000 May; 55:694–699.
31. Boeken Kurger AE, Schröder FH, Thomas C, et al. (1999) Selective and specific assay of human kallikrein 2 (hK2) in serum improves prostate cancer diagnosis. *J Urol* 161 (no 4 Suppl):317, Abstract 1222.
32. Koning de HJ, Auvinen A, Berenguer-Sanchez A, Calais da Silva f, Ciatto S, Denis J, et al. (1999) Large-scale randomized prostate cancer screening trials: program performances in the ERSPC- and PLCO-trials (European Randomized Study of Screening for Prostate Cancer and Prostate, Lung, Colorectal and Ovary cancer trials), submitted.
33. Bangma CH, Kranse R, Blijenberg BG, Schröder FH. (1995) The value of screening tests in the detection of prostate cancer. Part I: Results of a retrospective evaluation of 1726 men. *Urology* 46:773–778.
34. Bangma CH, Kranse R, Blijenberg BG, Schröder FH. (1995) The value of screening tests in the detection of prostate cancer. Part II: Retrospective analysis of Free/Total Prostate-Specific Analysis ratio, age-specific reference ranges, and PSA density. *Urology* 46:779–784.
35. Ciatto S, Bonardi R, Mazzotta A, Lombardi C, Santoni R, Cardini S, Zappa M. (1995) Comparing two modalities of screening for prostate cancer: digital rectal examination and transrectal ultrasonography vs prostate specific antigen. *Tumori* 81:225–229.
36. Denis LJ. (1996) Clinical Assessment: digital rectal examination, in *Textbook of Benign Prostatic Hyperplasia.* (Kriby R, McConnell J, Fitzpatrick J, Roehrborn C, Boyle P eds.), Isis Medical Media Ltd., Oxford, pp. 149–154.
37. Blijenberg BG, Kranse R, Eman I, Schröder FH. (1996) Some Analytical considerations on the measurement of prostate-specific antigen. *Eur J Clin Chem Clin Biochem* 34:817–821.
38. Bangma CH, Rietbergen JBW, Schröder FH. (1996) PSA as a screening test: experience in The Netherlands. *Urol Clin North Am* 24:307–314.
39. Rietbergen JWB, Kranse R, Kirkels WJ, De Koning HJ, Schröder FH. (1997) Evaluation of prostate specific antigen and transrectal ultrasonography in population-based screening for prostate cancer: improving the efficiency of early detection. *Br J Urol* 79(Suppl 2):57–63.
40. Bangma CH, Rietbergen JBW, Kranse R, Blijenberg BG, Pettersson K, Schröder FH. (1997) The free/total prostate-specific antigen ratio improves the specificity of PSA in screening for prostate cancer in the general population. *J Urol* 157:2191-2196.

41. Bangma CH, Kranse R, Blijenberg BG, Schröder FH. (1997) The free to total serum prostate specific antigen ratio for staging prostate carcinoma. *J Urol* 157:544–547.

42. Aus G, Ahlgren G, Hugosson J, Pedersen KV, Rensfeldt K, Söderberg R. (1997) Diagnosis of Prostate Cancer: Optimal Number of Prostate Biopsies Related to Serum Prostate-Specific Antigen and Findings of Digital Rectal Examination. *Scand J Urol Nephrol* 31:541–544.

43. Schröder FH, Van der Maas PJ, Beemsterboer PMM, et al. (1998) Evaluation of Digital Rectal Examination (DRE) as a screening test for prostate cancer. *JNCI* 90(23):1817–1823.

44. Beemsterboer PM, Kranse R, de Koning HJ, Habbema JD, Schroder FH. (1999) Changing role of 3 screening modalities in the European randomized study of screening for prostate cancer (Rotterdam). *Int J Cancer* 84:437–441

45. Zappa M, Ciatto S, Bonardi R, Mazzotta A. (1998) Overdiagnosis of prostate carcinoma by screening: an estimate based on the results of the Florence screening pilot study. *Ann Oncol* 9:1297–1301.

46. Rietbergen JBW, Hoedemaeker RF, Boeken Kruger AE, Kirkels WJ, Schröder FH. (1999) The changing pattern of prostate cancer at the time of diagnosis: Characteristics of screen detected prostate cancers in a population-based screening study. *J Urol* 161:1192–1198.

47. Lodding P, Aus G, Bergdahl S, Frösing R, Lilja H, Pihl CG, Hugosson J. (1998) Characteristics of screening detected prostate cancer in men 50 to 66 years old with to 4 ng/mL PSA. *J Urol* 159:899–903.

48. Hoedemaeker RF, Kranse R, Rietbergen JBW, Boeken Kruger AE, Schröder FH, Van der Kwast ThH. (1999) Evaluation of prostate needle biopsies in a population-based screening study: the impact of borderline lesions. *Cancer* 85:145–152.

49. Kranse R, Beemsterboer PMM, Rietbergen JBW, Habbema D, Hugosson J, Schröder FH. (1999) Predictors for Biopsy Outcome in the European Randomized Study of Screening for Prostate Cancer (Rotterdam region). *Prostate* 39:316–322.

50. Schröder FH, Cruijsen-Koeter I van der, Kranse R, Kirkels WJ, Koning HJ de, Vis A, Kwast Th van der, Hoedemaeker R. (2000) Prostate cancer detection at low prostate specific antigen (PSA). *J Urol* 163:806–812 (Ramon Guiteras lecture, AUA 1998).

51. Schröder FH, Cruijsen-Koeter I van der, Vis A, Kwast Th van der, Kirkels WJ, Kranse R. (2000) PSA based early detection of prostate cancer–validation of screening without rectal examination. *Urology*, in press.

52. Beemsterboer PMM, Kranse R, Koning HJ de, et al. (1999) Changing role for 3 screening modalities in the Euopean Randomised Study of Screening for Prostrate Cancer (Rotterdam). *Int J Cancer* 84(4):437–441.

53. Stenman UH, Hakama M, Knekt P, Aromaa A, Teppo L, Leinonen J. (1994) Serum concentrations of prostate-specific antigen and its complex with $\alpha 1$-antichymotrypsin before diagnosis of prostate cancer. *Lancet* 334:1594–1598.

54. Parkes CJ, Wald NJ, Murphy P, et al. (1995) Prospective observational study to assess value of prostate specific antigen as screening test for prostate cancer. *BMJ* 311: 1340–1343

55. Mettlin DJ, Murphy GP. (1998) Why is the prostate cancer death rate declining in the United States? *Cancer* 1998; 82: 249–251.

56. Schröder FH, Van der Maas PJ, Beemsterboer PMM, et al. (1998) Evaluation of Digital Rectal Examination (DRE) as a screening test for prostate cancer. *JNCI* 90:1817–1823.
57. Bartsch WH, Klocker H, Oberaigner W, et al. (2000) Decrease in prostate cancer mortality following introduction of prostate specific antigen (PSA) screening in the federal state of Tyrol, Austria. *J Urol* 163 (no. 4 Suppl):88, Abstract 387.
58. Oliver SE, Gunnett D, Donovan JL. (2000) Comparison of trends in prostate-cancer mortality in England and Wales and the U.S.A. *Lancet* 355(9217):1788–1789.

Index

About the CD

CAPRI software installation instructions:

>CAPRI software is compatible with WINDOWS 95/98/2000/NT. No other operating system is currently supported.

>Installation option one: At the Windows desk top, Click the start icon on the tool bar located at the bottom of the desk top. Click on the Run option. Within the Run window type the drive reference that is assigned to the CD-ROM followed by Setup and press return: Example: F:/Setup [carriage return]. Follow Setup Instructions.

>Installation option two: At the Windows desk top, click the Start icon on the tool bar located at the bottom of the desk top. Click on the Programs option. Click on Windows Explorer. Locate the drive reference for the CD-ROM. Click on the drive reference, which will bring up the contents of the installation CD. Locate the file Setup.exe and double click on this file. Follow Setup Instructions.

>Questions regarding installations, comments, or to register for future versions of the CAPRI currently in development can be made to capri@texas.net

Warning: Opening the CD package makes this book non-returnable.